Craft in Art Th

Craft in Art Therapy is the first book dedicated to illustrating the incorporation of craft materials and methods into art therapy theory and practice.

Contributing authors provide examples of how they have used a range of crafts including pottery, glass work, textiles (sewing, knitting, crochet, embroidery, and quilting), paper (artist books, altered books, book binding, origami, and zines), leatherwork, and Indian crafts like mendhi and kolam/rangoli in their own art and self-care, and in individual, group, and community art therapy practice. The book explores the therapeutic benefits of a range of craft materials and media, as well as craft's potential to build community, to support individuals in caring for themselves and each other, and to play a valuable role in art therapy practice.

Craft in Art Therapy demonstrates that when practiced in a culturally sensitive and socially conscious manner, craft practices are more than therapeutic—they also hold transformational potential.

Lauren Leone, DAT, ATR-BC, LMHC, is an assistant professor of art therapy at Lesley University, maintains a private practice, and facilitates a community-based art therapy group. Her research interests include the therapeutic benefits of craft activism and how emancipatory pedagogy informs art therapy practice and education.

Craft in Art Therapy

Diverse Approaches to the Transformative Power of Craft Materials and Methods

Edited by Lauren Leone

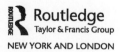
Routledge
Taylor & Francis Group

NEW YORK AND LONDON

First published 2021
by Routledge
52 Vanderbilt Avenue, New York, NY 10017

and by Routledge
2 Park Square, Milton Park, Abingdon, Oxon, OX14 4RN

Routledge is an imprint of the Taylor & Francis Group, an informa business

© 2021 Taylor & Francis

Library of Congress Cataloging-in-Publication Data
Names: Leone, Lauren, editor.
Title: Craft in art therapy : diverse approaches to the transformative
   power of craft materials and methods / edited by Lauren Leone.
Description: New York, NY : Routledge, 2020. | Includes bibliographical
   references and index.
Identifiers: LCCN 2020006186 (print) | LCCN 2020006187 (ebook) |
   ISBN 9780367506148 (hardback) | ISBN 9780367343163 (paperback) |
   ISBN 9781003050513 (ebook)
Subjects: LCSH: Art therapy. | Handicraft—Therapeutic use.
Classification: LCC RC489.A7 C73 2020 (print) | LCC RC489.A7 (ebook) |
   DDC 616.89/1656—dc23
LC record available at https://lccn.loc.gov/2020006186
LC ebook record available at https://lccn.loc.gov/2020006187

ISBN: 978-0-367-50614-8 (hbk)
ISBN: 978-0-367-34316-3 (pbk)
ISBN: 978-1-003-05051-3 (ebk)

Typeset in Minion
by Apex CoVantage, LLC

Contents

Figures and Tables

Tables

Color Plates

Acknowledgments

Thank you to Alex Kapitan, for your enthusiasm, expertise, and thoughtful editing.

Thank you to all of the contributors to this book for sharing your passion for craft in art therapy and your valuable experience. I have so much gratitude for your wisdom and hard work.

Thank you to my parents, Don and Madeleine, for your unwavering support.

Thank you to my husband Mike for your support, encouragement, genuine and ongoing interest in my research, and always being willing to review "one last thing" for me.

And finally: thank you Brenda, Christine, Donna, Francisca, Leslie, Sarah, and Yohanna—my collaborators in the *Crafting Change* craft activism group. Without you, the research that inspired this book wouldn't have been possible. I thank each of you for your enthusiasm, wisdom, strength, and humor. And for being open to finding our way together.

Contributors

Mikey Anderson, MAAT, is a Queer artist-art therapist who graduated from the School of the Art Institute of Chicago with a BFA in fine art and an MA in art therapy and counseling. Their art practice is informed by a community-driven art therapy practice, which incorporates fiber crafts, Queer theory, and activism. Their artworks range from embroideries and quilts to comics and a handmade plush toy line they call "Yarnies." Their artworks are soft, cuddly, and invite participation. These artworks entice people to come closer, where the underlying message about Queer advocacy becomes evident. Their art therapy practice has spanned multiple age groups, from children, adolescents, and young adults to elders. Their practice is grounded in Relational-Cultural Theory and a social justice focus, as implemented through radical collective crafting. Mikey believes that collectively we create inclusive spaces that are communal, participatory, and open-ended through crafting. These spaces provide the opportunity for constructing alternative narratives that reject the dominance of heteronormativity. They strive to broaden Queer representation by way of both their art and art therapy practices. Through the sessions they run, the community-based art projects they facilitate, and the Yarnies they create, they are committed to Queer advocacy.

Stephanie Clark, ATR-BC, LCPC, is an art therapist for the Road Home Program, The National Center of Excellence for Veterans and Their Families. Stephanie provides both individual and group art therapy services to veterans and their family members in both the Intensive Outpatient Program and the Outpatient Program. A graduate of Southern Illinois University in Edwardsville, Stephanie has been working as an art therapist in the Chicago area, working with children, adolescents, and adults in various not-for-profit social service agencies. Stephanie has also served on the Illinois Art Therapy Association's board of directors since 2014 and is the current president.

Alison Etter, MM, MT-BC, received a Bachelor of Music in Music Therapy from Southern Methodist University and completed her clinical internship at San Antonio State Hospital. She received a Master's in Music Therapy from Colorado State University. She has worked at Kerrville State Hospital for over seven years. She has also worked as an adjunct instructor at Schreiner University. In 2014 she received the Harmony award for Clinical Practice from the Southwestern region of the American Music Therapy Association. She represents the Southwestern region on the technology committee for the American Music Therapy Association and has served for over six years. She has presented at the following conferences and events: Kerrville State Hospital Forensic Networking Conference (2013, 2014, 2016), Central Texas Music Therapy Association Conference

(2014), Music Therapy Awareness Weekend hosted by Mu Tau Omega at Sam Houston State University (2016), the Southwestern region of the American Music Therapy Association Conference (2013, 2015, 2018), the American Music Therapy Association Conference (2015), the American Art Therapy Association Conference (2016), Dartmouth's New Hampshire Hospital (2018), the Canadian Association for Music Therapists conference (2018), and the International Art Therapy Practice/Research Inaugural Conference in London (2019). Her work on collaborative arts interventions for the forensic population has been published in the Canadian Art Therapy Association Journal.

Lisa Raye Garlock, ATR-BC, ATCS, LCPAT, has worked with adults, adolescents, and children in hospitals, schools, community-based organizations, and shelters. She is an assistant professor, clinical placement coordinator, and art therapy gallery manager at the George Washington University Graduate Art Therapy Program in Washington, DC. She encourages art therapy students to use textiles in their work and teaches a class in Story Cloths and Art Therapy. She has created the Storycloth Database, an online resource that highlights collections of story cloths that focus on human rights issues. Her own story cloth work focuses on immigration and environmental issues. Lisa works with the international non-profit, Common Threads Project, co-training therapists in using story cloths, along with art therapy, mind/body awareness and psychoeducation to help women recover from the trauma of gender-based violence. She has done Common Threads training in Bosnia and Herzegovina and facilitated Survivor workshops in Geneva, Switzerland through the Mukwege Foundation.

Marilyn Holmes, MA, began pursuing her Master's in art therapy counseling at Southern Illinois University Edwardsville in 2017 and graduated in May 2020. She received a Bachelor's in both studio art and psychology from Morehead State University in Morehead, KY. While pursuing her education, Marilyn also serves as a graphic designer for the Louisville Family Justice Advocates, an organization focused on advancing policies and practices for families with incarcerated loved ones in Louisville, KY. Holmes's research interests revolve around exploring the experience of Black art therapists suffering from racialized stress. Currently, she works as an outpatient community counselor in East Saint Louis while pursuing her counseling license and art therapy credentials.

Eliza S. Homer, PhD, ATR-BC, LAC, NCC, is an educator, a registered, board-certified art therapist, and licensed counselor, who has worked with a range of under-served populations, including youth, adults with severe mental illness, incarcerated males, and Native American communities. She holds a doctorate in Expressive Therapies and a master's degree in Counseling Psychology and Expressive Art Therapy. Her counseling practice emphasizes utilizing creative modalities to address trauma and increase resilience. Eliza presents extensively at local, state, national, and international levels on a variety of practice and research topics related to trauma treatment, art therapy, diversity, and working within interdisciplinary teams. Eliza resides in Mexico, where she is focused on exploring the role of textiles and other folk-art traditions for healing and well-being.

Ephrat Huss, PhD, chairs an MA in arts therapy for social work at Ben-Gurion University of the Negev in Israel. She has published over 65 articles—two theoretical—and two edited books on art therapy and arts based research within social contexts. She has also received competitive grants in this field. She is currently working on experiences of marginalized Bedouin youth in Israel, crafts as empowerment for Bedouin women, use of arts in the women for peace movement, and arts as salutogenic coping for medical staff and for recovering oncological patients in healthcare. Her overall areas of research are the interface between social theories and arts therapy, as well as the use of arts in high context social situations and in healthcare contexts.

Mahesh Iyer, MA, is an art psychotherapist working for Extra•Ordinary People, a non-profit organization providing services for individuals with special needs in Singapore. Prior to his training, Mahesh completed his BSc in Psychology and volunteered as an art teacher for children with special needs in Abu Dhabi, UAE. His experience at the center induced him to take up postgraduation in art psychotherapy. During his training, Mahesh gained experience working with older adults at a sheltered home in Singapore. The collective exposure to multi-cultural populations naturally gravitated his research interests towards the complex inter-play of culture, ethics and practice. Mahesh has since then developed and presented his research at several professional art therapy conferences, including the recent International Art Therapy Practice/Research Inaugural Conference 2019 in London, UK.

Krupa Jhaveri, PhD candidate, CAGS, TIEAT-C, MPS, is an international art therapist, art director, artist, and founder of Sankalpa: Art Journeys based in Auroville, South India. With graduate training in art therapy from SVA-NYC (2008), she has experience working with children and women with HIV/AIDS, in child protection, as a certified Trauma-Informed Expressive Arts Therapy consultant, cross-cultural exchanges, mindful and nature-based art-making, and the combined practice of art and yoga. Krupa is a TEDx Women speaker and Ambassador to India for Art Therapy Without Borders, with specialized research on the therapeutic experience of traditional Indian art forms. Born in the US and of Indian ethnic origin, she is a living bridge between cultures through art and Krupa travels, presents, and teaches regularly throughout Asia, America, and Europe. She is a CAGS graduate and currently a PhD candidate at the European Graduate School in Switzerland, documenting her work within Expressive Arts: Therapy, Coaching, Consulting & Education, Conflict Transformation & Peacebuilding. www.sankalpajourneys.com.

Lynn Kapitan, PhD, ATR-BC, HLM, is a professor of graduate art therapy, research advisor, and founding director of the Doctor of Art Therapy at Mount

Mary University in Milwaukee, WI. A former executive editor of *Art Therapy: Journal of the American Art Therapy Association* and a past president of the Association, she has authored a seminal text on art therapy research and several articles on the subjects of social action in art therapy, multicultural and professional issues, advances in research, and leadership. The practice of crafting in the contemplative tradition of the artist book form has accompanied her professional life for many years. She currently consults with a non-governmental organization in Central America as a member of a community-based, cross-cultural research team.

Michal Katoshevski, MBA, is a social activist. Her research at Ben Gurion University focuses on work-empowerment of marginalized Bedouin women. She has an BA in Hebrew Literature and African studies and an MBA in Social Leadership and NGO Management.

Lauren Leone, DAT, ATR-BC, LMHC, is an assistant professor of art therapy at Lesley University. She works with art therapy participants in private and community-based settings, and her research interests include the unique therapeutic benefits of craft materials and methods for art therapy practice and how DIY practices and craft activism can support art therapy participants in being agents of social change and how craft can provide a medium for engaging in art therapy with social justice aims. Lauren maintains an active fiber arts practice and has exhibited her work nationally. Lauren holds a BA from Tufts University, a BFA from the School of the Museum of Fine Arts, a MA in clinical mental health counseling with a specialization in art therapy from Lesley University, and a Doctorate of art therapy from Mount Mary University.

Joe Mageary, PhD, LMHC, is a licensed mental health counselor in the state of Massachusetts, an experienced educator, and an active musician. He holds a PhD in transformative studies from the California Institute of Integral Studies and is the current director of field training—and an assistant professor—in the Division of Counseling and Psychology at Lesley University. Throughout his career, Joe's clinical work has been rooted in efforts to decrease stigma associated with chronic mental illness through providing community-based and collaborative- and recovery-oriented services. His clinical approach is influenced by tenets of Narrative Therapy, trauma-informed approaches, critical psychology, and brief therapies as well as by transdisciplinary thinkers such as Gregory Bateson and Edgar Morin. Joe has published and presented on topics ranging from the transformative potential of social justice-oriented hardcore punk rock culture to the role that technology plays in working with teens. In 2015, Joe led a team that developed the *Visual Reflection Team* model: an arts-based version of the Reflecting Team technique used in Family Systems and Narrative therapies.

Joshua Kin-man Nan, PhD, is a potter, art therapist, social worker, and spiritual worker. With the training background of social work (BSW, Hong Kong Baptist

University), divinity (MDiv, Regent College, Canada), art therapy (St Mary-of-the-Woods College, USA), and social sciences (PhD, The University of Hong Kong), Joshua has rich experiences of providing workshops, talks, psycho-therapy, and training by weaving various disciplines together. Joshua has many years of experience of applying arts to work with a wide range of populations. In the recent years, he has actively investigated the Expressive Therapies Continuum (ETC) by integrating it with the use of clay in the approach of Clay Art Therapy (CAT). He has applied CAT to work with adults and adolescents in treating mood disorders and other mental health challenges. His areas of interests include Clay Art Therapy, emotion regulation and neurological processes, youth work, spirituality, Jungian psychology and art, art for social care, and life—death education/palliative care. He has presented his art therapy research projects in many different international conferences, including the American Art Therapy Association Annual Conference and has published articles in different international journals. Joshua is currently an assistant professor and the 4-Year PhD program director in the Department of Social Work, Hong Kong Baptist University: http://sowk.hkbu.edu.hk/inner_people.php?type=1&lang=1.

Jaimie Peterson, MAAT, ATR, LPC-Intern, received her BFA in painting from the Kansas City Art Institute and her MAAT at the School of the Art Institute of Chicago. She has worked as an art therapist at Kerrville State Hospital, a forensic psychiatric facility for over ten years. She has also been an adjunct art instructor at Alamo Colleges since 2012. In 2015 she received the Friends of Music Therapy Award from the Southwestern region of the American Music Therapy Association. Her work focuses on creating community and shattering stigma through art. She has presented on her work and writing at the Texas Forensic Networking Conference (2010, 2011, 2012, 2013, 2014) American Art Therapy Association Conference (2009, 2014, 2015, 2016, 2017) American Music Therapy Association Conference (2015), Dartmouth's New Hampshire Hospital (2018), the Canadian Association for Music Therapists conference (2018), and the Inaugural International Art Therapy Conference in London. (2019). Her work on collaborative arts interventions for the forensic population has been published in the Canadian Art Therapy Association Journal.

Jessica Woolhiser Stallings, DAT, ATR-BC, LMHP, LPC, is a mental health clinician at a therapeutic school providing art therapy and counseling. Jessie adjuncts for the Emporia State University (ESU) Art Therapy and Counseling Masters programs where she previously served as an associate professor. She maintains a part time private practice at the Center for Mindful Living working with teens and adults. A graduate of the ESU MS in Art Therapy (2005) and Mount Mary Doctorate of Art Therapy (2019), Jessie has researched use of art therapy with individuals with autism and written on a variety of topics in the field. She has served on the Kansas Art Therapy Association board for eight years and is a past president. Jessie also serves on the Nebraska art therapy licensure coalition.

Savneet Talwar, PhD, ATR-BC, is a professor and chair in the graduate art therapy program at the School of the Art Institute of Chicago. She is a member of the Critical Pedagogy in the Arts Therapies think tank. Her current research examines feminist politics, critical theories of difference, social justice, and questions of resistance. Using an interdisciplinary approach, she is interested in community-based art practices; cultural trauma; and performance art and public cultures as they relate to art therapy theory, practice, and pedagogy. She is the author of *Art Therapy for Social Justice: Radical Intersection* and has published in *Arts in Psychotherapy*, *Art Therapy: Journal of the American Art Therapy Association*, and *Gender Issues in Art Therapy*. She is also the founder of the CEW (Creatively Empowered Women) Design Studio, a craft, sewing, and fabrication enterprise for Bosnian and South Asian women at the Hamdard Center in Chicago. She is the past associate editor of *Art Therapy: Journal of the American Art Therapy Association*.

Rachel Wallis, MA, is a self-taught crafter, artist, and activist. She is interested in transgressing the lines between fine art and craft and engaging in questions of identity, labor, and value when it comes to the creation and appreciation of art. Her work focuses on collaborative community quilting projects addressing issues of race and social justice. Past projects have included *Gone But Not Forgotten*, a community quilting process creating a memorial quilt for individuals killed by the Chicago Police Department, and *Inheritance: Quilting Across Prison Walls*, a project using quilts to help rebuild relationships divided by incarceration. Rachel completed an MA in art and social practice at Moore College of Art and Design in 2016. Her work has been featured in the Chicago Tribune, the Chicago Sun Times, the Journal of Surface Design, and "Art Therapy for Social Justice: Radical Intersections." She has taught classes or served as artist in residence at the School of the Art Institute, A Studio in the Woods, Lillstreet Art Center, and the Coffee Creek Women's Correctional Center.

Chun-shan (Sandie) Yi, MAAT, MFA, ATR, received a MA in art therapy from the School of the Art Institute of Chicago and MFA from the University of California Berkeley. She is a disabled artist and disability culture worker whose work, Crip Couture, focuses on wearable art made for and with disabled people. Yi is a PhD candidate in disability studies at the University of Illinois at Chicago. Her research interests include Disability Arts and Culture; disability fashion; accessibility design and programming for arts and cultural venues; and social justice-based art therapy. Her publications include, Res(Crip)ting Art Therapy: Disability Culture and Art as a Social Justice Intervention; Art for Social Impact: Aging & Disability Research in Taiwan; Disablement and Sexuality: Crip aesthetics of the disabled body and Disability Culture; Social Justice and Power in Museum Service and Accessibility Practices and *Materials & Media in Art Therapy: Critical Understandings of Diverse Artistic Vocabularies*.

Editor's Note

Please note that parts of the preface, introduction and Chapter 10 have been excerpted and adapted from the Editor's doctoral thesis, and parts of Chapter 10 have been adapted from Leone, L. (2019). *Crafting change: Craft activism for community-based art therapy.* In H. Mandell (Ed.), *Crafting dissent: Handicraft as protest from the American Revolution to the Pussyhats* (pp. 247–262). Lanham, MD: Rowman & Littlefield.

Preface

On my birthday in 2003, a friend gave me an embroidery kit, and I was immediately engaged. The slow, meditative process of stitching and the comforting nature of the materials captivated me. The deliberate process provided a sense of control, and the slow tempo allowed for reflection. I began to use embroidery as a medium to tackle emotionally charged content within my own art making. This new experience was part of what led me to pursue a career in art therapy.

About a decade later I learned about craftivism (craft activism) when I attended a workshop entitled "The Wandering Uterus Project: Craftivism Meets Art Therapy" at the 2014 American Art Therapy Association conference. Led by art therapists Angela Lyonsmith, Melissa Raman Molitor, and Savneet Talwar, the workshop offered information about a community-based art project the presenters had developed to encourage dialogue about reproductive justice. Using a variety of craft materials, workshop attendees were asked to create an image of a uterus, which was accompanied by storytelling on the topic of women's reproductive health. For me, the exercise connected a personally meaningful art form with an activist context. As a means of combining my political beliefs, personal art making, professional work, and teaching, the project enlivened me. It deepened my interest in bringing social justice perspectives as well as the use of craft into my art therapy practice.

After attending that workshop, I began incorporating craft practices such as embroidery, needle felting, and knitting into in my private and community art therapy practice, and I led craftivism workshops in my community. I found craft to be a fulfilling and approachable medium for participants and craftivism to be a creatively stimulating way to engage groups in the issues that matter to them.

As I explored these techniques in my practice, I looked to the art therapy literature for more context on the use of craft and realized that there wasn't much available. I found that craft has historically been underrepresented in art therapy literature and that craft media were absent from many of the texts that are used in art therapy training programs to teach theory and practice. This suggested to me that craft may be undervalued in art therapy practice in general.

Although embroidery was foundational in my personal art making and influential in my becoming an art therapist, I realized only in hindsight that I had used it very little while studying art therapy in graduate school. I also had never thought to use it in my work during several art therapy internships and early jobs. Reflecting on my graduate school experience, I realized that I had felt the presence of an implicit standard that materials of the "fine arts" (e.g., pastels and paints) were the expected tools of a professional art therapist. This bias was never explicitly stated—and I *can* remember a few instances in which professors provided less conventional materials—but, nevertheless, I had come away with a strong impression of what art therapy "looked like," and this impression did not include craft.

I conducted my doctoral research in an effort to learn more about craft activism and how it could inform art therapy theory and practice. My research focused on the use of craftivism in a community-based art therapy setting in order to gain more knowledge about how craft could support art therapy participants in being change agents. I facilitated a participatory action research project with members of an existing art therapy group (as well as friends and family that they invited to join us) at a community health center in Boston. The project took the physical form of a collaborative quilt addressing issues of gentrification and displacement in the participants' community. Upon its completion, participants shared the quilt with the community in a range of different settings through a travelling exhibition. This research project solidified my belief that craft deserves more attention in art therapy theory and practice and that craft can serve as a powerful and transformational tool for both art therapists and art therapy participants.

Fortunately, craft practices, especially textiles, have recently begun to see greater representation in the art therapy literature. This exciting trend may indicate that art therapists are becoming more receptive to incorporating craft into their practices. This book aims to build on this growing interest in craft by bringing attention to the value of craft materials and methods and functions as an invitation for art therapists to widen our conception of what approaches we can use with the individuals and communities with whom we work. The authors in the pages that follow illuminate not only the therapeutic potential of a range of craft materials and media—from quilting to pottery, artist books to glass work, leatherwork to embroidery—but also demonstrate the potential of craft to help us build community, care for ourselves and each other, and play a valuable role in a socially just art therapy practice.

Introduction

Defining Craft

"Craft" is a word that resists easy definition. It has meant many things to many different civilizations over tens of thousands of years of human history, so what people mean when they say "craft" often depends on the specific context they are exploring. Interestingly, in a number of languages, including Old English, Middle English, German, Dutch, and several Scandinavian languages, the word "power" has been used to define craft.

This book's title comes from Bratich and Brush's (2011) vision of craft as power—"the ability or capacity to act"—emphasizing the potential of craft practices for social and political action (p. 233). Being a craftsperson is a "state of being engaged," wrote Sennett (in Langlands, 2017, p. 11)—"how we interact materially, with each other and our immediate surroundings" (p. 11). In his book *Making is Connecting*, sociologist and media theorist David Gauntlett (2011) described craft's essential dimensions as being "the inherent satisfaction of making; the sense of being alive within the process; and the engagement with ideas, learning, and knowledge which come not before or after but *within* the practice of making" (pp. 24–25). This description of craft parallels important tenets of art therapy theory and practice—that it is *within* the creative process that we make connections to ourselves, to others, and to our understanding of the world around us.

Craft modalities provide unique benefits to art therapy practice on individual and community levels, offer accessible and culturally resonant art therapy experiences for marginalized groups with strong craft traditions, and possess the potential for collective action and social justice in art therapy contexts. However, craft has historically been devalued in art therapy training and literature, and misconceptions about craft affect its perceived value, with the result that many art therapy participants have not had access to materials and processes that could benefit them greatly.

As Moon (2010) noted, "The field of art therapy has been operating within an unnecessarily constricted visual vocabulary" (p. xvi), and it is time to critically examine the materials and methods we use in art therapy practice with the "same intentionality and cultural competence applied to other aspects of the therapy encounter" (p. xv). She further explained that the field of art therapy hasn't paid adequate attention to material theory and practice, and that the field's views on art haven't evolved over the course of its history, leaving art therapists today to "often operate on the basis of outdated and restricted knowledge of contemporary art practice, a situation that would never be collectively tolerated in relation to knowledge of contemporary psychotherapy theory and practice" (Moon, 2010, p. xv).

Crafts such as textiles, woodcraft, book and paper crafts, pottery, glasswork, and metalwork should be seen as legitimate and foundational to art therapy practice as media that are equally valuable and have just as much therapeutic potential as drawing, painting, and sculpture. But before we can adopt this perspective, we have to understand the history behind why art therapists have not yet fully embraced the value of craft into our practices.

The Social Construction of Art Versus Craft

To understand art therapy's relationship with craft, one must first explore the boundaries that have historically divided "art" and "craft," how those boundaries evolved, and how such divisions have been subtly or overtly constructed along gender, racial, and class lines. The division between art and craft is a Western concept, with associated values and hierarchies; it is "a symptom of cultural colonization" (Han Sifuentes, 2017, para. 6). The "fine arts," usually referring to painting, sculpture, and architecture, have historically been valued over "crafts" such as pottery, woodcraft, textiles, and glasswork. "Fine arts" as a term has not merely served to distinguish between materials; it also has functioned as a default description of what fundamentally constitutes "art" and as an ideal—grounded in European standards—to which art created by the rest of the world is compared. Yet art is created in all cultures, and defining and measuring those cultures' art based on how it aligns with white, Eurocentric values is ethnocentric. Broude and Garrard (1982) argued that, in a broad historical context:

> When the small trickle of "high art" activity that has occurred in a few centuries at our own end of the historical spectrum is measured against the millennia in which weaving and pot-making were among the world's principle forms of art-making, one may conclude that it is not the crafts and traditional arts, but the fine arts, that are history's aberration.
>
> (pp. 12–13)

Within the Western world, art created by white men with formal training has been exalted, whereas works created for functional uses or using skills passed on outside of formal academies have been disregarded (Dunn, 2014). Mainardi (1982) argued that museums, art education, and art history are largely controlled by white men, who have "used their power to gerrymander the very definition of art around the accomplishments of all those who are not white and male" (p. 344). She elaborated that this resulted in the creation of terms such as "primitive art," "folk art," and "decorative art" to describe what is created outside of the "fine arts" realm and that these terms serve to "reveal more about the prejudices of the art historians than the art itself" (p. 344). Berger (2005) argued that the implications of Western divisions of art and craft had the greatest consequences for non-white people who didn't live in Europe or the United States, as they often had not created categories for art based solely on aesthetics. He posited: "Fine art was a Western test of cultural development that non-Western people had little hope of passing" (p. 100).

Prior to the Renaissance there was no distinction between art and craft in the Western world. Anything made by hand—whether for utility, decoration, or ritual—was considered a craft object (Lucie-Smith, 1981). During the Renaissance, as art education shifted from craft-based workshops to guilds and academies, a distinction between *artist* and *artisan* emerged, which also marked the beginning of the split between fine arts and craft (Parker & Pollock, 2013). A subsequent historical marker occurred during the industrial revolution: things that were handmade were now considered craft, and those made by machines were objects (Langlands, 2017; Lucie-Smith, 1981). This split also served to move the conception of craft from something functional to something decorative: as objects such as clothing and furniture were increasingly created by machines, home crafting focused on decorative and folk arts (Lucie-Smith, 1981).

The industrial revolution also resulted in the Arts and Crafts movement that originated in Britain in the late 19th century and subsequently spread to Europe and North America (Krugh, 2014). This movement was founded on active resistance to machine-made objects and a reverence of the handmade. Proponents sought to unite craftspeople with artistry and bring back a sense of pleasure to craftwork. However, although craft practices rose in society's regard, this was likely due to the involvement of tradespeople and industrial designers. In fact, divisions between art and craft throughout history have virtually always reflected social divisions; for example, even in the Arts and Crafts movement women artisans and textile crafts were perceived as less important to society (Callen, 1985; Lippard, 1978).

In the modern era, Western artists and art historians have continued to reinforce race, class, and gender biases through the art genres and activities that have been promoted or downgraded (Berger, 2005). These biases are interdependent and have been expressed in intersecting ways through the art/craft divide. For example, Browne (1994) pointed out that the art/craft hierarchy is rooted in the marginalization of groups with strong craft traditions, such as Latinx and Native American peoples in the United States. The same has been argued about Black women (e.g., Han Sifuentes, 2017). Citing Lippard (1995),

Kapitan (2011) posited that these same biases manifest in art therapy, stating that "in discounting craft, art therapy inadvertently participates in the history of economically deprived people who, denied access to the art world, had to channel their creative drives into art that was not considered 'art'" (p. 95).

Another example of how social bias plays out in the art/craft divide is through the repeated association of certain crafts with women. "Women's work" has historically been defined as the largely unpaid labor that women are expected to perform and that is often devalued and mostly associated with child-rearing and managing the home. Brown (1970) posited that compatibility with child-rearing, in fact, is what delegated certain types of labor to a woman's domain, including activities that can be easily resumed after interruptions, don't require much concentration, can be done at home, and don't put children in danger. This work has often taken the form of women making clothing and linens for their families while men worked outside of the home and earned wages. As such, craft practices such as knitting, sewing, and quilting have been labeled as "women's work" (Barber, 1994). "For millennia women have sat together spinning, weaving, and sewing," noted Barber (1994, p. 29), and these communal groups were where many women learned crafting skills, in lieu of the formal educational settings that emphasized fine art practices (Dunn, 2014). "Women's work," thus, has historically taken place in the private sphere and garners secondary status to professional work done in the public sphere.

The association of certain kinds of craft, namely textiles, with "women's work" has had implications for the art world. From a reading of Western art history it is clear that utilitarian and functional objects have long been devalued, whereas objects made for contemplation and exhibition have tended to be elevated in the eyes of the public. Similarly, some art historians have posited that the gendered division of hierarchies in art reflected not what was made but rather where the production took place: fine arts were considered professional and public, whereas crafts were thought to be made in the home by women for their families (Lippard, 1978; Parker & Pollock, 2013). However, the feminist art movement of the 1960s and 70s and Postmodern art of the mid- to late 20th century paved the way for post-disciplinary practice in contemporary art, where the borders between art and craft no longer exist (Adamson, 2010) in which the contemporary art world has become more accepting of crafts (e.g. Jefferies, 2011; Smith, 2016). This is leading to what curator and historian Glenn Adamson (2010) referred to as "an end to the old 'craft versus art' debate because in an undifferentiated field of practice, no one activity has any more right to be called art than another" (p. 586).

"Contemporary" Craft

The 21st century has seen a resurgence in the popularity of so-called domestic crafts, as evidenced, for example, in the growing interest in knitting, quilting, and other textile crafts by young people (Bratich & Brush, 2011; Minahan &

Wolfram Cox, 2007; Pentney, 2008). Another example is the rise of maker culture, defined as "a worldwide movement of individuals using a mix of digital fabrication, open hardware, software hacking and traditional crafts to innovate for themselves, underpinned by an ethos of openness and skill sharing rather than commercial benefit" (Taylor, Hurley, & Connolly, 2016, p. 2). Maker spaces illustrate how the renewed interest in crafting is often coupled with civic and community facets. Some have argued that the renewed popularity of many crafts may be a reaction to globalization, climate change, the growth of terrorism, and alienation in the Information Age (Minahan & Wolfram Cox, 2007), as well as a shift toward collectivity that fulfills a need for social connection. Another reason for the resurgence of crafts that traditionally have been considered "women's work" may be directly related to third-wave feminism's focus on "choice": people of all genders may now feel that they can freely choose to engage in textiles rather than being forced to practice these crafts thanks to the hard work earlier feminists did to gain distance from being relegated to "women's work" and to increase women's access to other spheres of work (Pearl-McPhee, as cited in Pentney, 2008). Some contemporary crafters even seek to directly challenge the domestic and gendered nature of textile practices, leading to a reclamation, redefinition, and repurposing of media traditionally associated with "women's work" as activism (Chansky, 2010; Goggin, 2014).

As craft practices become more popular another assumption needs to be addressed: that of craftwork as a "leisure" activity. Contemporary crafting in the Global North is generally uncritically conceived of as being by and large a leisure activity pursued by those who can afford the time, energy, and materials to engage in it. Hollenbach (2019) reminded us of the importance of "analyses that investigate the intersections of the craftsperson's identity (gender, race, economic privilege or deprivation, geographic location, and so on) as well as the social, economic, political, and ideological circumstances of craft's creation and its appreciation and consumption" (para. 2).

In reality, crafts that many people engage in as leisure activities constitute poorly paid jobs or unpaid labor for poor and working class people and people of color throughout the world (Portwood-Stacer, 2007; Robertson & Vinebaum, 2016); for example, factory labor and clothing manufacturing. Robertson and Vinebaum (2016) found that although contemporary craft and craft activism may draw attention to oppression, exploitation, and other social issues, the practice also has been "associated with ideals of utopian labor that often obscure real, exploitative, and gendered conditions of production" (pp. 8–9). Again, it is important to note that many discussions of the merits of craft do not address the race and class biases inherent in the assumption that craft can be utilized as a form of leisure for everyone, thus revealing an ethnocentric bias. It is essential to remember that "crafting has traditionally been an activity of leisure for white women but a means of survival for people of color" (Ivey, 2019, p. 312). Thus, there exists the potential for racist and classist behaviors if we do not acknowledge that leisure is inherently a privilege—applied to crafting, doubly so.

Another way in which class, racial, and gender biases manifest within discourse about crafts is that even within the realms of North American craft, a modernist hierarchy exists. This division results in criteria that have functioned to "gatekeep and exclude craft objects and practices that did not fit with a materially and conceptually restricted program," such as "craft made by non-western people [and] indigenous makers, naïve folk art by rural and oftentimes impoverished craftspeople, and women's domestic handicrafts made from patterns and kits" (Hollenbach, 2019, para. 6). Therefore, art therapists who seek to incorporate craft practices into their work need to be mindful of assumptions about leisure and labor, culturally resonant practices, and which materials and methods we continue to tacitly value and devalue. Art therapists must also be conscious not to replicate problematic cultural appropriation that exists in the contemporary crafting industry, where designs created by Native American, African American, Latinx, and Asian American crafters based on their heritage are appropriated by white people (Ivey, 2019). Crafts created by the "other" have throughout history been primitivized, fetishized, appropriated, stolen, and stripped of their context (Han Sifuentes, 2017, para. 1), and art therapists need to guard against perpetuating colonized frameworks when incorporating crafts into personal and professional practices.

The Therapeutic Properties of Craft

Crafts have long been understood to be beneficial even if these benefits haven't been fully understood or embraced by art therapy. Specifically, crafts have kinesthetic and sensory properties, they can be a more accessible art form for those who do not consider themselves artistic, they allow for a range of skill levels and subsequent sense of agency through mastering new skills, and they offer the potential for greater socialization than many other art forms.

Most of the research on the therapeutic potential of crafts has focused on textiles. Collier (2011, 2012), a clinical psychologist and Reynolds (1999, 2000, 2002, 2004a, 2004b, 2009), a health psychologist, have conducted significant research on the therapeutic properties of textiles. Collier (2011, 2012) learned that many of her clients independently sought to creatively use textile arts for psychological reasons and, in response, conducted several qualitative and quantitative studies that affirmed the value of craft to her clients. Working with textiles allowed participants to calm and center themselves, gain a sense of control over their lives, benefit from social interaction, and connect with a pleasurable sensory experience.

Collier (2011, 2012) also found that participants in her study derived a healing pleasure from both the tactile properties of textile crafts and the rhythm of the repetitive motion involved. Subsequently, Collier and von Károyli (2014) explored how textile handcrafters experienced rejuvenation—that is, a state of mood improvement that persisted after completion of their crafting activity. The researchers related the textile crafters' feelings to *flow state*, as named by Csikszentmihalyi (1990) in reference to a state of relaxed productivity that individuals achieve through engaging in tasks that balance focus with a sense of mastery. A subsequent study by Collier, Wayment, and Birkett (2016) determined that "a textile art-making activity that was high in arousal, engagement, and positive mood and low in rumination and negative affect" was an effective approach to mood repair (p. 178). The finding that crafts can support affect regulation and promote positive moods was supported in a large international survey of knitters conducted by occupational therapists Riley, Corkhill, and Morris (2013) that found significant psychological and social benefits of knitting. These included "a significant relationship between knitting frequency and feeling calm and happy" as well as "higher cognitive functioning" (p. 50). And in a study of women textile crafters, Pöllänen (2015) found that crafting contributed to well-being and a sense of empowerment through mastery over materials, a sense of control over emotions, and the social and cultural dimensions of craft.

Some art therapists have also observed the therapeutic benefits of textiles. For example, Homer (2015) described the use of fabric collage in the treatment of trauma and noted the importance of the medium's relational and rhythmic properties, as well as how the sensory experience of working with textiles proved soothing and nurturing to her clients. Garlock (2016) also mentioned the importance of the sensory and kinesthetic properties of textiles in her research on the use of story cloths with women who had experienced trauma. She explained that the slow process of sewing allowed time to work through "difficult or deep emotions" (p. 58). Talwar (2015) and Garlock (2016) both posited that fiber arts that use both hands may promote bilateral stimulation of brain functions and therefore may serve an integrating function when people recount traumatic experiences. In describing art therapy with survivors of domestic violence, Miller and Malchiodi (2012) highlighted the self-soothing properties that repetitive practices such as sewing, quilting, knitting, and weaving possess. They observed how these media provided comfort through their kinesthetic properties and also by fostering a sense of psychological safety, due to being media that were not usually analyzed or judged on the merits of their aesthetic qualities.

According to research by Reynolds (1999, 2000, 2002, 2004a, 2004b, 2009), craft textile processes can positively affect people with physical and mental health problems. She found that textile arts provided women with chronic illnesses with a means to fill time productively, gain social contacts based on mutual interests rather than caregiving relationships, discover symbolic expression, experience a sense of mastery, and express spiritual values. Over the course of their illnesses, participants who engaged in textile arts transformed their feelings and strengthened their sense of identity (Reynolds, 2002, 2004a,

2004b). Reynolds (2000) also found that participants with depression identified textile work as mentally and physically relaxing and that crafting increased self-esteem, restored a sense of control, bolstered energy, and provided social support and a way to structure time.

Coupled with its individual therapeutic aspects, craft's "social power" (Talwar, 2015) gives it unique therapeutic potential. In contrast with many fine arts practices, crafting often involves socialization and collective activity, as seen in quilting bees, sewing and knitting circles, woodworking and hot glass shops, and pottery studios. When people come together to participate explicitly in community building through crafting, craft may serve as a focal source for solidarity, which for a distressed community is essential to mending the social fabric (Goggin, 2014). When crafting occurs in a community setting, there is an opportunity for sharing experiences in which individuals can gain support and validation (Leone, 2018).

As part of a decade-long participatory action research study with older African American women transitioning out of homelessness, Moxley, Feen-Calligan, Washington, and Garriott (2011) created a quilting project, in part for its community-building potential. The researchers found that quilting simultaneously functioned as a form of advocacy for participants who exhibited the quilts to the public and as a form of social support. They concluded that "quilting affirms a group's experience and offers its members opportunities for reflection, reframing of experiences, and mutual support" (Moxley et al., 2011, p. 114). Nainis (2005) also investigated the community-building benefits of quilt making during a hospital oncology care team retreat focused on self-care and communication. She found that a quilt, as something that brings separate pieces together to create an aesthetically pleasing and functional piece of work, served as a powerful metaphor to participants, along with providing associations of warmth and protection. The social benefits of crafting in a group were also found in a study of knitters who reported that knitting in a group has significant influence on a sense of happiness, increased social contact, and improved communication with others (Riley et al., 2013).

Although some crafts are easily accessible, such as knitting, others have historically been reserved for certain people based on class and gender—but the increased popularity of crafting is offering a wider range of people access to craft practices. For example, woodworker Sarah Marriage (2018) started A Workshop of Our Own, "an educational woodshop created by and for women and non-binary people" as one of many activist woodshops emerging in recent years that are working to "change expectations and encourage greater participation in the field" (para. 9). As part of a similar trend in community glass crafts studios, Project FIRE, co-created by a glass blowing artist and a clinical psychologist, "combines glassblowing, mentoring, employment, and leadership opportunities for youth injured by violence" (Project FIRE, n.d.). The program also provides participants psychoeducation about trauma, along with case management and medical treatment.

Another way that mutual support can emerge in community crafting is through storytelling. When crafting occurs in groups, relaxed conversation typically emerges. Garlock (2016) posited that when people are encouraged to tell their stories while they sew, they find support, social connection with others, and group validation of their individual experiences and feelings. She elaborated that many people who have experienced trauma feel shame and isolation and may be afraid to think or talk about their trauma and that sewing groups can serve as an "antidote" to those emotions (p. 58). A powerful example of using craft for storytelling is the Combat Paper Project (n.d.), a papermaking workshop program for military veterans. Participants transform their old uniforms by cutting them up and learning to make paper from them, on which they recount personal stories of military service through images and words. They then engage in exhibitions and community dialogue involving veterans, activists, and artists "about their collective responsibilities and understanding of war" (The Combat Paper Project, 2013, p. 96).

Crafting in groups also merges the dichotomies of private/public and individual/collective. For example, Moxley et al. (2011) noted that creating quilt squares in a group allowed participants to choose to work alone in the group and/or collaboratively. Because individuals often hold their crafts in or near their laps, the experience may engender a sense of privacy and intimacy while still providing the benefit of group support. This idea of craft as containing an element of intimacy relates to the fact that many forms of crafting have primarily taken place in the domestic sphere, away from the public eye and in close proximity to loved ones.

The communal nature of many crafts lends them to models of collective care rather than individual care, which can disrupt the norm of individual therapy. Art therapist Talwar is the project director of Creatively Empowered Women Design Studio (n.d.), which provides a space for refugees and immigrant women to gather and craft together with the goals of empowerment, building social connections and support, and earning income through selling creations made at the studio. Talwar (201b) explained that the studio "expands the focus on art therapy and wellbeing through crafting to increase the social capital and self-efficacy of its members" (p. 21). She also described how "the joyful act of crafting and community collaboration can play a critical role in envisioning 'new paradigms of care' that cultivate a sense of community, wellbeing, and social capital" (Talwar, 2019a, p. 180).

Similarly, the international Men's Shed movement (Culph, Wilson, Cordier, & Stancliffe, 2015; Taylor et al., 2016) is creating communal workspaces where older men who may be experiencing isolation due to retirement, bereavement, or health issues congregate to work on woodworking and metalworking projects, among other crafts. Taylor et al. (2016) found that in participants with depression, the social focus combined with the crafting resulted in decreased self-reports of symptoms of depression, concluding that Men's Sheds provide social contact and a sense of purpose without foregrounding the mental health issues that many participants may not be comfortable directly addressing due to stigma.

Taking into consideration the renewed interest in craft practices accompanied by the proliferation of public crafting, feminist scholars have proposed that participatory cultures of making are a way for "people to reclaim power in their everyday lives" and have even led to what some refer to as a shift from DIY (do-it-yourself) to DIT (do-it-together; Chidgey, 2014, p. 104). The 21st-century craft movement is taking place in community spaces—or "third places" (Oldenburg, 1997)—more and more. Oldenburg (1997) asserted that "social well-being and psychological health depend upon community" and even suggested that the rise of helping professions in the United States was directly related to the destruction of community support due to suburban planning (p. 7). This belief in the interrelatedness of individual and community health is at the core of community psychology, which asserts that well-being is not reliant on an individual's health but is rather something that takes place between individuals and their environments (Nelson & Prilleltensky, 2010).

"Third spaces" can provide fertile settings for socially just art therapy practice. Unlike home, work, and institutional spaces where many therapy practices are located, third spaces act as sites for individuals to address community issues within their communities (Timm-Bottos, 2016, 2017) and a community model of art therapy can support "concepts of belonging and wellbeing as a collective endeavor" (Talwar, 2019a, p. 183). Thus, the community setting is witness to actions individuals can take and possibly sustain collectively, beyond their individual issues.

Given the social power of craft, when groups of people who are marginalized or oppressed gather together to craft, both process and product can become an awareness-raising tool and even a method of resistance to social and/or political oppression. And throughout the world and across history, craft has indeed been used as form of activism to resist social and political oppression—from abolitionist quilts created before and during the U.S. Civil War (Lufkin, 2019) to embroidered banners made by British suffragists (Parker, 2010; Wheeler, 2012), from truth-telling *arpilleras*—or story cloths—created by Chilean women during Augusto Pinochet's dictatorship (Agosín, 2008) to the *AIDS Memorial Quilt*.

Attention to Craft in Art Therapy

Although there has been a recent increase in research about the use of textile arts in art therapy practice, craft is underrepresented in the art therapy literature overall. Particularly noteworthy is the general absence of craft from art therapy training literature, especially texts on theory and practice, which demonstrates a pattern of privileging the fine arts. In my survey of commonly used introductory texts (e.g., Case & Dalley, 2014; Dalley, 1984; Hogan & Coulter, 2014; Malchiodi, 2012; McNiff, 1981, 1998, 2004; Rubin, 2011, 2016; Wadeson, 2010), the term *art* is used to connote drawing, painting, or sculpture; *craft* is rarely mentioned. Likewise, when art therapy texts feature images of client artwork, they rarely if ever show craft. For example, Rubin's (2001) *Approaches to Art Therapy* includes over 100 images of client artwork, and none of them veer from drawing, painting, or sculpture. Wadeson's (2010) *Art Psychotherapy* features hundreds of images of drawings and paintings, and a few sculptures. Hinz's (2009) *Expressive Therapy Continuum*, based on Lusebrink's (1990) organization of "media interactions into a developmental sequence of information processing and image formation from simple to complex" (p. 4), describes a range of art materials based on their properties (from fluid to resistive), and the experiences they may elicit has been central to many art therapists' understanding of material use. However, there is no mention of craft materials in the 2009 edition, and in the second edition (Hinz, 2020) there is only a short section about textiles, along with the recognition that they are still considered unconventional materials in art therapy practice but are being used more frequently. Because these and other texts that offer formative instruction for art therapy students who are entering and being socialized into the profession model the language and images used by established professionals to describe art therapy practice, the omission of craft from such foundational art therapy texts undoubtedly influences students' beliefs, perceptions, and attitudes regarding the "art" involved in art therapy.

Although there are some exceptions when authors do mention craft in art therapy texts, such instances typically appear as warnings against the limitations of craft. For example, in *The Art of Art Therapy*, Rubin (2011) stated that unstructured materials such as paint, clay, and pastels allow individuals to find their own expressive styles, whereas paint-by-numbers, clay molds, and looms for creating pot holders do not constitute art therapy activities because they do not allow individuals to "find their own imagery and in doing so find their authentic selves" (p. 5). Rubin goes on to describe the properties of various art materials without exploring craft materials beyond the conception of them as formulaic or "pleasant activities" (2011, p. 5). Craft materials can be used alone, of course, rather than only through kits or patterns, and they indeed contain expressive properties. In addition, Kapitan (2003) explained that even when we as artists do use someone else's pattern, we don't merely imitate but "bring to it our own particularities or personality something from us that joins with the other, the living material in our hands" (p. 72).

Prevailing beliefs about craft's limitations may have their roots in early art therapists' perceptions of craft. Kramer (1975), for example, held that craft resulted in useful objects whereas art resulted in a product that had symbolic value, and therefore craft's therapeutic potential was limited. "Only when art is freed from its decorative function can it become fully expressive," she wrote, going on to claim that "truly expressive art is sometimes out of reach for children who are very constricted, or fearful, or empty" and that "there is a need, therefore, for projects which allow a child to succeed in making something with his own hands simply by following a logical procedure that does not tax his limited capacities beyond endurance" (Kramer, 1975, p. 107). These statements reveal the implicit and likely cultural bias of the historical moment in which Kramer was writing, which viewed craft as formulaic, not requiring or engaging in creativity and to be used only with clients whose functioning is limited.

Additionally, early art therapists focused on the importance of the unconscious and felt that the skills needed to engage in crafts would inhibit this process (Talwar, 2019b). Art therapy pioneers Ulman, Kramer, and Kwiatkowska (1977) even directly called for art and craft to take place in different physical areas from one another, describing them as "distinct realms" (p. 9). This was most likely part of an effort to legitimize art therapy and create a distinction between art therapy and occupational therapy, which recognized the therapeutic potential of arts and crafts (Moon, 2010; Talwar, 2019b). Art therapists may also have felt an implicit need to ally themselves with "fine arts" media in academic and psychological contexts to distinguish themselves from art educators working exclusively with children. This need to distinguish the art therapy field from other allied professions persists today, continuing to limit art therapy's adoption of craft practices (Kaimal, Gonzaga, & Schwachter, 2017; Talwar, 2019b).

Regardless of their origins, there are many misconceptions about crafts. Until recently, mentions of craft in art therapy literature primarily were found in texts on adapting art therapy for children and individuals with exceptional education or rehabilitative needs. These biased assumptions about craft have the inadvertent effect of constraining art therapy participants from access to craft materials and processes that could benefit them greatly. As Huss (2010) explained, "An important conceptual shift for art therapists is one that understands all art forms, not just traditional fine arts practices, as potentially expressive of personal and cultural values" (p. 220).

Craft practices have begun to see greater representation in more recent art therapy literature and conference presentations. Textiles have the greatest representation (e.g., Collier, 2011; Collier & von Károyli, 2014; Collier et al., 2016; Garlock, 2016; Homer, 2015, 2019; Huss, 2010; Leone, 2018, 2019; Moxley et al., 2011; Napoli & Kirby, 2019; Ravichandran, 2019; Talwar, 2019a, 2019b), along with media such as glass arts (Horovitz, 2018; Somer & Somer, 2000; Parker-Bell, 2019; Stallings, Wolf Bordonara, Miller, & Clark, 2019), ceramics (Nan, 2015; Nan & Ho, 2017), zines (Houpt, Balkin, Broom, Roth, & Selma, 2016), jewelry (Horovitz, 2018; Ravichandran, 2019), body adornments (Yi, 2010), and upcycled fashion (Timm-Bottos, 2011).

This increased interest in crafting may reflect the larger culture of the United States. In their call to art therapists to incorporate craft practices in their work, Kaimal et al. (2017) cited their secondary analysis of data from the National Endowment for the Arts' 2012 Survey of Public Participation in the Arts, which found that:

> There are more individuals engaged in crafting than visual arts activities, indicating that crafting and intentional engagement with crafting traditions

can be a means for art therapists to break the dominion of Western artistic traditions and paradigms and engage with artisanal approaches.

(p. 88)

Themes of This Book

The many diverse voices and craft media represented in this book provide further evidence of the individual and collective benefits of craft, leading the way toward a future art therapy field in which the power and potential of craft is fully appreciated, valued, and utilized. The book's chapters are organized around the objective of demonstrating how craft practices can serve as valuable and culturally resonant practices in art therapy contexts. Craft's value is illustrated through themes such as collaboration, care, and community, revealing what Ravestz, Kettle, and Felcey (2013) referred to as "craft's fundamentally social and relational character" (p. 13).

Contributing authors provide examples of how art therapists have incorporated a range of crafts including pottery, glass work, textiles (such as sewing, knitting, crochet, embroidery, and quilting), paper (such as artist books, altered books, book binding, origami, and zines), leatherwork, and traditional Indian crafts like mendhi and kolam/rangoli in their own art practice, self-care, and art therapy practice with individuals, groups, and communities. At the time of writing this book, I was unable to find the work of art therapists who incorporate woodworking or metalsmithing in their practice, but I hope to be able to include these and other crafts in subsequent editions as the use of craft in art therapy increases.

Craft as a Tool for Transformation and Self-Care

Craft practices transform raw materials into objects that serve a purpose, whether aesthetic, functional, or both. Transformation can take place through reworking, revising, reforming, adjusting, or altering—all processes that hold symbolic value and thus have unique therapeutic potential. In Chapter 1, Lynn Kapitan shares how the contemplative practice of crafting artist books has paralleled an unfolding and transforming understanding of art therapy for her. She describes how this embodied craft can allow the maker to process the trauma of living in a world in need of human touch and caring and demonstrates that *how* things are made—with exquisite care, loving touch, and attention—matters and is worthy of attention. In another take on transformation, Jessica Woolhiser Stallings and Stephanie Clark describe their experiences incorporating glass fusion and glass blowing in art therapy practice in Chapter 2, demonstrating the metaphorical properties of glass art and highlighting its potential for cathartic and mindful experiences. And in Chapter 3, Joshua Nan describes his experience establishing a pottery studio at a social service agency in Hong Kong, illustrating how the alchemical process of transforming clay into ceramic, along with the constructing, destructing, and reconstructing processes of clay art making, can provide a parallel inner alchemical process of transformation for art therapy participants.

Two authors directly address the use of craft in self-care practices. In Chapter 4, Chun-shan (Sandie) Yi challenges existing self-care strategies in the field of art therapy by calling into question the field's Western, individualistic focus. Through describing her process of sewing wearable art objects about the lived experiences of disabled activists, Yi examines the metaphor of sewing and the meaning of repair, illustrating the need for a sustainable self-care practice for art therapists who have experienced disability and/or illness. And in Chapter 5, Marilyn Holmes discusses a method of self-care she developed to contain the complex feelings caused by the toxic racial stress she experiences as a Black woman in higher education. She explains how creating small crocheted animals helps her unpack, contain, and externalize her responses to microaggressions she has experienced in the classroom or in her practicum work.

Craft as Culturally Resonant and Accessible

As discussed earlier, utilizing only "fine arts" media in art therapy not only cuts participants off from many media that could be uniquely beneficial to them, it is also ethnocentric. "One size fits all" approaches that assume that the materials that have been privileged throughout the course of the field's short history are the best and only ones to use negatively affect people whose cultural traditions are not reflected in such approaches. Incorporating culturally resonant craft practices into art therapy can honor participants' cultural context, history, and knowledge. In Chapter 6, Eliza Homer discusses an arts-based research study she conducted in Central Mexico to explore if using traditional Mexican craft could serve as a culturally appropriate art therapy tool. She describes how the link between artisan craft and well-being can increase cultural connection and create a bridge between folk healing and Western mental health treatment, with the potential of increasing engagement in services.

In Chapter 7, Krupa Jhaveri describes her incorporation of the traditional Indian art forms of mendhi and kolam into her art therapy practice, demonstrating how traditional Indian crafts can be sensitively adapted within art therapy practice to help restore participants' relationships to their roots. Mahesh Iyer, in Chapter 8, discusses his cross-cultural integration of rangoli (a regional variation of kolam), within a group art therapy setting of predominantly Chinese elderly residents at a sheltered home in Singapore. He identifies the range of therapeutic benefits the group experienced through the themes of cultural integration and reconnection with their personal, local, and cultural identities. Finally, in Chapter 9, Michal Katoshevski and Ephrat Huss use an intersectional feminist perspective to illustrate how contextualizing embroidery in traditional

Bedouin culture provides art therapists with an example of how to use crafts to support art therapy participants within their social realities.

Craft as Empowerment and Activism

Incorporating craft processes into art therapy practice can support individuals in experiencing empowerment and agency, expressing their individual and collective realities, and even working together to resist marginalization and oppression. In Chapter 10, I describe a collaborative craft activism project I facilitated with a group of senior women aimed to raise community awareness around the gentrification and displacement impacting their neighborhood. In this community model of art therapy, collaborative craft activism built individuals' capacity to address an issue affecting their community, and developing these skills served a therapeutic function. In Chapter 11, Joe Mageary shows how zines, as a form of do-it-yourself activism and identity empowerment, promote learning, healing, and an association with supportive communities, particularly within marginalized groups. He demonstrates that zines provide a fertile ground for art therapists and art therapy participants to co-construct both meaningful acts of resistance to oppression and connection to experiences of empowerment.

In Chapter 12, Lisa Raye Garlock explores how narrative textiles may start as personal stories that need to be told and then become important statements about universal human rights and social justice issues. Through examining individual and group story cloth making, she demonstrates how narrative textiles and art therapy work powerfully together to express what needs to be known and heal on individual and collective levels. In Chapter 13, Jaimie Peterson and Alison Etter describe how art mentorship through peer-led craft workshops result in reducing stigma, creating community, and providing valuable social roles for the individuals they work with in a forensic psychiatric hospital. They describe how their experience can inform art therapists who work with individuals with stigmatized and/or marginalized identities in a range of settings.

In Chapter 14, Mikey Anderson presents a call to action for art therapists to push the field toward a truly inclusive space for Queer people through centering Queer voices and experiences. By centering collaborative and individual art making focused on quilting, comics, and other fiber crafts, Anderson engages in a reflective, intersectional exploration of Queer experience, ultimately proposing the practice of Queering art therapy as a political act. Finally, in Chapter 15, Savneet Talwar and Rachel Wallis examine social practice through an art therapy lens and use an ethics of care methodology to contextualize "radical empathy" in public crafting spaces. Their description of a collaborative quilting project that took place across prison walls demonstrates how artists and art therapists can engage in community-based settings and socially engaged art in ethical and affectively responsible ways.

In sum, this book invites art therapy students, practitioners, and educators to widen our conception of what approaches we can use with the individuals and communities with whom we work. The examples in this book of how craft can be integrated into art therapy theory and practice show that when practiced in a culturally sensitive and socially conscientious manner, crafts practices are more than uniquely therapeutic—they also hold transformational potential.

References

Adamson, G. (2010). *The craft reader*. New York, NY: Berg.

Agosín, M. (2008). *Tapestries of hope, threads of love: The* arpillera *movement in Chile* (2nd ed.). Lanham, MD: Rowman & Littlefield.

Barber, E. W. (1994). *Women's work: The first 20,000 years: Women, cloth, and society in early times*. New York, NY: W. W. Norton.

Berger, M. A. (2005). *Sight unseen: Whiteness and American visual culture*. Berkeley, CA: University of California Press.

Bratich, J. Z., & Brush, H. M. (2011). Fabricating activism: Craft-work, popular culture, gender. *Utopian Studies, 22*(2), 233–260. doi:10.5325/utopianstudies.22.2.0233

Broude, N., & Garrard, M. D. (1982). *Feminism and art history: Questioning the litany*. New York, NY: Harper & Row.

Brown, J. K. (1970). Notes on the division of labor by sex. *American Anthropologist, 72*(5), 1073–1078.

Browne, K. (1994). The future perfect: Activism and advocacy. *Metalsmith, 14*(Spring), 34–39.

Callen, A. (1985). Sexual division of labor in the arts and crafts movement. *Woman's Art Journal, 5*(2), 1–6. doi:10.2307/1357958

Case, C., & Dalley, T. (2014). *The handbook of art therapy* (3rd ed.). New York, NY: Routledge.

Chansky, R. A. (2010). A stitch in time: Third-wave feminist reclamation of needled imagery. *Journal of Popular Culture, 43*(4), 681–700. doi:10.1111/j.15405931.2010.00765.x PMID:20645475

Chidgey, R. (2014). Developing communities of resistance? Maker pedagogies, do-it-yourself feminism, and DIY citizenship. In M. Ratto & M. Boler (Eds.), *DIY citizenship: Critical making and social media* (pp. 101–113). Cambridge, MA: MIT Press.

Collier, A. F. (2011). The well-being of women who create with textiles: Implications for art therapy. *Art Therapy: Journal of the American Art Therapy Association, 28*(3), 104–112. doi:10.1080/07421656.2011.597025

Collier, A. F. (2012). *Using textile arts and handcrafts in therapy with women: Weaving lives back together*. London, England: Jessica Kingsley.

Collier, A. F., & von Károyli, C. (2014). Rejuvenation in the "making": Lingering mood repair in textile handcrafters. *Psychology of Aesthetics, Creativity, and the Arts, 8*(4), 475–485. doi:10.1037/a0037080

Collier, A. F., Wayment, H. A., & Birkett, M. (2016). Impact of making textile handcrafts on mood enhancement and inflammatory immune changes. *Art Therapy: Journal of the American Art Therapy Association, 33*(4), 178–185. doi:10.1080/07421656.2016.1226647

Combat Paper. (n.d.). *About*. Retrieved from www.combatpaper.org/about

The combat paper project. (2013). *The Iowa Review, 43*(1), 96–100. doi:10.17077/0021-065X.7307

Creatively Empowered Women Design Studio. (n.d.). *Home*. Retrieved from www.creativelyempowered women.com/

Csikszentmihalyi, M. (1990). *Flow: The psychology of optimal experience*. New York, NY: Harper & Row.

Culph, J. S., Wilson, N. J., Cordier, R., & Stancliffe, R. J. (2015). Men's sheds and the experience of depression in older Australian men. *Australian Occupational Therapy Journal, 62*(5), 306–315. doi:10.1111/1440-1630.12190

Dalley, T. (1984). *Art as therapy: An introduction to the use of art as a therapeutic technique*. New York, NY: Routledge.

Dunn, R. (2014). The changing status and recognition of fiber work within the realm of the visual arts. In M. Agosín (Ed.), *Stitching resistance: Women, creativity, and fiber arts* (pp. 43–53). Kent, England: Solis Press.

Garlock, L. R. (2016). Stories in the cloth: Art therapy and narrative textiles. *Art Therapy: Journal of the American Art Therapy Association, 33*(2), 58–66. doi:10.1080/07421656.2016.1164004

Gauntlett, D. (2011). *Making is connecting: The social meaning of creativity, from DIY and knitting to YouTube and Web 2.0*. Cambridge, England: Polity Press.

Goggin, M. D. (2014, September). *Threads of feeling: Embroidering craftivism to protest the disappearances and deaths in the "war on drugs" in Mexico*. Textile Society of America 2014 Biennial Symposium Proceedings: New Directions: Examining the Past, Creating the Future, 937. Retrieved from http://digitalcommons.unl.edu/tsaconf/937

Han Sifuentes, A. (2017, April 23). Steps towards decolonizing craft [Blog post]. *Textile Society of America*. Retrieved from https://textilesocietyofamerica.org/6728/steps-towards-decolonizing-craft/

Hinz, L. D. (2009). *Expressive Therapies Continuum: A framework for using art in therapy*. New York, NY: Routledge.

Hinz, L. D. (2020). *Expressive Therapies Continuum: A framework for using art in therapy* (2nd ed.). New York, NY: Routledge.

Hogan, S., & Coulter, A. M. (2014). *The introductory guide to art therapy: Experiential teaching and learning for students and practitioners*. New York, NY: Routledge.

Hollenbach, J. (2019). Moving beyond a modern craft: Thoughts on White entitlement and cultural appropriation in professional craft in Canada. *Studio Magazine: Craft and Design in Canada, 14*(1), 24–27.

Homer, E. S. (2015). Piece work: Fabric collage as a neurodevelopmental approach to trauma treatment. *Art Therapy: Journal of the American Art Therapy Association, 32*(1), 20–26.

Horovitz, E. G. (2018). *A guide to art therapy materials, methods, and applications: A practical step-by-step approach*. New York, NY: Routledge.

Houpt, K., Balkin, L. A., Broom, R. H., Roth, A. G., & Selma. (2016). Anti-memoir: Creating alternate nursing home narratives through zine making. *Art Therapy: Journal of the American Art Therapy Association, 33*(3), 128–137.

Huss, E. (2010). Bedouin women's embroidery as female empowerment: Crafts as culturally embedded expression within art therapy. In C. H. Moon (Ed.), *Materials and media in art therapy: Critical understandings of diverse artistic vocabularies* (pp. 215–230). New York, NY: Routledge.

Ivey, D. (2019). Reshaping the narrative around people of color and craftivism. In H. Mandell (Ed.), *Crafting dissent: Handicraft as protest from the American Revolution to the Pussyhats* (pp. 309–318). Lanham, MD: Rowman & Littlefield.

Jefferies, J. (2011). Loving attention: An outburst of craft in contemporary art. In M. A. Buszek (Ed.), *Extra/ordinary: Craft and contemporary art* (pp. 222–240). Durham, NC: Duke University Press.

Kaimal, G., Gonzaga, A. M. L., & Schwachter, V. (2017). Crafting, health and wellbeing: Findings from the survey of public participation in the arts and considerations for art therapists. *Arts & Health, 9*(1), 81–90. doi:10.1080/17533015.2016.1185447

Kapitan, L. (2003). *Re-enchanting art therapy*. Springfield, IL: Charles C Thomas.

Kapitan, L. (2011). Close to the heart: Art therapy's link to craft and art production. *Art Therapy: Journal of the American Art Therapy Association, 28*(3), 94–95. doi:10.1080/07421656.2011.601728

Kramer, E. (1975). Art and craft. In E. Ulman & P. Dachinger (Eds.), *Art therapy in theory and practice* (pp. 106–109). New York, NY: Schocken Books.

Krugh, M. (2014). Joy in labour: The politicization of craft from the arts and crafts movement to Etsy. *Canadian Review of American Studies, 44*(2), 281–301. doi:10.3138/CRAS.2014.S06

Langlands, A. (2017). *Craeft: An inquiry into the origins and true meaning of traditional crafts*. New York, NY: W. W. Norton & Company.

Leone, L. (2018). *Crafting change: Craft activism and community-based art therapy* (Doctoral dissertation). Mount Mary University. Retrieved from www.worldcat.org/oclc/1035718897

Leone, L. (2019). Crafting change: Craft activism for community-based art therapy. In H. Mandell (Ed.), *Crafting dissent: Handicraft as protest from the American Revolution to the Pussyhats* (pp. 247–262). Lanham, MD: Rowman & Littlefield.

Lippard, L. R. (1978). Making something from nothing (toward a definition of women's "hobby art"). In G. Adamson (Ed.), *The craft reader* (pp. 483–490). Oxford, England: Bloomsbury Academic.

Lippard, L. R. (1995). *The pink glass swan: Selected essays on feminist art*. New York, NY: New Press.

Lucie-Smith, E. (1981). *The story of craft: The craftsman's role in society*. Ithaca, NY: Cornell University Press.

Lufkin, F. (2019). The Underground Railroad quilt code myth and the culture of crafted experience. In H. Mandell (Ed.), *Crafting dissent: Handicraft as protest from the American Revolution to the Pussyhats* (pp. 77–94). Lanham, MD: Rowman & Littlefield.

Lusebrink, V. J. (1990). Art therapy and the brain: An attempt to understand the underlying processes of art expression in therapy. *Art Therapy: Journal of the American Art Therapy Association, 21*(3), 125–135.

Mainardi, P. (1982). Quilts: The great American art. In N. Broude & M. D. Garrard (Eds.), *Feminism and art history: Questioning the litany* (pp. 330–346). New York, NY: Harper & Row.

Malchiodi, C. A. (2012). *Handbook of art therapy* (2nd ed.). New York, NY: Guilford.

Marriage, S. (2018, January 8). *Sisterhood is powerful*. Retrieved from https://craftcouncil.org/magazine/article/sisterhood-powerful

McNiff, S. (1981). *The arts in psychotherapy*. Springfield, IL: Charles C Thomas.

McNiff, S. (1998). *Trust the process: An artist's guide to letting go*. Boston, MA: Shambhala.

McNiff, S. (2004). *Art heals: How creativity cures the soul*. Boston, MA: Shambhala.

Miller, G., & Malchiodi, C. A. (2012). Art therapy and domestic violence. In C. A. Malchiodi (Ed.), *Handbook of art therapy* (2nd ed., pp. 335–348). New York, NY: Guilford.

Minahan, S., & Wolfram Cox, J. (2007). Stitch'n Bitch: Cyberfeminism, a third place and the new materiality. *Journal of Material Culture, 12*(1), 5–21. doi:10.1177/1359183507074559

Moon, C. H. (Ed.). (2010). *Materials and media in art therapy: Critical understandings of diverse artistic vocabularies*. New York, NY: Routledge.

Moxley, D. P., Feen-Calligan, H., Washington, O. G. M., & Garriott, L. (2011). Quilting in self-efficacy group work with older African American women leaving homelessness. *Art Therapy: Journal of the American Art Therapy Association, 28*(3), 113–122. doi:10.1080/07421656.2011.599729

Nainis, N. A. (2005). Art therapy with an oncology care team. *Art Therapy: Journal of the American Art Therapy Association, 22*(3), 150–154. doi:10.1080/07421656.2005.10129491

Nan, J. K. M. (2015). *Therapeutic effects of Clay Art Therapy for patients with depression* (Doctoral dissertation). The University of Hong Kong, Hong Kong.

Nan, J. K. M., & Ho, R. T. H. (2017). Effects of clay art therapy on adult outpatients with major depressive disorder: A randomized controlled trial. *Journal of Affective Disorders, 217*, 237–245.

Napoli, M., & Kirby, M. (2019). Crafting the "Vulva Quilt": A community response to being silenced. In H. Mandell (Ed.), *Crafting dissent: Handicraft as protest from the American Revolution to the Pussyhats* (pp. 279–290). Lanham, MD: Rowman & Littlefield.

Nelson, G., & Prilleltensky, I. (2010). *Community psychology: In pursuit of liberation and well-being* (2nd ed.). New York, NY: Palgrave Macmillan.

Oldenburg, R. (1997). Our vanishing third spaces. *Planning Commissioners Journal, 25*, 6–10.

Parker, R. (2010). *The subversive stitch: Embroidery and the making of the feminine*. New York, NY: Palgrave Macmillan. (Original work published 1984).

Parker, R., & Pollock, G. (2013). *Old mistresses: Women, art and ideology*. London, England: I.B. Taurus.

Parker-Bell, B. (2019). *Strong of heart: Designing a fused glass project to support student resilience*. Paper presented at the 50th Annual Conference of the American Art Therapy Association, Kansas City, MO.

Pentney, B. A. (2008). Feminism, activism, and knitting: Are the fibre arts a viable mode for feminist political action? *Thirdspace: A Journal of Feminist Theory and Culture, 8*(1). Retrieved from http://journals.sfu.ca/thirdspace/index.php/journal/article/viewArticle/pentney/210

Pöllänen, S. (2015). Elements of crafts that enhance well-being: Textile craft makers' descriptions of their leisure activity. *Journal of Leisure Research, 47*(1), 58–78.

Portwood-Stacer, L. (2007, May). *Do-it-yourself feminism: Feminine individualism and the girlie backlash in the "craftivism" movement*. Paper presented at the annual meeting of the International Communication Association, San Francisco, CA. Retrieved from http://citation.allacademic.com/meta/p169635_index.html

Project FIRE. (n.d.). *Our story*. Retrieved from https://www.projectfirechicago.org/our-vision

Ravestz, A., Kettle, A., & Felcey, H. (2013). *Collaboration through craft*. New York, NY: Bloomsbury Academic.

Ravichandran, S. (2019). Radical caring and art therapy: Decolonizing immigration and gender violence services. In S. K. Talwar (Ed.), *Art therapy for social justice: Radical intersections* (pp. 144–160). New York, NY: Routledge.

Reynolds, F. (1999). Cognitive behavioral counseling of unresolved grief through the therapeutic adjunct of tapestry-making. *The Arts in Psychotherapy, 26*(3), 165–171.

Reynolds, F. (2000). Managing depression through needlecraft creative activities: A qualitative study. *The Arts in Psychotherapy, 27*(2), 107–114.

Reynolds, F. (2002). Symbolic aspects of coping with chronic illness through textile arts. *The Arts in Psychotherapy, 29*, 99–106.

Reynolds, F. (2004a). Conversations about creativity and chronic illness II: Textile artists coping with long-term health problems reflect on the creative process. *Creativity Research Journal, 16*(1), 79–89.

Reynolds, F. (2004b). Textile art promoting well-being in long-term illness: Some general and specific influences. *Journal of Occupational Science, 11*(2), 58–67.

Reynolds, F. (2009). Taking up arts and crafts in later life: A qualitative study of the experiential factors that encourage participation in creative activities. *British Journal of Occupational Therapy, 72*(9), 393–400.

Riley J., Corkhill, B., & Morris, C. (2013). The benefits of knitting for personal and social wellbeing in adulthood: Findings from an international survey. *British Journal of Occupational Therapy, 76*(2), 50–57. doi:10.4276/030802213X13603244419077

Robertson, K., & Vinebaum, L. (2016). Crafting community. *Textile, 14*(1), 2–13. doi:10.1080/14759756.2016.1084794

Rubin, J. A. (2001). *Approaches to art therapy: Theory and technique* (2nd ed.). New York, NY: Routledge.

Rubin, J. A. (2011). *The art of art therapy: What every art therapist needs to know* (2nd ed.). New York, NY: Routledge.

Rubin, J. A. (2016). *Approaches to art therapy: Theory and technique* (3rd ed.). New York, NY: Routledge.

Smith, T. (2016). The problem with craft. *Art Journal, 75*(1), 80–84. doi:10.1080/00043249.2016.1171544

Somer, L., & Somer, E. (2000). Perspectives on the use of glass in therapy. *American Journal of Art Therapy, 38*, 75–80.

Stallings, J., Wolf Bordonara, G., Miller, K., & Clark, S. (2019). *Healing with fire: Glass fusion in clinical practice*. Paper presented at the 50th Annual Conference of the American Art Therapy Association, Kansas City, MO.

Talwar, S. K. (2015, April). *Stitch by stitch: DIY citizenship and the politics of the "therapeutic".* Keynote presentation at the Spring Art Therapy Symposium, Mount Mary University, Milwaukee, WI.

Talwar, S. K. (Ed.). (2019a). *Art therapy for social justice: Radical intersections.* New York, NY: Routledge.

Talwar, S. K. (2019b). Feminism as practice: Crafting and the politics of art therapy. In S. Hogan (Ed.), *Gender and difference in the arts therapies: Inscribed on the body* (pp. 13–23). New York, NY: Routledge.

Taylor, N., Hurley, U. K., & Connolly, P. (2016). *Making community: The wider role of makerspaces in public life.* Retrieved from http://usir.salford.ac.uk/id/eprint/38669/

Timm-Bottos, J. (2011). Endangered threads: Socially committed community art action. *Art Therapy: Journal of the American Art Therapy Association, 28*(2), 57–63. doi:10.1080/07421656.2011.578234

Timm-Bottos, J. (2016). Beyond counseling and psychotherapy, there is a field. I'll meet you there. *Art Therapy: Journal of the American Art Therapy Association, 33*(3), 160–162. doi:10.1080/07421656.2016.1199248

Timm-Bottos, J. (2017). Public practice art therapy: Enabling spaces across North America (La pratique publique de l'art-thérapie: Des espaces habilitants partout en Amérique du Nord). *Canadian Art Therapy Association Journal, 30*(2), 94–99. doi:10.1080/08322473.2017.1385215

Ulman, E., Kramer, E., & Kwiatkowska, H. (1977). *Art therapy in the United States.* Craftsbury Commons, VT: Art Therapy Publications.

Wadeson, H. (2010). *Art psychotherapy* (2nd ed.). Hoboken, NJ: John Wiley & Sons.

Wheeler, E. (2012). *The political stitch: Voicing resistance in a suffrage textile.* Textile Society of America 13th Biennial Symposium Proceedings: Textiles and Politics, 758. Retrieved from https://digitalcommons.unl.edu/tsaconf/758/

Yi, C. S. (2010). From imperfect to I am perfect: Reclaiming the disabled body through making body adornments in art therapy. In C. H. Moon (Ed.), *Materials and media in art therapy: Critical understandings of diverse artistic vocabularies* (pp. 103–117). New York, NY: Routledge.

I
Craft as a Tool for Transformation and Self-Care

1

Crafting the Artist Book as Embodied, Relational Practice

LYNN KAPITAN

Introduction

I pick up a hand-crafted book, hold it gently in my hands, feel a subtle shift as I open it—and cross into a miniature world within its covers. It moves me through an ever-changing experience of time and space appearing and slipping away with the rhythm of each turning page. Not simply a holder of words and images, the book is a physical object that requires touch to experience it (Smith, 1993). When each element—page, pictures, text, page turnings and display, and binding—is carefully conceived and composed to foreground a theme, a reader cannot help but have an intimate relationship with it (Tretheway, 2006). In its subversive form, a book can upend expectations of what it should be and how we, as readers or viewers, should interpret or respond to it.

The *artist book*, which is an artwork created solely in book format, straddles the art–craft spectrum, with book artists falling "where they may" along it (Niffenegger, 2007, p. 13). Drucker (2007) connected the interest that women in particular have in the craft to traditionally sanctioned pursuits of keeping diaries and journals, sewing, needlework, decorating, and the careful preservation of familial and collective memory. The space of a book, she observed, is both intimate and public: it mediates *enclosure* for private reflection with *exposure* for public communication. Those who craft books from the material of their lives and imaginations find a balance here that gives voice to their own concerns on their own terms.

I have been a maker of books for decades now, having first experimented with the form during the 1970s heyday of guerilla presses that proliferated in the political unrest of the times. I met and fell in love with my spouse in the letterpress studio of the campus art department where I set love poems into movable type one letter at a time, positioned into blocks caressed with oily brayers of ink, and pressed into luscious sheets of papers to be folded, scored, and gently bound together with loving hands. In the years since, I have crafted all manner of artist book: from a single folded page to elaborate codices; accordioned and fan folded, tunneled into and embellished with pop-ups and swivel tabs; as miniature books, altered books, flip books, cloth and paper scrolls, visual journals; and more recently as sculptures that only obliquely evoke the *bookness* (Drucker, 2004) of their origins.

Making in the contemplative craft tradition of the book, for me, has paralleled in so many ways my unfolding understanding of art therapy. Both offer the paradox of the contained yet dynamic space that holds endless possibilities. In this chapter I will draw out these parallels and reflect on the handcrafted artist book as a reminder to us that everything exists in relationship: text and image, content and form, object and subject, time and space, and with a reader/viewer to make these connections. As they craft, construct, and subvert meaning with folded and bound papers, art therapists and their clients may perceive a cultural purpose as well: to process the trauma of living in a world in desperate need of human touch and caring. Book craft helps us make sense of day-to-day experiences, interrupt narratives and injustice, and claim the knowledge that crafting—with exquisite care, loving touch, and attention—matters and is worthy of our attention.

The Crafted Book

In a brilliant reflection on the expressive power of the artist book Keith Smith (1993, pp. 17–25) distilled its essential properties. Fold a sheet of paper in half, he explained, and you are no longer in the two-dimensional world of the single picture plane. The fold creates a *book* in its simplest form: two connecting picture planes that now arc in space on either side of the fold. Turn the sheet over and the "front" becomes a "back," offering four interrelated surfaces for expression. Because these pages cannot be seen simultaneously, they are experienced in time, like a play in four acts or a symphony in four movements. Marks move across the space of one surface only to disappear into the hinge and reappear with the next surface coming forward. These are among the qualities that make a book *relational* and "so ephemeral that it exists as fragments in now-time," fully seen only after the act of viewing (Smith, 1994, p. 59).

From long familiarity with mass-produced books, we are conditioned to think of them as mere containers for information arranged horizontally, row by row, in a flat field. But, Smith (1993) argued, this is not how a book should be experienced. The problem for the craftsperson is in approaching it "as if it were many single pictures, and it is not" (1994, p. 15). To treat a book this way denies the animated movement of fronts into backs, the eye and hand absorbing one page and then changing with the next and the next (p. 18). Each successive image depends upon—in fact, grows, unfolds, and emerges from—what came before it. An artist book, thus, is a wonderful play upon the action of turning a page. Conceptual, visual, and physical elements of the book all unfold meaning in time and space.

The book's structure is determined by its folds or binding. Take a single sheet and fold it in alternating directions. Now you have an *accordion* of surfaces to play with or a concertina binding into which additional pages can be inserted (Figure 1.1). Folding the paper so that its two edges meet and open out like French doors inspires face-to-face interactions of text and imagery. More possibilities arise when something can be hidden by closing the folded pages. And if the pages are arranged to fan out or telescope open like a tunnel and then collapse shut? A partial image on one page can be completed by its remainder on another (Figure 1.2). Pages, text, and imagery can be interwoven, with hinges or pockets added or cut through to reveal images below. Myriad ideas can be adhered or sewn together in this way, as well as folded, bound, and layered into sheets, texts, covers, and images. By understanding these innovative

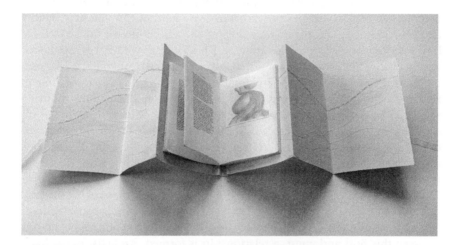

Figure 1.1 Concertina book with inserted pages

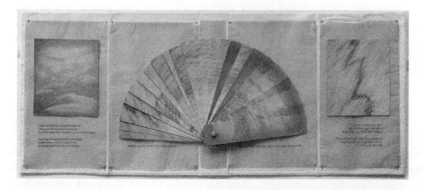

Figure 1.2 Fan book

structures, the book maker can arrange them into relationships that convey meaning through their interaction (Drucker, 2014; Smith, 1993).

Smith wrote that "without discipline, there is no freedom" and "without play, craft is sterile" (1993, p. 37). Never treat a book as merely an empty vessel to stick things into—he advised—or as a pretty but meaningless object. Learn to see the book for its power and potential as an entity in itself. Take another sheet of paper and consider that what you say with it reveals who you are. "Think of what you are holding. Think as you are folding. Think as *you*. Think" (p. 25).

Materiality, Time, and Space

The hand-held book is a material object that demands touch and effort to see it completely (Smith, 1994). Every book invites a journey through time, space, and consciousness. Like the therapy session, there is within the book's pages a little interior world of protected intimacy. Until I engage with it, I do not know what will arise in the openings and structure of its pages—only that it will lead me from opening to journeying and finally to arrival. As in art therapy, I might find that I am taking a linear path, moving step-by-step through the intimate spaces of the encounter, pausing at intervals to absorb what is happening—or spiraling ever inward toward a central point of complete focus, only to travel outward again from the source to its very edge. I close the book or leave the session and return to ordinary experience, still resonating with what just transpired.

There is a parallel in the idea of art therapy as an enactment of the ancient practice of hospitality (Kapitan, 2003). The therapist, as host, opens the door to the client or guest. The client stays long enough to rest and recover, and, between this host and guest, a relationship is formed. An artist book, likewise, is a "habitable structure" (Oliveira, 2017, p. 42), where embodied selves and the world intertwine (Küpers, 2011). Both the book and therapy house thoughts and memories, a before and an after, and an inside and an outside (Figure 1.3). There must be a stable, grounding base on which to layer imagery and build these relationships. The size, shape, and proportion of the book's pages protect and enclose the interior realm; book covers shelter like a roof. Openings in the pages provide door-like access or window-like enlightenment.

Turning the pages, breathing in and breathing out, we pace our interactions in the space–time of the book much as we do with our sensory and body-mind awareness in therapy. Thus, we "think with the materiality of the world" rather than presume that we already know everything we need to understand it (Laidlaw, 2012, as cited in Gilroy, Linnell, McKenna, & Westwood, 2019, p. 14). With its marks flowing dynamically across the spatial planes, the book reveals narrative and imagery through their continuous contact with the reader's mind.

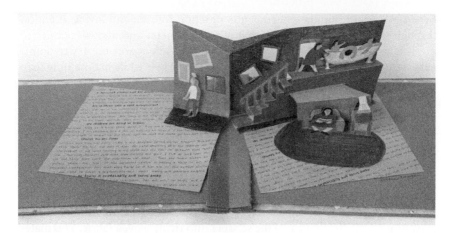

Figure 1.3 Diorama book of a dream image

Craft as Loving Touch

At its essence, craft is an intimate dialogue with the materials and objects that surround us (Lawlor, 1994). When awake to my material surroundings, I cannot help but see creative potential everywhere. Book-making thoughts constantly accompany me, glimpsed in the veins of a banana leaf, for example, or in tangled reeds I might chance to see along the riverbank after a flood. "What kind of book could I make with this?" I wonder. Books move me materially in a language that paper, fabric, ink, and thread understand. I listen carefully with my hands as I touch rice paper, handmade paper, creamy printmaking paper; notice flecks of coconut husk or flower petals caught in the fibers; or ponder the possibilities of translucent tissue and glassine.

Cutters and boards, needles, thread, stick-flat paste spreading over paper, the balanced heft of the folding bone—I know these tools as my body knows itself. Nothing can be rushed or shaped against its will. My attention is held by how the straight-edge ruler must align with the paper as I mark with a pin prick where to cut or fold, knowing that a pencil dot is fat enough to throw off the measurement and ruin the whole piece. I'm aware that the book's memory easily records the marks of hand or tool. If I am angry and irritated while crafting it, the book will be bound in anger and irritation. If am distracted, my thread will tangle up. Thus does my craft teach me to still myself and listen to its material nature and to sense the openings between us. This calm, relational "being-presence" in the moment is a practice of great care and loving touch.

I remember watching a salesperson carelessly flip up the corners of a stack of paper I had selected in order to count them. She handled that paper so roughly, her mind elsewhere and paying no attention to what her hands were doing.

Even in the most mundane therapeutic practice, we transmit loving attention through the "touch" of presence that absorbs contact and allows energies to meet. Likewise, a book maker knows not to leave any marks nor try to dominate the materials. My hand gently gives with the paper while maintaining firm contact, even as I cut delicate sheets into pages, stack and align their edges, and sew multiple pages together. Despite these many actions, the result shows no evidence of being handled at all. No dents, no dings. Bound with a craft person's loving care, the book's pages are allowed to settle in with each other in a way that maintains their true nature.

Well-crafted therapy, as with artist books, requires an evenly hovering, suspended process of listening and noticing, setting aside inattention and, over time, transforming memories and perceptions into new consciousness. We must suffer the process of creation as well, such as in the line drawn across pristine paper or the first cut of the scissors into richly woven fabric. *This* material, as with *this* client, is alive—with a history, a character, and certain needs or capacities. Whatever arises in the encounter is animate and seeking transformation (Kapitan, 2003).

Making Sense: The Crafted Book in Art Therapy

I return to the essence of the book as a time–space medium that helps me, an art therapist and craftsperson, "make sense" through the interplay of object and subject, material, form, and symbol. Something in me knows but has forgotten; thinking can only take me so far. When thoughts weigh upon my mind and I need to work out what is roiling within me, I turn to my craft to show it to me. I have to make a book—if only to see what the book sees. For example, a barbed-wire fence I'd seen had "haunted" me for months. When I finally turned my attention to it, I discovered the memory wanted to be a book. With sudden insight, I saw the whole concept, all of a piece, in my mind's eye. That image spoke to me of something I was experiencing and needed to say, without my knowing how or why.

As an art therapist, I always strive to become a more attuned instrument of the psychological, emotional, and spiritual forces passing through me in my work with people in need. The practice of a craft "makes me available" by putting me in right relationship with these forces. To house the haunting image and give space to its disturbance, I created *All These Sharp Edges* (Figure 1.4). Repeating images of the fence are pinned to book boards covered in soft black wool. Then a line of tiny, beaded pins. They hold small, translucent flags to "carry the feeling of sacrifice and wounding, of being strung up along the fence," I later journaled "or memorials of roadside accidents. Or the disappeared." The accordion-style book is wired together with metallic thread and held upright with tree branch supports. Once my book was complete, the disturbance transformed and, like a guest, moved on. I was at peace again.

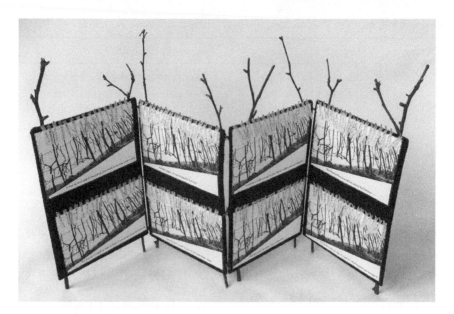

Figure 1.4 All These Sharp Edges

As Carroll and Dickerson (2018) observed, an artist book is a material object, a product of creative processes, and a container for aesthetic expression. However, they also highlighted the book's *epistemic properties* as valuable for embodied, tacit knowing—what we know but cannot say. Artist books, by virtue of their unique form, can draw attention to the easily forgotten nature of texts and "make them vivid again" (p. 43). The crafting–thinking process is a kind of sense-making that can be deployed to interrupt the narratives we or our clients tell and to consider them anew. Visual journaling can support art therapists in their own contemplative practices. For clients as well, the crafting of a book can support the retrieval and building up of fragments of memories, constructing and reconstructing narratives, and engaging intertwined actions of making, viewing, embodied thinking, and exchange.

But sometimes we make books simply for the sheer tactile and sensory pleasures of inking, printing, drawing, collaging, pasting, folding, and assembling. Many variations on the form offer expressive possibilities in art therapy (Table 1.1). Perhaps this slow, body-led craft serves to counteract our over-intellectualized age and the disembodied cacophony of imagery that bombards us daily. Craft takes us into the physicality of focused thought, creating a space of "silence" from distracting thoughts in one's interior being, allowing a journey beyond the rational and into a book's quiet intuitive spaces.

Table 1.1 Common Book Structures and Their Expressive Potential

Book type	Description	Expressive potential
Codex	Standard print format for mass-produced books, pages are folded and sewn into signatures and then bound together along one edge.	Can be created as a blank book to fill with writing and imagery. Paper or fabric can be cut into various shapes and sizes and embellished with tabs or cut-outs. A portfolio of existing artwork or collection of images can be bound together as a codex.
One-page	Composed of a single paper folded into eighths, cut in the center, and then re-folded to form a smaller, eight-page book.	Made with simple materials, compact and easy to make. Can be used as a journal, story book or timeline, individual or group pass-around book, zine, or documentation of an event or narrative. Can be oversized or miniature.
Accordion	Constructed by continuously folding one or more papers in alternating directions to form pages. The "venetian blind" variation laces the folded pages together on a cord. Accordion folds also can serve as binding with sheets inserted into the folds. When two texts are rotated 90 degrees and inserted into an accordion binding, a "dos-a-dos" book is created.	Versatile format and simple binding, with rich potential for pictorial sequencing, as images unfold or progress from the front to back. May be read like a book or stood upright to view all pages at once. Standing accordions can form scenes or backgrounds, silhouettes, and dioramas. Shaping or cutting into and through the pages reveal layering effects when the pages are stacked or unfolded. Dos-a-dos or alternating colored pages can express polarities or different perspectives.
Step and flip books	Overlapping folds or pages of staggered size are stapled or sewn together at the top edge. Each page flips up to reveal another page beneath it. In the fan book variation pages are stacked and attached on one side to fan out when opened.	Easily made with a few pieces of paper, the top of each page can be viewed together as a single image or scene or as a narrative broken into steps on each page. Good for pass-around group poetry or for breaking down a narrative into steps. Partial images of the whole can be viewed to varying degrees when a page is flipped or fanned out.

Book type	Description	Expressive potential
Scrolls	Paper or fabric of any size is attached to a rod on one or both edges and then wound around it and secured with a cord.	As an ancient form that predates the codex, scrolls lend ritual, sacred, honorary, or special treatment to their contents. Can be used to mark occasions or accomplishments. May be read horizontally or vertically.
Tunnel books and dioramas	Created by attaching single pages to an accordion binding that form a three-dimensional scene when the book is opened.	3-D vivifies an image and gives it focal power, volume, and form. Can be used to study the relationship of elements in one image, story, scene, or event. A tunneling effect is made by layering pages with progressively larger or smaller openings surrounding the images.
Shadow box	A codex-like book opens to reveal a hollow space where miniature objects and texts can be assembled in lieu of pages.	Created to house found objects, photos, and ephemera in meaningful relationships. As in dioramas, can vivify focal concerns and memorialize important people and events.
Flag book	Variation on the accordion and flip book, paper tabs are attached to alternating sides of accordion folds, and move the imagery in opposite directions when the book is opened.	Complex and innovative, they offer a good structure for material display of photos and images. Involves puzzle-like, creative problem solving.
Altered book	Pre-existing printed book is used as a structure for collaging, adding or deleting pages, folding or carving into the text, and other changes to its original form.	Rich metaphoric potential for expressing change in one's "template" of life expectations or experiences. Used primarily for visual journaling; also supports working through by selecting pages randomly or returning to earlier altered pages to develop them anew.

Border Crossings

"All real living is meeting."

—Buber (1958, p. 25)

I have long been fascinated with the entrances and exits between, among, and through the liminal spaces of the book form. The *līmen* refers to a threshold between two different existential planes (Küpers, 2011). The "place where edges meet" always brings focus and shifts in perception. As in therapy, by linking the external to the internal a book carries a portal-like sense of opening up and closing away. Blank pages at the beginning of a book, called endsheets, function to clear the mind and prepare for stepping into an imagined world across the threshold that is a "once in a while genuinely magical" (Moore, 2000, p. 34) experience.

In my earliest artist books, I sought a sanctuary from the stresses of day-to-day experience. I crafted them in a state of free-floating "relaxed expectancy" that lent specialness to the experience (Schaverien, 1992, p. 68). But while some thresholds invoke familiarity, comfort, and play, others are fraught with ambiguity and difficulty. *Prayer to the Gods of Death* (Figure 1.5) marked a changing consciousness in me from therapeutic bystander to engaged witness willing to leave comfort behind to risk the rupture of her own certainties (Watkins, 2015). The impetus for the book's starkly black and white imagery was my compassion for mothers whose children are lost to the politics of fear and hate. In place of book covers I positioned two bleached jaw bones to sanctify and enclose the

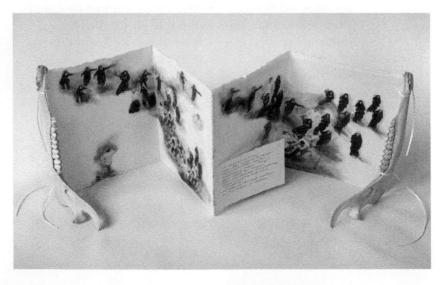

Figure 1.5 Prayer to the Gods of Death

central, unfolding scene. In creating this piece, I had accepted the stance of an artist being "inside the world to feel its hurts and wounds" and yet "outside enough to recognize these outrages and shape them creatively into new images that are less untrue to our reality" (Gilkey, 1996, p. 191).

Craft persons have long described the feeling of being shaped by the very materials in their hands that invite them to participate in their own process of transformation (Tracol, 1991). As both entryway and boundary marker, the threshold between the inner and outer worlds of the books that I was crafting were challenging my notions of *third spaces* (Soja, 2000) of cultural contact I was encountering in my art therapy practice at the time. Anzaldúa (2007) called these fluid, liminal places *borderlands* created from the "emotional residue" of a boundary in constant transition (p. 25). In making me more open and porous, my craft was guiding me to critically examine who and where I was and how I was interacting with the world as a result.

Boundary crossing is difficult yet necessary, according to hooks (1990), to understand how things came to be defined the way they are. She cautioned not to expect borders to be "safe" places; "one is always at risk," she wrote (p. 149). How could it be otherwise? The making of artist books has accompanied my gradual abandonment of art therapy's safe, separate enclosures and movement into the borderlands and the structural roots of distress that I encounter. I believe this was due to the ability of books to *emplace* multiple realities and voices on multiple planes—cognitively, emotionally, and sensually—while testing the reflexivity of one's responses. Moreover, books are participants: as physical objects they can pass through multiple hands, exchange memories and histories, and cross different times and geography in ways that connect or accentuate social and cultural differences. A single book can interrupt conventional thinking, de-mythologize personal and social fictions, and make space for re-symbolizing the world.

Un-Making and Re-Making Narratives

Even with the complex and labor-intensive process that goes into them, interest in artist books endures, despite the proliferation of digital media that have taken the place of physical books for so many people. Their old-school appeal might be connected to the power of books to confer authority as sacred, secular, and cultural icons. Because books represent "the body of human thought," when we deliberately re-configure them in unusual ways, we are transgressing or "messing with that body" (Niffenegger, 2007, p. 13). Consider, for instance, the deference given to "book learning" or the complaint of disobedience and disrespect people direct at artists who, in the genre of altered books, enjoy cutting up library books on band saws to make their creations.

My awareness of the subversive power of the book grew in parallel fashion to my evolving practice of art therapy as a form of social action; I don't know which came first. Perhaps critical theory, which examines taken-for-granted assumptions underlying interpretations of human experience (Tyson, 2006), has become for me a particularly valid art therapy lens because of what I've learned from the craft of books. Both develop the ability to see connections—in time, location, space, and relationship—we didn't see before or even knew existed. These include connections between what we think is common sense and "normal," how we hear and interpret text and narratives, and what we see and have internalized to see based on the ideologies we have been taught or subscribe to. As argued elsewhere in this text, critically important shifts in consciousness emerge when people use their craft making to resist, subvert, and/ or challenge the categories, labels, and roles they have been subjected to or consigned (Wexler, 1970, as cited in Fay, 2011).

La Frontera/Wall (Figure 1.6, Color Plate 1) was created from the rupture I felt in the aftermath of the 2016 U.S. presidential election. Like many white, professional class, and politically liberal people, the outcome shook me out of a kind of unseeing trance. What were the narratives I had told myself about my country, and where did these narratives originate? To pierce denial, I threw myself into crafting, seeking understanding through the disruptive interplay of a book's layers and meanings. The base of this artist book is a *codex*—that ubiquitous, iconic print format of conventional books, which alludes to literate, "civilized" people and the dominant narratives passed down in books as history or as laws that govern and protect us from the Other. Dusky covers open to reveal illegible markings that form an image of a wall across the interior space, interrupted by the central hinge where eight small pages have been inserted. Instead of text these translucent pages create overlapping images of multiple, disembodied hands reaching through the wall and toward the viewer. By substituting text with such imagery, the expectation of language is subverted and denied; absent voices are replaced with clamoring bodies demanding the viewer not look away.

Art therapy awakens new ways of thinking and imagining that change is possible, whether for individuals or within the systems that structure our lives.

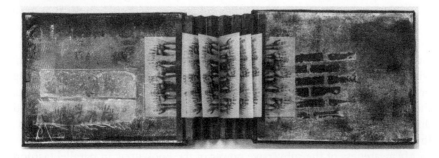

Figure 1.6 La Frontera/Wall

Those practitioners who are interested in creating artist books to inform an anti-oppressive practice might tackle questions (adapted from Strega, 2005, p. 199) such as: How can I best capture the complexities and contradictions of the experiences I encounter daily? Whose voices do I represent in my work? Whose interests does my work serve? How do I know that my practice is ethically valid or sound? A craftsperson learns that various ways of working have greater or lesser validity for a given circumstance (Kapitan, 2018). To succeed, one must learn to be patient, forgiving, and humble and able to give full attention to the craft as well as study the effects of each action taken. Craft steers the crafter–therapist toward a different kind of "being-present"; that is, of bringing presence to what is difficult and allowing it to matter, to affect oneself, and thereby alter one's course (Watkins, 2015). Thus do we and our clients disrupt narratives and unmake, break up, and remake old bonds to create our world once again.

Re-Claiming: Culture and Community

In times of political, technological, and social upheaval, art therapists are called to build and affirm resilience against intolerance, hatred, and violence. As my own history with crafting suggests, we might desire instead to turn away and search for spaces where we can feel protected from unpredictable, often horrifying events in the world. However, choosing to ignore political reality does not remove oneself from politics; it merely draws attention away from prevailing power structures (Tyson, 2006). I have grappled with this paradox directly as a cross-cultural art therapist with Cantera, a Nicaraguan organization that has collectively advanced hundreds of capacity-building projects aimed at systemic social change. To support the community on its own terms, I've learned to function very much like the material in a crafter's hands: as a malleable, maximally responsive resource to be used by others in crafting their lives (Kapitan, Litell, & Torres, 2011). Collaboration has meant continuously ceding control of the agenda while moving into, within, and across the borderlands of difference. As a result, my practice—and very identity—have been reoriented toward accompanying the work of community by drawing on collaborative imagination and action to address social change.

The practice of critical inquiry that I've learned from Cantera over many years revealed its power and significance only slowly, due to my own culture and social location. In Latin America *accompaniment*, which has a rich history among mental health professionals there, involves "an invited dialogical relationship that becomes close and continuous" through "listening, witnessing, and the offering of specific, flexible, and strategic support" to counteract oppression (Edge, Kagan, & Stewart, 2003, as cited in Watkins, 2015, p. 327). A crucial element, according to Watkins's (2015) study, is reliable presence: to be an accompanier, I show up—fully and not as a bystander. I don't disappear when things get inconvenient or risky. My showing up must be practiced with cultural humility and respect. When accepted as trustworthy, I am invited again and again into deep hospitality.

Last year, in the spring of 2018, this work was abruptly caught up in the worst political crisis in a generation to hit Nicaragua. Hundreds of protesters lost their lives in brutal clashes with police and paramilitary forces, throwing the country into traumatizing chaos, fear, and deep despair. Although I was an outsider with freedoms my partners did not possess, I had long ceased to be a stranger. I had a duty to assist. First through online conferencing and later in face-to-face collaboration, we crafted interventions to help hard-hit communities emerge from the violence and strategize their own survival. *Managua, December 2018* (Figure 1.7) is an artist book I created in reflection on an art therapy retreat that not only acknowledged the community's suffering but also its enduring strength, beauty, and resilience. Constructed in the sacred form of a scroll, the imagery illustrates a tender moment when we were silently painting together by candlelight, as a process of finding hope in the darkness, lighted by the collective spirit of community.

The scroll hangs unfurled, vertically on the wall. A hand-colored photograph is framed above and below with fragments of darkened, nearly unreadable text hand-stitched together with bright red thread. The text itself is a fragment in Spanish of a local newspaper report on the deaths of more than 350 Nicaraguans during the first three months of the violence and the disappearance and exile of many thousands more. Viewed by audiences in the U.S. where I live, the broken, untranslated text underscores the obscure, near invisibility of the crisis in my own country and challenges indifferent, easily abandoned viewing. Through the power of paper, thread, facts, and memory, the book lays the matter out and engages multiple senses. As audiences take in the book, the community's empowerment is evoked in that relationship, despite that the community is not presently able to act on it.

Injustice persists, in part, because voices at the margins go unheard. We cannot escape the differing locations we find ourselves in, but we can listen closely with our hearts and share our realities, reaching through and beyond words and images. Although the artist books I've described here have served my private contemplative needs, books also can be created collectively to assist exchange and dialogue in the therapeutic process. For example, a book can be constructed by passing it from one member of a group to another to take home, read and reflect upon, and add to with their own layered and embellished imagery and narratives. However, rather than focus on the "how-to-do" of book craft in community, I want to call attention to the *place-attentive* practice (Fenner, 2012) that the medium can facilitate. Crafting can be a powerful form of being present in the physical company of one another and may, perhaps, build alliances and bridge the tragic divides of privilege, separation, and passive bystanding. We build community when we craft together. We commit to crafting a more just world.

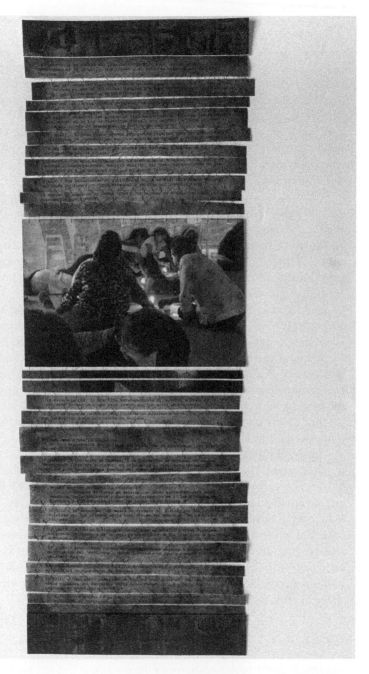

Figure 1.7 Managua, December 2018

Conclusion

In meeting a craft's demands we develop strength to meet the demands of life, as well as balance who we are in relation to forces that are greater than us (Kapitan, 2011). Therein lies a crucial role of craft in art therapy. Book craft presents rich possibilities for therapeutic work. As a medium that bridges time and space, hand-crafted books allow their makers to be authors of their own lives by shaping stories and experiences into knowledge and then memory (Drucker, 2007). Life offers up rich materials for crafting an ongoing autobiography of revelation, evolution, and transformation. Artist books thus become co-collaborators and accompaniers to a life.

Because books are relational objects, they invite the reader to cross into imagined worlds that may resonate or disturb, affirm or disrupt meaning and expectation. Craftpersons can exploit the activist potential of such an experience by challenging or subverting a viewer's taken-for-granted perceptions. The book's enduring power has carried sacred and secular authority through the ages; it is therefore rich with possibility for presenting differently imagined or voiced realities that demand we do not turn away from them unseeing. Books invite dialogic relationship and critical consciousness.

Books also are participating "travelers" that synthesize and house individual and collective memory in material form. I was recently reminded of this role when sorting my late parents' personal effects. Their books had journeyed with them from place to place and across time as marked with collections of treasured children's books, dusty school primers, and their own parents' and grandparents' family Bibles that had accompanied their crossing from the old country to the new, through cultures, histories, and many lives. Such objects are cherished for their ability to connect us—physically, emotionally, and spiritually— to our pasts, present, and hoped-for future.

Finally, crafting is, importantly, a way of loving the world through human touch (Kapitan, 2011). It is this direct link to the human heart that is the essence of the craftperson's need to gather up materials, to envision their possibilities, and to turn them into beloved objects for contemplation, sharing, and exchange. When we, in turn, take the hand-crafted object into our own hands, we are able to feel the traces of the human heart on them. Art therapists who practice a craft stand to gain important insights into the always delicate matter of how to offer hospitable help that relieves suffering and validates resilience and strength. The hand-crafted book, as one such craft, can bring all of these aspects together and move us anew with each turning of a page.

References

Anzaldúa, G. (2007). *Borderlands/la frontera: The new Mestiza* (3rd ed.). San Francisco, CA: Aunt Lute.
Buber, M. (1958). *I and thou* (2nd ed., R. Gregory Smith, Trans.). Edinburgh, Scotland: T. & T. Clark.

Carroll, M., & Dickerson, A. (2018). The knowing of artists' books. *Journal of Artist Books*, *43*, 10–13.

Drucker, I. (2004). *The century of artists' books*. New York, NY: Granary.

Drucker, J. (2007). Intimate authority: Women, books, and the public private paradox. In K. Wasserman (Ed.), *The book as art: Artists' books from the National Museum of Women in the Arts* (pp. 14–17). New York, NY: Princeton Architectural Press.

Drucker, J. (2014). Concepts of production. *Afterimage: The Journal of Media Arts and Cultural Criticism*, *42*(1), 2–5. doi:10.1525/aft.2014.42.1.2

Fay, J. (2011). Let us work together: Welfare rights and anti-oppressive practice. In D. Baines (Ed.), *Doing anti-oppressive practice: Social justice social work* (pp. 64–78). Winnipeg, MB: Fernwood.

Fenner, P. (2012). What do we see? Extending understanding of visual experience in the art therapy encounter. *Art Therapy: Journal of the American Art Therapy Association*, *29*(1), 11–18. doi:10.1080/07421656.2012.648075

Gilkey, L. B. (1996). Can art fill the vacuum? In D. Apostolos-Cappadona (Ed.), *Art, creativity, and the sacred: An anthology in religion and art* (pp. 187–192). New York, NY: Continuum.

Gilroy, A., Linnell, S., McKenna, T., & Westwood, J. (2019). *Art therapy in Australia: Taking a postcolonial, aesthetic turn*. Leiden, England: Brill Sense.

hooks, b. (1990). *Yearning: Race, gender and cultural politics*. Boston, MA: South End Press.

Kapitan, L. (2003). *Reenchanting art therapy: Transformational practices for restoring creative vitality*. Springfield, IL: Charles C Thomas.

Kapitan, L. (2011). Close to the heart: Art therapy's link to craft and art production. *Art Therapy: Journal of the American Art Therapy Association*, *28*(3), 94–95. doi:10.1080/07421656.2011.601728

Kapitan, L. (2018). *Introduction to art therapy research* (2nd ed.). New York, NY: Routledge.

Kapitan, L., Litell, M., & Torres, A. (2011). Creative art therapy in a community's participatory research and social transformation. *Art Therapy: Journal of the American Art Therapy Association*, *28*(2), 64–73. doi:10.1080/07421656.2011.578238

Küpers, W. (2011). Dancing on the limen: Embodied and creative inter-places as thresholds of (be) coming: Phenomenological perspectives on liminality and transitional spaces in organizations and leadership. *Tamara: Journal for Critical Organizational Inquiry*, *9*(3–4), 45–59. doi:10.1177/1742715013485852

Lawlor, A. (1994). *The temple in the house: Finding the sacred in everyday architecture*. New York, NY: Putnam's Sons.

Moore, T. (2000). Neither here nor there. *Parabola*, *25*(1), 35–37.

Niffenegger, A. (2007). What does it mean to make a book? In K. Wasserman (Ed.), *The book as art: Artists' books from the National Museum of Women in the Arts* (pp. 12–13). New York, NY: Princeton Architectural Press.

Oliveira, M. (2017). Weaving the archive: Some notes on the books of Louise Bourgeois. *Journal of Artists Books*, *42*, 24–28.

Schaverien, J. (1992). *The revealing image: Analytical art psychotherapy in theory and practice*. London, England: Routledge.

Smith, K. A. (1993). *Non-adhesive binding* (3rd. ed.). Rochester, NY: Keith Smith.

Smith, K. A. (1994). *Structure of the visual book* (3rd. ed.). Rochester, NY: Keith Smith.

Soja, E. W. (2000). *Postmetropolis: Critical studies of cities and regions*. Oxford, England: Blackwell.

Strega, S. (2005). The view from the poststructural margins: Epistemology and methodology resistance. In L. Brown & S. Strega (Eds.), *Research as resistance: Critical, indigenous, and anti-oppressive approaches* (pp. 199–235). Toronto, ON: Canadian Scholars' Press.

Tracol, H. (1991). Birth of a sculpture. *Parabola*, *26*(2), 68–70.

Tretheway, A. (2006). A study of book arts: Form as integral to content. *How2*, *2*(4).

Tyson, L. (2006). *Critical theory today: A user-friendly guide* (2nd ed.). New York, NY: Routledge.

Watkins, M. (2015). Psychosocial accompaniment. *Journal of Social and Political Psychology*, *3*(1), 324–341. doi:10.5964/jspp.v3i1.103

2

Healing With Fire

The Use of Hot Glass in Art Therapy

JESSICA WOOLHISER STALLINGS AND STEPHANIE CLARK

James, a young adult with autism, reported that he did not feel confident making art and was hesitant to enter the glass studio. However, he agreed to enter on the condition that he would not have to make anything. James observed his peers, with and without autism, working with the glass media and decided to try it. Two weeks later when James saw his completed glass fusion piece for the first time, he proudly shared it with anyone who would listen. James frequently requested returns to the glass studio and went on to become a practicing glass artist after his participation in art therapy programming discontinued.

Luis, an adolescent attending individual and group counseling, was artistically inclined and volunteered himself for the glassblowing group. Luis appeared almost instantly comfortable with glassblowing and was drawn to the molten glass. Before long he was gathering his own glass from the furnace and forming shapes with tools and little help from the instructors. Time in the hot shop was a reprieve from difficult life situations that often caused him stress. He formed positive, playful relationships with the adult male instructors and peers in the program. One evening Luis arrived at the hot shop with a hospital band on his wrist and when asked about it he replied, "Oh, I had to go to the hospital today [to treat my chronic illness] and I told them I had to be discharged so I could go to the glass group." He then stated, "I couldn't miss it."

*Note: cases based on actual art therapy participants with some details changed to protect confidentiality.

Introduction

Hot glass is an enticing art medium enthralling both artists and viewers since before the Common Era, with a history that can be traced to ancient Rome (Frank, 1982) and ancient Egypt (Reynolds, 1987). Hot glass craft ranges from blown glass used to make glassware, sculptures, and chandeliers among other things to glass fusion utilized in making jewelry and glassware. The Corning Museum of Glass in Corning, NY which displays 50,000 glass craft pieces spanning 3,500 years, highlights the persistence of glass media throughout modern history (Corning Museum of Glass, 2002). Additional evidence of the endurance of glass is demonstrated in the multitude of high school, university, and craft school programs across the United States where students learn various hot glass techniques. These courses attract a wide variety of individuals with a wide variety of backgrounds.

Prior to the late 19th century, women were often discouraged from or not allowed to have longer apprenticeships, which limited their skills, participation, and pay (Bardhan, 2012). However, more recently Cromwell (2017) interviewed glass blower Leib, who encouraged women to become glass artists despite history of unequal pay, stating she felt glassblowing was becoming more "egalitarian." Truman and Minter (2016) reflected upon Truman's experience as a female glass blower, emphasizing the importance of supporting one another both in aiding in the hot shop and buying glass products made by women. Although glass craft was for centuries a male-dominated field, in recent years women have been able to enter it in greater numbers—as evidenced most recently by the reality show *Blown Away*, a glassblowing competition (Bicketon, 2019) and notable female crafters such as Leib and Truman (Cromwell, 2017; Truman & Minter, 2016).

Glass as a Therapeutic Medium

Although introducing glass requires considering client appropriateness, closely monitoring participation, and considering the use of safety contracts, especially for participants experiencing suicidal ideation, (Moon, 2010; Somer & Somer, 2000), Somer and Somer (2000) and Horovitz (2018) have argued that glass craft provides far more benefit than harm. Where Horovitz emphasized need of first aid kits and suggested precutting materials to minimize danger and Somer and Somer cautioned not to utilize glass in groups due to needed therapist vigilance, our experience is contrary to this as we have both successfully utilized glass arts in group settings, described later.

Moon (2010) and Somer and Somer (2000) suggested that therapeutic glass participants are drawn to the use of glass because of its metaphorical potential. Somer and Somer explored the use of glass heating and blowing and stained glass, drawing specific attention to the potential for cathartic release in the breaking of glass. The potential to make something new out of something broken also provides a powerful therapeutic metaphor. Properties such as "transparence, translucence, and reflectance" are concepts intrinsically related to the therapeutic process (Somer & Somer, 2000, p. 79). The use of fire in art making can also be healing through representing cleansing and new beginnings (Woodruff, 2015).

Additionally, despite requiring intense focus, glassblowing and glass fusion produce pleasing products at high success rates even with novice crafters, encouraging feelings of self-efficacy (Minson, 2002). Minson (2002) and Woodruff (2015) have explored not only the traditional therapeutic potential of glass arts but also the commercial potential in teaching glass art as an entrepreneurial skill. Minson produced a film on the use of hot glass as a part of art therapy, illustrating how torch work (similar to glassblowing but done with a blow torch) can be turned into an adaptive skill to produce saleable craft products for participants in need of income.

The level of concentration and care necessary in glass arts promotes exclusive focus on the media and art form, lending some support to the idea of glass as a flow-producing medium (Csikszentmihalyi, 1990). Nainis et al. (2006) found creating stained glass useful as a pain-relieving activity; however, they instituted nontraditional glass painting rather than traditional glass scoring and soldering in making stained glass pieces. In our experience flow can occur with traditional hot glass media as well.

Examples of glass craft in art therapy often focus on cold glass. Horovitz (2018) and Dean (2016) discussed alternatives to hot glass, such as painting on existing glass products and the potential for integrating glass into mixed media as embellishment. Dean underlined the ceremonial use of glass beads as inspiration for use in art therapy. Hinz (2009) examined the use of traditional stained glass, describing the experience of neuroanatomist Jill Bolte Taylor, who after a stroke used stained glass to assist in rehabilitation by teaching her brain hemispheres to again work together.

Horovitz (2018) explored the use of hot glass, specifically the use of glass fusion in her practice with adults and in her own artwork. She highlighted the use of specialized photo paper to personalize participants' crafts and emphasized the creation of wearable glass fusion pieces.

Additionally, one can find examples of therapeutic glassblowing programs across the United States, often involving veterans, that provide an opportunity for participants to engage in "an exciting, challenging and collaborative art medium offering a powerful vehicle for social emotional learning" (Ignition Community Glass, n.d.; Woodruff, 2015). One such program, Operation Zen, was founded by U.S. Marine veteran Christopher Stowe after his experience with art therapy at the National Intrepid Center of Excellence (National Endowment for the Arts, n.d.; Zen Glass Studio, n.d.). Stowe noted that the art therapy program "helped him explore his artistic side and express his emotions in a positive way" (Zen Glass Studio, n.d., para. 1). He founded Operation Zen to assist others like himself.

We explore uses of glass craft in art therapy through our experience and that of other art therapists in the pages ahead. We share our experiences with glass fusion and glass blowing, respectively and explore safety and accessibility issues related to glass media to encourage use in your practice. Our use of glass is rooted in the centuries of experience that have come before, contributing to the continuation and diversification of glass craft practice by increasing exposure and accessibility through inclusion in art therapy services.

Glass Fusion in Art Therapy

Glass fusion (Figure 2.1) is related to traditional stained glass in that it involves scoring and breaking glass into smaller pieces that are assembled into a finished product. Glass fusion specifically refers to the process of layering and bonding glass in a kiln (Glass Fusing Basics, 2014). This technique has the potential to

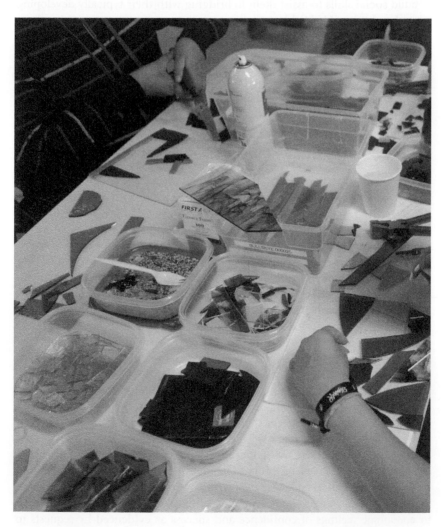

Figure 2.1 Youth cutting and layering glass for glass fusion

incorporate the metaphors and concepts pointed out earlier, as well as metaphors related to layers (Stallings & Clark, 2018). Gutsch (n.d.-a) reported: "I was introduced to glass fusion as a part of art therapy for a traumatic brain injury and a new way of self expression emerged" (para. 1). Gutsch (n.d.-b) now identifies as a glass fusion artist, following this therapeutic experience.

I (Jessica) found glass fusion by accident. In 2006, I was a young art therapist serving as lead clinician for the recreation therapy-based social skills program for individuals with autism at the Munroe Meyer Institute of the University of Nebraska Medical Center (UNMC) in Omaha. I was tasked with completing individual sessions with middle- and high-school-aged adolescents with autism to build social skills to assist them in bridging with their typically developing peers. In addition, I led field trips with participants to facilitate practicing these skills and to promote social acceptance among peers.

I needed to find field trip options that would interest a wide variety of participants. While searching, I happened upon an art studio called Adventure in Art in the Benson neighborhood of Omaha, which offered workshops in glass fusion. Although Adventure in Art has since closed, the experience I shared with my staff and participants there has been very influential in my art therapy practice. The artist and teacher Kristi Pederson welcomed our groups and taught us the basics of glass fusion, beginning with the creation of small projects such as pendants and working up to larger projects such as coasters and collaborative wall hangings. Kristi worked with my adolescent groups and also with my adult groups when programming later expanded. The studio provided a social setting with a fun, challenging, and rewarding art form as a focus. Having the focus on the art making assisted in lessening the social pressure inherent in the structure of the group, giving group members a focus for conversational practice and the formation of friendships. The group provided an atmosphere like an extracurricular activity, an experience many of the participants with autism had not experienced. The program I facilitated was able to safely implement glass fusion with groups due to our heavy staffing ratios—one staff to two adolescents—which provided for adequate supervision.

Although glass fusion workshops started out as an extracurricular field trip, I quickly saw the potential of glass fusion (see Figure 2.2, 2.3, Color Plate 2) as a medium for art therapy. Among my observations were that glass fusion provided opportunities for rapport and relationship building, feelings of mastery and confidence with a potentially dangerous art process, and a sense of pride in the product created; I observed these outcomes in staff and participants alike, and although they are anecdotal I feel these observations are useful for other art therapists to consider. The shared experience of handling glass and mastering its use to create art pieces provided common experiences leading to further social communication and feelings of trust among clinicians, staff, and participants. This sense of mastery of a complex, often-inaccessible medium appeared to encourage feelings of confidence and success as evidenced by requests to return to Adventure in Art for future field trips. Finally, despite the complexity

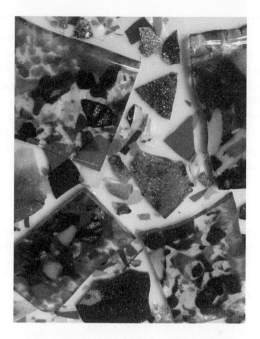

Figure 2.2 Rejoinder (before of repurposed broken pieces)

Source: Jessica Woolhiser Stallings

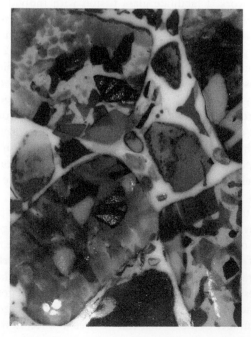

Figure 2.3 Rejoinder (after of repurposed broken pieces)

Source: Jessica Woolhiser Stallings

of the media and the delicate process in the creation of pieces, the glass fusion process resulted in visually pleasing and interesting pieces nearly 100% of the time. Participants often made gifts for friends and family, which facilitated continued social initiation through the glass craft. Most notably I recall a participant making a cross-shaped suncatcher for his parents, as their family life centered around their church. Due to the process involved in glass fusion—a minimum of four hours in a hot kiln of approximately 1000° and the bi-weekly nature of our field trips—participation from start to finish for our participants and staff was typically two to four weeks before the receipt of the art product. This delay promoted excitement and social opportunities between groups to discuss the previous field trip.

It is important to note that this opportunity would not have been possible without partnering with Adventure in Art, nor without a generous grant from the Autism Action Partnership that paid for my salary, our trips to the studio, and other programming. Without these partnerships we would not have had access to the equipment and supplies to do glass fusion. I would be remiss to leave out that it cost approximately $35 per person to access the studio time, instruction, supplies, and equipment, and this cost is on the low end of what it can cost to access glass fusion opportunities. This cost makes the medium inaccessible for many art therapists and their clients.

I left my position at UNMC in 2008 but never forgot this experience with glass fusion. When I entered private practice in 2011, I prioritized purchasing a glass kiln so I could integrate this art form into my practice. In my private practice work, I facilitate glass fusion with individual participants and small groups (five or fewer) to help ensure adequate supervision and safe use of supplies. I have continued to utilize glass fusion with individuals with autism, generally individuals with Level 1 or Level 2 diagnoses due to increased safety issues with individuals with a Level 3 diagnosis. I have also utilized glass fusion in sessions with individuals with depression and anxiety, in family therapy, in art therapy supervision with supervisees, and in personal self-care and examination. In these instances we worked with metaphors of layers and self-discovery. Additionally, I have even implemented glass fusion with individuals with histories of self-harm. In cases of those who self-harm, participation in glass art serves as a celebration of progress in recovery from self-harm behaviors, creating a visual tangible representation of their progress.

However, for those wishing to integrate this craft into their private practice, cost can be an even greater barrier. Glass kilns generally range in price from $400 to $1400 as of this publication, and this cost is prohibitive for many. There is also the cost of glass fusion supplies, which can be prohibitively expensive. So how can art therapists make glass fusion available widely to their participants and communities? Fortunately microwave kilns are available for as little as $40 and the cost of access to a microwave oven of appropriate size. A microwave kiln limits the number of pieces that can be fired at once; however, because it is safest to use glass fusion in individual or small group settings anyway, this is generally not an issue.

Additionally, in my own practice I have obtained scrap glass from stained glass artists and purchased large lots of scrap glass from other fusion artists in online sale sites at substantial discounts. It is important to know that glass fusion works best when the glass all melts at the same coefficient of expansion, so it is essential to inquire about this when accepting donations or buying scrap glass. Further, one has less control of the colors and design of glass when sourcing supplies in this way. However, I have found this to be an asset in my practice, encouraging additional metaphors of rebirth through the use of discarded supplies. Using a microwave kiln and discarded supplies from other glass artists drastically reduces the cost of glass fusion to pennies or a few dollars rather than $35 per person. However, as in all art forms, the art therapist must master the medium first in order to be able to most effectively engage participants and anticipate safety and other issues in its use.

Glassblowing in Art Therapy

Glass blowing is "the art of shaping a mass of glass that has been softened by heat by blowing air into it through a tube" (Glassblowing, n.d.). The collaborative nature of the medium and the concentration and skill required to manipulate glass offers participants a unique experience. Glassblowing requires at least one partner to blow into a pipe, provide protection from the heat, or gather a specific tool while the artist sits on the bench balancing the glass on the other end of the pipe. The glass must be manipulated before it hardens, so artists must work quickly, with intention, and communicate their needs to the partner helping with the piece.

If you've ever blown glass or watched a glassblowing demonstration, you understand how mesmerizing it can be. Unlike traditional art therapy materials, hot glass requires a hot and cold studio, expensive tools, and an experienced glassblower. The molten glass is heated to about 2,000 degrees Fahrenheit in a furnace. It is then gathered at the end of a pipe, shaped with specialized tools, and reheated in a second furnace called a glory hole to remain pliable so that it can be further manipulated. When the glass piece is completed, it is knocked off the pipe and placed in an annealing oven to cool slowly in order to prevent cracking and breaking. Cooled glass pieces are then polished in the cold shop with a belt sander or grinder to remove any sharp or rough edges.

For these reasons, glassblowing is often inaccessible to artists or crafters who are not directly connected to the glassblowing field. Owning and operating a glass studio is expensive, and so it can be difficult for the average person to try glassblowing or even find a studio. Most glassblowing facilities are in larger, well-developed urban areas accessible only to those who live nearby (Friedman, 2015). Private lessons or classes are costly, averaging $150 per hour for private instruction.

One can see why art therapists underutilize this medium within their practice. In the city of Chicago, however, there are multiple ways for art therapists to incorporate glassblowing into therapy. Several Chicago-based glass arts programs are making this possible by providing underserved individuals the opportunity to learn glassblowing with experienced artists who understand the healing aspects of this medium.

One such program, Project FIRE (Fearless Initiative for Recovery and Empowerment), "combines glassblowing, mentoring, employment, and leadership opportunities for youth injured by violence" in addition to "trauma psychoeducation, case management, and medical treatment" (Our Story, n.d.). This program was the brainchild of glassblowing artist Pearl Dick and clinical psychologist Bradley Stolbach, both of whom recognized the healing power of glass arts with populations experiencing trauma symptoms. The program is a collaborative with ArtReach, an arts and glass studio and Healing Hurt People-Chicago, a violence intervention program (Our Story, n.d.). Project FIRE works with mostly young victims of gun violence in Chicago, but the organization has also provided programing to veterans in the Road Home Program at Rush University Medical Center in Chicago.

Another hot glass studio offering reduced rate programming to underserved youth is Ignition Community Glass (IGC). ICG is a community nonprofit organization supporting the mission to "leverage the power of hands-on glass making to foster positive youth development and offer youth from Chicago's under-resourced communities; and youth who traditionally have not had access to glass making, access to this powerful art form" (Support Our Mission, n.d.).

I (Stephanie) have been a fan of glassblowing since I attended the pre-art therapy program at Emporia State University in Emporia, Kansas. Though I didn't learn glassblowing while attending school, I formed relationships with the instructors and many of the glassblowing students. I sat in the hot shop watching my friends form shapes with molten glass, mesmerized by the process and the metaphorical aspects of the medium. The idea of a material being melted, shaped, melted again, and hardened in an annealer for hours only to potentially break, is alluring. It represents so much of what art therapists are about: the process of art making, not the product.

In 2014 I was working as an art therapist for Youth Outreach Services, a social service agency in Chicago serving youth with substance use problems and exposure to trauma and other stressors. I was able to provide art therapy services to many of our youth using traditional art therapy materials. However, I noticed a need for a more exhilarating, enticing medium through which the youth could express themselves. Many of the youth had experienced trauma, ranging from gun violence, family separation, and bereavement to poverty, abuse, and sexual violence. Sitting still in an office was difficult for them. Through my glassblowing connections, I knew there was a glassblowing program providing an opportunity for youth to learn the medium. I reached out to Pearl Dick, who was working for ICG, and we piloted a program during the summer of 2014.

The partnership between ICG and Youth Outreach Services lasted a year and included ten-week summer, winter, and spring sessions. Youth who participated were between the ages of 14 and 19 and were identified for the group if they had difficulty engaging in traditional individual and group therapy, if they struggled to interact respectfully with peers and adults, or if they had a propensity for artistic expression. The group met weekly for four-hour sessions and included glassblowing instruction, small group work, and verbal processing time where participants were encouraged to reflect on the art-making process.

None of the youth in the program had any previous experience with glassblowing, nor did many of them know each other very well or have familiarity with the facility in which the program took place. The instructors began the program with a safety lesson and demonstration, and soon the youth were able to begin making their own glass pieces with the aid of the instructors and their peers. Once they became comfortable with the medium, the youth developed more autonomy in the hot shop and began helping each other and working collaboratively. A sense of trust formed between group members as they navigated the space together and learned how to safely offer help shaping the glass with tools or anticipate the need for protective equipment to block the heat.

I collected data throughout each session to document the possible benefits of this type of art therapy program with the youth. The types of data collected included observations of the youth interacting with the glass, each other, and the instructors; photographic documentation of the youth learning glass safety and technique; and self-report surveys that youth completed at the beginning and end of each session. The first noticeable observation was the youth's apparent formation of positive relationships with each other and with the glassblowing instructors (see Figure 2.4, Color Plate 3). The youth began to laugh with each other and the instructors and discuss personal topics about their lives.

The attention and focus required to blow glass can also encourage mindfulness, as there are major safety concerns for those who aren't paying attention. I observed the youth being able to maintain focus for longer periods of time. I also noticed an increase in self-confidence and heard positive self-statements about their abilities to manipulate the glass in a way they hadn't been able to in the weeks before. I heard statements such as "I'm a glassblower" and "This is my favorite part of the week." These statements led me to believe it was a positive and therapeutic experience for the participants.

The pre- and post-program surveys included a ten-question Likert scale that measured principles of the Positive Youth Development model (Positive Youth Development, n.d.)—connection, confidence, character, competence, contribution, and caring—as well as open-ended qualitative questions about the participants' experiences in the program. The youth self-reported an increase in

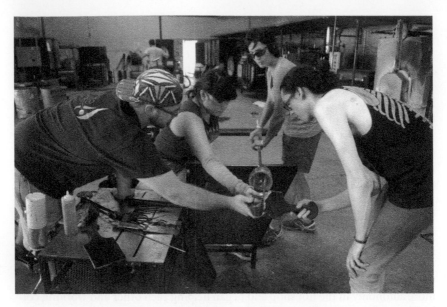

Figure 2.4 Three glassblowing instructors helping youth shape molten glass

knowledge of glass studio safety and glass techniques, an increase in confidence working with others, an increase in mindfulness, and an increase in being able to express themselves artistically.

Qualitative statements from the youth in the program included:

> "I enjoy going to the glass group. I would go everyday if I could. I learned I'm more capable of creating things than I thought."
>
> "I had an amazing experience. I was able to use glassblowing to distract myself from anything bad that I was going through or thinking. I learned that I can push myself to expand my artistic abilities if I try."
>
> "It was a bit scary at first working with glass because there was the risk of burning myself or others. However I was very proud of myself when I found I could in fact handle glass and manipulate it."

One of the participants in the program strongly identified as a glass artist after completing the summer, winter, and spring glass sessions. "Natalie" attended eighth grade in a Chicago area school. She was referred for art therapy to resolve conflict with her father, increase self-esteem, and resolve problems with peer relationships. Natalie was artistically inclined and made progress expressing herself in art therapy. I recommended her for the glass group because I thought the experience could help increase her self-esteem and improve peer relationships.

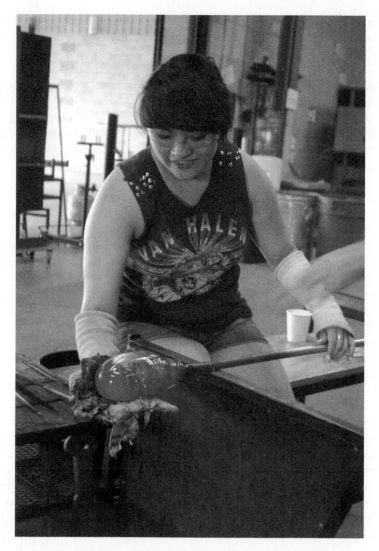

Figure 2.5 Youth working on glassblowing

Natalie excelled in the group, and her self-esteem, self-confidence, and self-efficacy flourished in a way that it hadn't in traditional art therapy. Though drawing, collage, and anger boxes could help her express her feelings about her family relationships and becoming a teenager, glassblowing allowed her an opportunity to build an identity. She connected with peers in the group who had similar experiences as her, and she formed a trusting relationship with one of the instructors.

For her eighth grade capstone project, Natalie wrote an autobiographical essay describing her identity as a glass artist. She titled it "Surprise! I'm a Glass Artist" and wrote:

> Glass blowing is a special form of art. It takes a certain kind of passion to work with glass. I love glass art and it's amazing for me to have an opportunity to work with it. I have a huge passion for it. I love going into the studio and feel[ing] the extreme heat. In glass art I can express myself and be free in my artwork. I was able to do glass blowing thanks to my therapist.

Glassblowing is a medium that provides a unique opportunity for youth who've experienced trauma and chronic stress to express themselves. Because of the innate danger of fire and molten glass, it is an engaging medium for many youth who find themselves able to focus on the process and nothing else (Bogira, 2015; Gilmore, 2018). Because the art form is collaborative, glassblowing can also help individuals learn to work and communicate with others and form safe, trusting relationships with their glassblowing partners (Bogira, 2015). It is a mindful, collaborative, and healing craft for many who find it difficult sitting at a table or in an office with more traditional art and talk therapies. New research also supports this type of trauma therapy, as it involves sensory and body-movement interventions that can help integrate experiences in the brain (Zulkey, 2018).

Another glassblowing community project occurred at a Midwestern university. This project was provided by an early childhood education program, in conjunction with a glassblowing studio on campus. I co-participated in this project with a client with autism and also assisted with an additional participant with co-occurring attention deficit hyperactivity disorder and autism, both eight years old. The structure of this program had the child first sculpt an imaginary creature in clay, then write a story about the creature, and finally a glassblowing student made that creature out of glass to the child's specifications. Although the children did not directly participate in the glassblowing process, they were encouraged to supervise the glass blowers and provide them feedback on the piece as it was created. For the children with autism, this provided an opportunity to co-participate with neurotypical peers with support from adults and control the process of creating a multi-step art piece that was subsequently displayed in a traveling art show. My client expressed feelings of mastery and satisfaction with his participation and stated he would like to participate again in such a project. The second child expressed similar feelings. Both children participated in an opening reception for the art show. My client elected to stay for only a short period, as he was overwhelmed by the crowd at the opening reception; however, the second child expressed feelings of pride and accomplishment and enjoyed giving autographs at the event.

Conclusion

Although historically art therapists have viewed glass as an inappropriate medium for use in art therapy (Moon, 2010; Somer & Somer, 2000), glass has been utilized effectively in art therapy practice, as illustrated earlier. Even though costs may be prohibitively high, thanks to community partnerships and creative resourcing, hot glass can be made accessible to a wide variety of populations. Moreover, glass fusion and glassblowing promote communication and social skills, feelings of confidence and self-efficacy, job skills, mindfulness, and engagement with powerful metaphors for art therapy participants. We hope that after reading about these experiences, art therapists will consider the potential of glass as a therapeutic medium and form relationships with local glass facilities to initiate collaborative programming as well as pursue further education in these powerful processes!

References

Bardhan, G. (2012, October 12). Breaking the glass ceiling: Women working with glass. *Corning Museum of Glass*. Retrieved from www.cmog.org/article/breaking-glass-ceiling-women-working-glass

Bicketon, M. (Director). (2019). *Blown away* [Netflix series].

Bogira, S. (2015). *Project Fire offers peace forged in the flame*. Retrieved from https://www.chicagoreader.com/chicago/glassblowing-childhood-trauma-alex-harris-brad-stolbach-ignite-glass-studios/Content?oid=18301180

Corning Museum of Glass. (2002). *About us*. Retrieved from www.cmog.org/about

Cromwell, C. (2017, January 31). How female glass blowers are breaking the glass ceiling. *Entity*. Retrieved from www.entitymag.com/blowing-glass-ceiling/

Csikszentmihalyi, M. (1990). *Flow: The psychology of optimal experience*. New York, NY: Harper and Row.

Dean, M. (2016). *Using art media in psychotherapy: Bringing the power of creativity to practice*. New York, NY: Routledge.

Friedman, B. (2015). *Project FIRE ignites passion for glass making*. Retrieved from https://news.wttw.com/2015/08/20/project-fire-ignites-passion-glass-making

Frank, S. (1982). *Glass and archaeology*. London, England: Academic Press.

Gilmore, E. (2018, September 14). *Project FIRE uses glassblowing as a form of healing from gun violence*. Retrieved from https://thetriibe.com/2018/09/project-fire-uses-glassblowing-as-a-form-of-healing-from-gun-violence/

Glassblowing. (n.d.). *In Merriam-Webster Dictionary online*. Retrieved from www.merriam-webster.com/dictionary/glassblowing

Glass fusing basics. (2014). Retrieved September 3, 2015, from www.bullseyeglass.com/education/fusing-basics.html

Gutsch, B. B. J. [B. Becker J. Gutsch] (n.d.-a). *Facebook* [Fan page]. Retrieved September 3, 2015, from www.facebook.com/pages/Becker-J-GutschRed-Dot-Glass-Art/208137948421?sk=info&tab=page_info

Gutsch, B. B. J. [B. Becker J. Gutsch] (n.d.-b). *Linked In*. Retrieved September 3, 2015, from www.linkedin.com/pub/b-becker-j-gutsch/13/366/991

Hinz, L. D. (2009). *Expressive therapies continuum: A framework for using art in therapy*. New York, NY: Routledge.

Horovitz, E. (2018). *A guide to art therapy materials, methods, and applications: A practical step-by-step approach*. New York, NY: Routledge.

Ignition Community Glass. (n.d.). Retrieved from https://icg-chicago.org/our-story/

Minson, J. (2002). *The arts as therapy with children: Glass art as therapy.* Films Media Group. Retrieved from www.films.com/ ecTitleDetail.aspx?TitleID=30432

Moon, C. H. (2010). *Materials and media in art therapy: Critical understandings of diverse artistic vocabularies.* New York, NY: Routledge.

Nainis, N., Paice, J. A., Ratner, J., Wirth, J. H., Lai, J., & Shott, S. (2006). Relieving symptoms in cancer: Innovative use of art therapy. *Journal of Pain and Symptom Management, 31,* 162–169.

National Endowment for the Arts. (n.d.). Creative forces: NEA military healing arts network. *Veteran's Voices: Christopher Stowe.* Retrieved from www.arts.gov/national-initiatives/creative-forces-nea-military-healing-arts-network/resources/veterans-voices-christopher-stowe

Our Story. (n.d.). Retrieved from www.projectfirechicago.org/our-vision

Positive Youth Development. (n.d.). Retrieved from www.hhs.gov/ash/oah/adolescent-development/positive-youth-development/index.html

Reynolds, G. (1987). *The fused glass handbook.* Scottsdale, AZ: Hidden Valley Books.

Somer, L., & Somer, E. (2000). Perspectives on the use of glass in therapy. *American Journal of Art Therapy, 38,* 75–80.

Stallings, J., & Clark, S. (2018, November). *Glass as therapeutic medium in art therapy.* American Art Therapy Association 49th Annual Conference. Hyatt Regency Miami, Miami, FL.

Support Our Mission. (n.d.). Retrieved from https://icg-chicago.org/support-our-mission

Truman, G., & Minter, H. (2016, April 22). A day in the life of a female glass blower. *The Guardian.* Retrieved from www.theguardian.com/ women-in-leadership/2016/apr/22/a-day-in-t he-life-of-a-female-glass-blower

Woodruff, L. (2015). *In urban glass.* Retrieved January 4, 2017, from www.urbanglass.org/glass/detail/hot-shop-heroes

Zen Glass Studio. (n.d.). *Operation Zen.* Retrieved from zenglass.com/operationzen

Zulkey, C. (2018). *Healing the hurt.* Retrieved from https://chicagohealthonline.com/healing-the-hurt/

3

From Clay to Ceramic
An Alchemical Process of
Self-Transformation

JOSHUA KIN-MAN NAN

Introduction: Nuwa Mended the Collapsed Skies With Clay

Clay is referred to as "the *prima materia* of man" (von Franz, 1980, p. 88), meaning that clay is the most fundamental material on earth. In the Biblical story of Genesis, the creator made the first man, Adam, out of clay. In the ancient alchemist's mind, clay is one of the basic, humble, and commonly used elements but is used to refine noble metals such as gold and silver (Cotnoir, 2006). Clay is a symbol of procreation (Eliade, 1956). In both Western and Eastern cultures, there are many myths and legends that center around clay or earth. One Chinese myth is about the goddess Nuwa (女媧)). There are various stories about Nuwa, but the most famous one is about how she repaired the collapsed skies with clay.

As the story goes, at one time, the four pillars that supported the skies broke and a massive earthquake occurred. Fires and floods hit the earth. As there was not enough food, animals began to eat humans. Those who were weak and old became prey. Nuwa, the goddess who created humans, could not bear to see the destruction of the whole world. However, to save the earth and all living beings, the skies had to be restored to their original state, which was a huge task. After contemplating for some time, Nuwa thought of a solution—but it would be extremely challenging. She had to refine thousands of five-colored stones in order to mend the holes of the skies and restore them to their original function. The five-colored stones were created from the primitive earth material—the five-colored clay—in a stove made from boulders using fire borrowed from the sun. She spent nine days and nine nights making 36,501 pieces of five-colored stones, of which 36,500 stone pieces were used to patch up the skies. The last unused, huge stone was left in the Tiantai Mountain in China. After Nuwa repaired the skies, she begged a giant turtle to use his four legs to create new pillars to support the skies. The turtle was willing to sacrifice his life, and the pillars were eventually constructed.

The Value of the Craftsmanship of Pottery Art

As an art therapy student in the past and as an art therapy educator now, I'm all too familiar with the prevalent belief within the art therapy field that the process of art making is more important than the art product. The production of functional objects through art training or practice also seems to be looked down upon, and its therapeutic potential overlooked. Similarly, investigation of the functions and values of art products also emerge in the wider world, such as the potters' circle. My sister Rita and I are both potters, and we are often bothered by the devaluation of crafting. We especially uphold the value of craftsmanship in pottery art and the rich values and meanings carried by handmade ceramic art pieces.

Art therapy literature explores a range of approaches for the use of clay in art therapy practice (Elbrecht, 2013; Henley, 2002; Sholt & Gavron, 2006). I have described the use of clay as a therapeutic medium in clinical practice, especially when integrated with the Expressive Therapies Continuum (Hinz, 2009; Lusebrink, 1990) for treating depression (Nan, 2016, 2017). The use of empirical science provides strong evidence for the therapeutic impact of clay art making (Nan & Ho, 2017). Nevertheless, the reductionist methods of quantitative research fall short of exemplifying the details of my approach. In this chapter, I reiterate the distinctive characteristics of clay—including the many possibilities for how to interact with it, such as wheel throwing, hand building, and glazing methods. The sensory nature and plastic texture of clay helps create positive psychophysiological effects, such as raising body awareness, creating a mindful state for the artist, and enhancing positive affective experience. The distinct life cycle of clay embodies and expresses the different stages of life. Stories from the pottery studio that I set up in Hong Kong describe how I developed and integrated Clay Art Therapy, a distinct art therapy approach using clay, into the local social work practice setting. These stories exemplify the constructing, destructing, and reconstructing processes of clay that are crucial to enable a clay piece to withstand the firing test prior to its transformation into ceramic. In a parallel manner, through a prolonged period of developing the craftsmanship of clay art making, the artist goes through an inner alchemical process of self-transformation. The essence of this transformation affirms one's discovery of one's ability to create and recreate beautiful ceramic art pieces through repetitive practices and offers insight into the possibility of reorienting one's life path, looking for more potential in oneself, and withstanding hardship with a transformative soul.

The Distinctive Transformation From Clay to Ceramic in Art Therapy

The Various Methods of Interacting With Clay

Art therapists and other mental health professionals were pioneers in identifying the various therapeutic features of clay (Brock, 1991; Brown, 1975; Henley, 2002; Sholt & Gavron, 2006; Winship & Haigh, 1998). As an art material, clay has distinctive features that make it an extraordinary art therapy medium. Clay art making involves a range of methods that facilitate choosing a unique and expressive manner in which to interact with it. The most typical form of clay work is wheel throwing, a method focusing entirely on centering a piece of clay slump on a wheel and making a symmetrical clay work. Other methods include hand building with pinching or clay slabs, casting, sculpting, or a mixture of these techniques. Another attractive and exciting clay art-making option is surface treatment or glazing bisque-fired clay products. The transformative process—from clay to the crystallization of glazes and a final ceramic piece shining with beautiful colors—can often surprise the creator. In fact, glazing can require knowledge that covers the advanced techniques of firing, such as wood and salt firing, as well as kiln-firing methods, such as *saggar* and Japanese *raku* firing. The unpredictable way color changes during the process of glazing can enchant some potters to the extent that some spend a lifetime practicing glazing methods and techniques.

The Sensory Experience of Clay Art Making

In the process of clay art making, the artist is required to directly and continuously touch the clay. Touch is a "haptic" sensation that involves "cutaneous sensation." The cutaneous sense is very rich in that it includes responses to pressure, vibration, and temperature (Carr, 2008), spatial sense (position/location, size, and shape), contact sense (e.g., rough/smooth, soft/hard, comfortable to touch or not), and the sense of pain (Elbrecht, 2013; Grunwald, 2008). Related to haptic sensation is "proprioceptive sensation" or "proprioception," a term referring to the awareness of spatial position via the body's "built-in" sensors in muscles, joints, tendons, ligaments, and the skin (Wilson, 1998). Proprioceptive perception allows people to be aware of their presence in space and interact with the surrounding physical environment appropriately. Sensory-rich processes and kinesthetic movements therefore help clay art making provide a profound effect on raising somatic consciousness (Stein, 1998) or body awareness in a physical space (Schutz, 2005) that also can create positive psychological effects, such as mindfulness. Also intriguing is that clay has a distinct feature of recording every print or touch of the artist. Therefore, it is rich in enhancing bodily based affective expression (Panksepp & Watt, 2011; Schore, 2009) through the direct touch with clay.

The Life Cycle of Clay

The texture and plasticity of clay varies depending on the composition of the different ingredients mixed with it, such as grog, water, minerals, and ash. When clay is wet, it is soft and very malleable. Interacting with wet clay can allow the artist to make more changeable three-dimensional products and express spontaneous inner movements. These spontaneous and intuitive expressions very often evoke predominantly affective experience (Nan & Ho, 2014). When clay is dry, it becomes resistive to changing its form, like wood or stone. Interacting with dry clay requires more organized and controlled procedures, in order not to destroy the material to an extent that it cannot be restored. Like wood or stone carving, every step of working on dry clay needs to be well-planned. Therefore, interacting with dry clay predominantly evokes more cognitive processes, such as planning, analyzing, organizing, and problem-solving skills (Nan, 2017). In a soft and tender form, clay can be molded into three-dimensional objects. At the other extreme, when clay is bisque-fired and becomes bone-dry, it is very fragile. After glazes are applied and fired, clay is transformed into ceramic. The firing of clay work is regarded as a test of whether it is well-built and strong enough.

Artists certainly want to create a well-crafted clay piece prior to putting it into the firing kiln or there is a risk that the work will crack and leave flaws in the surface of the ceramic. However, the artist cannot hold on to a clay slump and play with it for hours. When clay is over-built, the water adhered between the sand particles may dry up over time, and the cohesion between various ingredients inside the clay may also be destroyed. Eventually, the clay object may deform, which can be viewed as a metaphorical death. Given clay's rich-ness and unique malleability, the processes of clay art making can symbolize different stages and aspects of life. Clay products embody rich meanings at intrapersonal, interpersonal, and transpersonal levels (McGriffin, 2002).

Clay Art Therapy at the Mental Health Association of Hong Kong

The Story of the Pottery Studio

In 2010, I became the first and, so far, the only art therapist to work at the Mental Health Association of Hong Kong (MHAHK). This organization has a 65-year history of providing mental health services to individuals undergoing mental health rehabilitation. I was employed in one of the community-based outpatient centers. The members of the center were individuals participating in psychiatric rehabilitation, including services such as case and group social work services, interest classes, reemployment counseling, occupational therapy, psychiatric nursing, and psychiatric outpatient services from medical doctors.

Envisioning the potential of visual art as a therapeutic service in mental health rehabilitation, MHAHK obtained funds to establish an art therapy stu-dio as an innovative service. As the art therapist, I was responsible for setting up the studio, which included designing the layout of the studio and install-ing all required equipment. I decided to organize the space as a pottery studio because I found that there were very few art therapists who were familiar with clay work in Hong Kong. As I am a potter, this pottery studio would help to fill the service gap by providing art therapy services specializing in clay work.

However, this studio was also set up in a manner that could facilitate art making with a range of art materials. Therefore, the studio could facilitate multimedia art therapy services in group and individual art therapy services. The studio was large enough to accommodate 12 individuals taking part in clay art making (Figure 3.1). I purchased two wooden worktables (approximately 2 × 5 & 3.5 × 7.5 square feet) tailor-made for clay work, two electric wheels for clay throwing, and two electric kilns. The kilns, each able to fire up to two dozen clay works at a time, were stored in a separate room.

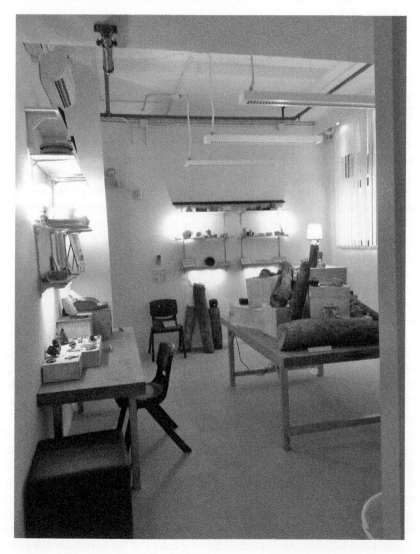

Figure 3.1 The pottery studio with an art show going on

As I developed new social services for MHAHK, I was privileged to try out various modes of art therapy services, including art therapy with clay. Apart from individual art therapy and the use of art training for professional colleagues, I facilitated short-term therapeutic groups for center members. These groups were open, in that all of the members of the center were welcome to join, with no need to be referred by social workers. As I led these groups periodically over the five years I spent working at this center, meeting at least once or twice per week, some of the frequent participants developed strong trust in me, as well as trust and friendship in one another, and I witnessed changes in them via clay art making.

I Am an Artist, Not a Patient

The art therapy group with clay (clay group) usually comprised two main groups of users. One of the groups was receiving social work casework services. These individuals could join a clay group via the referral and assessment of their caseworkers. Another group of users usually had full-time or part-time jobs. Their mental health was at a relatively stable point in the rehabilitation process. They could apply for a clay group as an interest class. Each clay group usually had six sessions, of two hours each. I would launch one or two groups in a week, depending on my schedule. After a group cycle was completed, some of the group members would request to join other classes or groups in the center. If some members wanted to continue to the next clay group, I would discuss this with them and set up some new goals or directions with them so that they could keep progressing with a focus. This mode of clay group could continually fulfill the needs of the service users of the center. Over time, about five to six individuals completed eight to ten group cycles or even more. As these members developed more advanced clay art-making skills, I would invite them to assist the new group members on a voluntary basis.

During the orientation session of a new clay group, I would introduce the pottery studio as follows: "Once you enter this studio door, you are an artist. I would love to invite you to care more about your involvement in the making of your clay products than your illness." I would give a brief orientation on the rules and regulations of the pottery studio. These norms created a container in which participants had the freedom to be themselves and to create as they pleased. During this initial phase, I would teach participants basic hand-building knowledge and techniques, such as understanding the features of clay and kneading and pinching techniques. A typical example of a group process would be making simple pinched works. The products were usually small containers at this stage.

Progressively, I would teach groups about various kinds of glazes and share my experiences of glazing techniques. Usually, glazes are in a fluid form, like yogurt, prior to firing. At this state, the true colors of the glazes are not seen. The glazed clay pieces would be put into a kiln to be fired up to a range of

900–1280 °C. After going through a melting and crystallization process, the clay works become as hard as rock, the glazes adhere to the surface of the clay, and the clay pieces are transformed into ceramic. There were always moments when everyone was enchanted when they saw how their tiny clay works were transformed into beautifully glazed ceramic art pieces. The sensory-rich experiences and intense process of clay art making were so engaging that these processes helped participants be mindful of the here-and-now and of every step of the creative process. In a sense, the pottery studio seemed to be a sacred space that gave participants a sense of tranquility and serenity.

Throughout the five years that I led these clay groups, I gradually integrated the practice with the Expressive Therapies Continuum (ETC) model (Lusebrink, 1990; Hinz, 2009), creating the approach of clay art therapy (CAT) (Nan & Ho, 2017). Whereas "clay art making" simply refers to the general approach of gaining the skills to work with clay as well as the hands-on practice of working with clay, clay art therapy integrates the framework and change mechanism of the ETC in assessing the needs of individuals and guiding them to interact with clay in the treatment process for achieving different therapeutic functions (Nan, 2016). The treatment goals and processes of CAT vary from one individual to another, depending on which ETC components the individual needs to develop and/or support, including the Kinesthetic/Sensory, Perceptual/Affective, Cognitive/Symbolic, and Creative levels (Hinz, 2009). A more complete treatment protocol of CAT can be found on the website of the American Art Therapy Association (Nan, 2016).

Clay Art Therapy: The Alchemical Process of Self-Discovery and Empowerment

The Capacity to Create

In an open group setting, participants in the pottery studio came and went. However, a group of members showed strong interest, dedication, and regular attendance in the CAT groups. Once participants acquired the fundamental techniques of pinching and clay-slab construction, they were free to follow their desires in pottery works creation. Very often, they enjoyed creating functional objects such as bowls, mugs, boxes, vases, or dishes, which they could use at home. The creative process and the ability to make these functional objects made them feel good. At other times, their ceramic works appeared more abstract and embodied their unforgettable life experiences, including fond memories and sad stories. Many participants' feedback to me was that CAT led them to a big discovery, a knowing in themselves—that they had capacity to create.

One participant, "Siu-ling," a woman in her fifties, once said to me, "Making something, a ceramic piece out of nothing, brought great satisfaction and happiness. The process of clay art making was like . . . pouring out something from my heart, somewhat like giving birth to a baby." Another middle-aged participant, "Mei-yee," remarked to herself after a group session, "Who said that I am useless? I can make this cute piggy!" No one in the group understood the true meaning of her words. Her social worker, who accompanied Mei-yee, told me afterward that after Mei-yee's son jumped from a building and died, every family member blamed Mei-yee and said that it was entirely her fault and that she was useless as a mother. However, the social worker was amazed by how clay art making had slowly helped Mei-yee rediscover her sense of self-worth and cheered her up, whereas the conventional treatment that Mei-yee had received for many years could only alleviate some symptoms of depression.

Outwardly, these artists gained benefits from CAT, such as alleviating the symptoms of mood problems, raising their sense of satisfaction in life, helping them to orient their direction in life, and helping them express their inner being embodied in the ceramic art pieces (Nan, 2015). Through the CAT process, they also gained more social support from other group members (Nan, 2015). Inwardly, the knowledge and techniques of clay work have guided them to discover their potential not just in the studio but also in their lives beyond the studio. Clay art making inspired them to create! This corresponds to the notion that existential psychologist Rollo May described in *The Courage to Create* (1994)—the possibility of life belongs to those who dare to create. There is a subtle but significant implication that with creative ability, many things are possible in life.

The Courage to Recreate

"Amanda" was in her fifties when she was diagnosed with depression. Amanda's husband had left her, and she did not know the real reason. This change also created distance between Amanda and her teenage son. After the divorce, her son stayed in his room all day. He and Amanda seldom spoke to each other. Amanda perceived that her life was a failure. When she was referred to join the CAT group, she commented that she was "bad," not only bad at art making but also other aspects of life.

Like all the other participants, Amanda created art pieces with flaws and made many mistakes in the steps of clay work. Despite numerous experiences of trial-and-error, she continued to practice hand-building techniques. With each session, Amanda's knowledge and skills progressed. From starting by creating pinched works as small as tiny snowballs, she eventually progressed to making large containers and, later, pottery works made from clay slabs. By continuously interacting with clay in various ways over time, Amanda immersed herself in clay art making. She embraced her mistakes in clay art making as she simultaneously learned to embrace her difficulties in life and soothed her broken emotions. The process of crafting clay paralleled the way she crafted her life—clay art making was soulcraft for her.

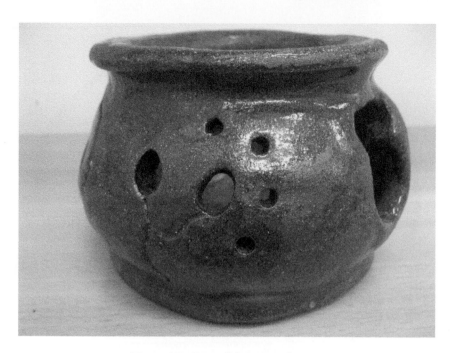

Figure 3.2 Amanda's incense burner

One day, before we engaged in the CAT session, Amanda told me there had been a tiny, marvelous change in the relationship between her son and her. I was both surprised and curious. She said that she had put out one of her nicest ceramic works at home, an incense burner (Figure 3.2). Her son gazed at the work and then asked Amanda if she had made it and she replied that she had. Though her son did not respond verbally Amanda perceived that her son's attitude toward her started to change when her ceramic art pieces became "adorable" or pleasing to the eye. We looked into each other's eyes and laughed loudly. We did not know exactly what her son was thinking. However, Amanda and I knew that her art products expressed her courage and intention to recreate her life. Figure 3.3 is a beautiful ceramic piece Amanda created at a later stage of her studio practice.

The Discovery Model

Individuals at MHAHK received various types of services during their psychiatric rehabilitation. Due to chronic mental health issues many members experienced diminished psychosocial functioning. The primary focus of rehabilitation was usually to assist individuals on their road to recovery for functioning in daily life, such as resuming self-care ability, regaining

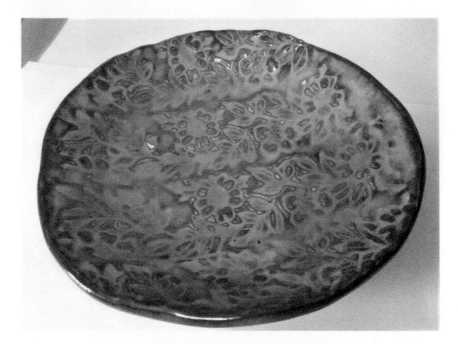

Figure 3.3 A dish created by Amanda at a later stage

employment, improving quality of sleep, and rebuilding social networks and/ or communication skills. In integrated clay art making with the Expressive Therapies Continuum, the approach of CAT supplemented conventional psychosocial care for rehabilitation on two levels.

On the first level, CAT aims at helping people integrate different inner processes, such as emotional and cognitive, with subjective and objective judgment (Hinz, 2009; Nan & Ho, 2017) and maintain a balance between them. On another level, the CAT approach facilitates artists in immersing themselves in clay art making and honing their artistry. In addition to strengthening abilities, the results of CAT include developing personal potential and creative ability. In this sense, the process of CAT is a voyage of self-discovery. In comparison, the recovery approach of rehabilitation (e.g. reduction of symptoms; reemployment) emphasizes resuming original functioning in the various aspects of life before illness. Figure 3.4 illustrates the different emphases of recovery and discovery approaches. The emphasis of the recovery approach is shown by the loop with blue font, whereas the emphasis of the discovery approach is shown by the orange line. CAT fosters the latter approach, helping individuals discover their potential in life; it emphasizes not only retaining or relearning lost abilities and strengthening old abilities but also learning new abilities for the future. The self-discovery

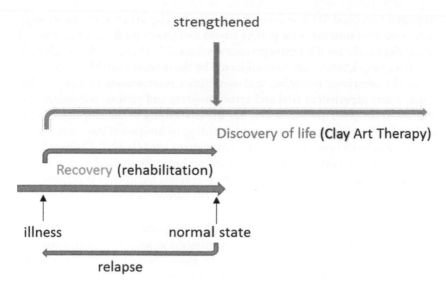

Figure 3.4 The approach of self-discovery in clay art therapy

Source: Adapted from Nan (2015)

approach has future-based implications in that it leads artists to adopt a pro-active attitude to envision and create their future.

The Transcendental Experience in Self-Discovery

An unexpected significance of the self-discovery approach was that through the process of self-discovery, the CAT group members shifted from being the targets of change to becoming the agents of change. This unanticipated outcome was very different from the rationale that I originally proposed in the CAT protocol that the art therapist plays an active role in assessing artists and guiding the treatment process. However, in the self-discovery approach, artists guide their own change. These artists can envision greater possibilities to create even more valuable and personally meaningful ceramic art pieces, which become metaphors for a brighter future. The CAT intervention becomes a transcendental experience for individuals to discover their own strengths. This self-discovery model contrasts sharply with the passive form of treating signs and symptoms of illness, which dampens the agency of individuals.

"Jenny," a woman in her forties, was a die-hard fan and a core member of the CAT groups. With a background in a creative industry, Jenny had lots of ideas for clay art making. However, she often insisted on trying advanced techniques that were very challenging or beyond her ability. From time to time, I needed to guide Jenny so that her clay art-making process wasn't so frustrating that it negatively impacted her mood. With an immense passion for clay in her heart, she strongly requested additional use of the pottery studio for extra hours for practice. I would usually let her do this if her extra practice sessions did not clash with the schedule of other group activities and were endorsed by the supervisor of MHAHK.

In the laborious, repetitive, and sometimes monotonous process of clay work, Jenny experienced trial and error, progress and retreat, and failure and success. Over time, she excelled in her understanding of the language of clay and had quite a firm grip on the hand-building techniques of clay work. Jenny became a powerful potter. Almost five years after I left MHAHK, I bumped into Jenny during my visit to the center. She enthusiastically showed me her recent ceramic pieces. I was fascinated by her ever-growing techniques in ceramic artistry. I asked her, "How did you do that?" Her response, a big smile, told me that it was no easy job (Figures 3.5–3.8).

Since I left MHAHK, the center has employed a potter to run clay art-making workshops as interest classes. Jenny has continued to join these workshops as a "Peer-Worker-with-Art" (PWA) for the past three years. In Hong Kong, in an effort to encourage individuals undergoing rehabilitation, a pilot project called

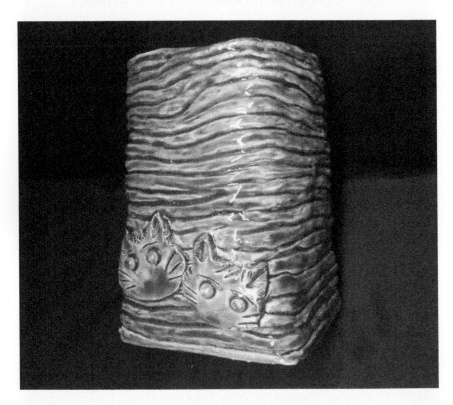

Figure 3.5 Selected works of Jenny

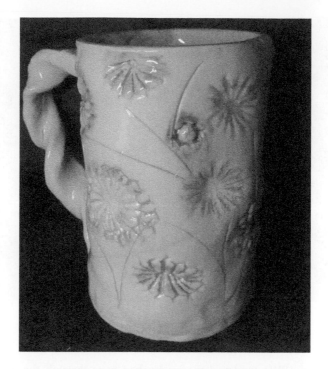

Figure 3.6 Selected works of Jenny

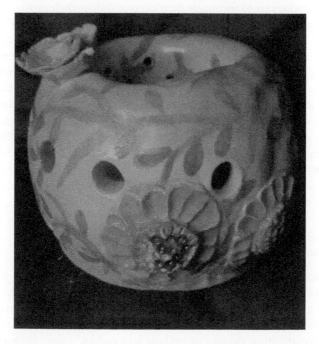

Figure 3.7 Selected works of Jenny

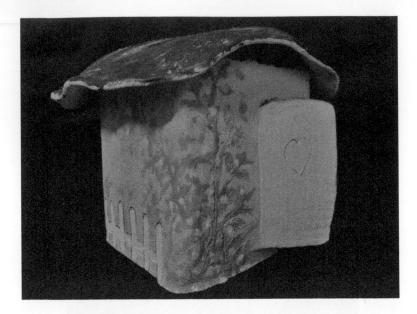

Figure 3.8 Selected works of Jenny

"Peer-Worker" (PW) employed those who had gone through the program to become peers of those still on the journey to recovery. The roles and responsibilities of peer workers are to encourage their peers and share their experiences on the recovery journey. MHAHK has also employed a few PWs in their centers for a few of the CAT participants who had developed quite sophisticated clay art-making knowledge and techniques. Jenny and another former clay group member have become PWs, but they are more. They have each become a "Peer-Worker-with-Art" (PWA)—demonstrating their clay art-making skills, encouraging participants to overcome the obstacles in the process, and assisting the potter in running the classes. Meanwhile, a few of my colleagues committed to continuing to use arts and crafts, especially clay art making, in their services. To enhance the professional competence of the social workers using art in their services, I launched a knowledge transfer project (August 2018—December 2019) in collaboration with MHAHK, aiming at providing more in-depth training, supervision, and application of the uses of art in their various social services (Nan, 2019).

Alchemical Process: Transforming From Construction and Destruction to Reconstruction of Life

The plasticity of clay, the many different ways of interacting with it, and the formation of the shining ceramic pieces remind us that there are many possibilities in art as there are in life. As one of the CAT members said, "You can make the clay into anything. The process is somewhat like your life. You can build your life into anything, depending on how you mold it" (Nan, 2015, p. 231).

The discovery of the ability to create and recreate symbolizes the many chances to make changes along the way at any time of one's life. In life, there are ups and downs as well as unpredictable frustration and failures. The construction and reconstruction processes of clay art making demonstrate that failures and frustration are inevitable parts of human existence. In the many endeavors to create a successful craft, the artist requires the courage and persistence to construct and reconstruct their clay work numerous times. At times, when the clay is overworked, the artist has to let it go and restart the whole work process again. As such, the construction and reconstruction processes subtly consist of a necessary step of destruction before reconstruction is made possible. Only through this reconstruction process can the clay work become strong enough to withstand the test of fire and transform into ceramic. It is parallel to the development of ego; through frustration and pain, ego can transform into a stronger state and become more resilient to adversity (Stein, 1998).

The process of constructing clay objects symbolizes various aspects of life on intrapersonal, interpersonal, and transpersonal levels. These rich meanings are embodied in the clay product (McGriffin, 2002). Externally, the construction and reconstruction process mends and reforms the clay work and makes it stronger. The firing of the clay work transforms it into ceramic. This process matches the alchemical process of transforming matter into a precious and durable material (Jung, 1983; Cotnoir, 2006). The alchemy of matter can be considered parallel with the alchemy of the inner self, which is transformed into a tougher state after each life challenge. As such, the transformation from clay to ceramic synchronizes with the transformation of the human psyche (Jung, 1983, 2011).

Reflections and Conclusions

Although clay is often regarded as a humble and lowly material, by going through complex crafting processes it is molded, refined, purified, and transformed into beautiful ceramic works. The crafting of clay comprises constant and disciplined practice alongside a mindful and patient heart. This process progressively establishes potters' knowledge and techniques in pottery work and their knowledge of their limits as well as those of the clay work they interact with (e.g., the time limit in the life cycle of clay). In the repetitive practices of clay art making, the artist gradually understands that life has many possibilities to be constructed and reconstructed through errors. This trial-and-error process is like the firing test on the clay work that ultimately transcends the soul to become more resilient to the adversities in life.

I started with the story of Nuwa repairing the collapsed skies. Nuwa used nine days and nine nights to conduct the strenuous and exhausting task of refining 36,500 pieces of five-colored stones from the five-colored clay. If we take the number as a metaphor, 36,500 can be compared to 365 days in a year, denoting a sense of completion. In Chinese tradition, the number nine has the same pronunciation as the word "long-lasting" or "everlasting"; thus, it is a lucky number. The legend conveys that this challenging but monotonous task was completed to perfection. It seems to not only boast of Nuwa's clay work

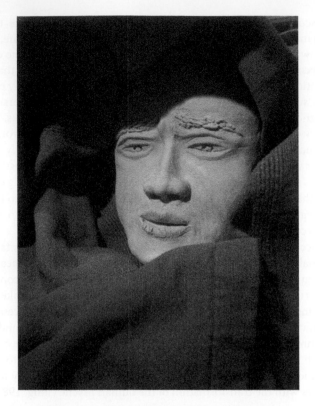

Figure 3.9 Agony & Ecstasy: The pilgrimage

Source: Joshua Nan

craftsmanship but also explain that Nuwa completed an alchemical process of self-transformation by conquering this extremely challenging work.

If Nuwa, as an archetype, represents every human being, the story in fact invites us all to take up the task to refine clay and to embark on this voyage of self-transformation. This voyage requires courage, diligence, and perseverance to craft the soul. An image of a pilgrim I created expresses this idea in a visual form (Figure 3.9). The image conveys that the voyage of self-transformation is like a pilgrimage of life—a journey filled with extreme emotions, with both agony and ecstasy.

References

Brock, M. (1991). The therapeutic use of clay. *British Journal of Occupational Therapy*, 54(1), 13–15.

Brown, E. V. (1975). Developmental characteristics of clay figures made by children ages three through eleven years. *Studies in Art Education*, 16(3),

Carr, R. (2008). Sensory processes and responses. In N. Hass-Cohen & R. Carr (Eds.), *Art therapy and clinical neuroscience* (pp. 43–61). London and Philadelphia: Jessica Kingsley.

Cotnoir, B. (2006). *The Weiser concise guide to alchemy* (J. Wasserman, Ed.). York Beach, ME: Red Wheel and Weiser.

Elbrecht, C. (2013). *Trauma healing at the clay field: A sensorimotor art therapy approach.* London and Philadelphia: Jessica Kingsley.

Eliade, M. (1956). *The forge and the crucible: The origins and structure of alchemy* (2nd ed.). Chicago, IL: University of Chicago Press.

Grunwald, M. (Ed.). (2008). *Human haptic perception: Basics and applications.* Basel, Switzerland: Springer Science & Business Media.

Henley, D. (2002). *Clayworks in art therapy: Playing the sacred circle.* Philadelphia, PA: Jessica Kingsley.

Hinz, L. D. (2009). *Expressive therapies continuum: A framework for using art in therapy.* New York, NY: Routledge.

Jung, C. G. (1983). *Alchemical Studies (Collected Works of C.G. Jung Vol. 13).* Princeton, NJ: Princeton University Press.

Jung, C. G. (2011). *Synchronicity: An acausal connecting principle (From Collected Works of C. G. Jung).* Princeton, NJ: Princeton University Press.

Lusebrink, V. B. (1990). *Imagery and visual expression in therapy.* New York, NY: Plenum Press.

May, R. (1994). *The courage to create.* New York, NY: W. W. Norton & Company.

McGriffin, M., S.P. (2002). *Reflections in clay.* Bloomington, IN: 1st Books Library.

Nan, J. K. M. (2015). *Therapeutic effects of clay art therapy for patients with depression* (Doctoral dissertation). The University of Hong Kong, Hong Kong.

Nan, J. K. M. (2016, August). *Mind-body-treatment for depression: Clay art therapy with the expressive therapies continuum.* At Annual Conference of the American Art Therapy Association, AATA, Baltimore, MD.

Nan, J. K. M. (2017, December). *Psychophysiological stress treatment: Comparing clay art therapy and mandala making: A randomized controlled trial.* At American Art Therapy Association Annual Conference, Albuquerque, New Mexico.

Nan, J. K. M. (2019, June). *Alternative medicine: Use of art for wellness & empowerment: A knowledge transfer project across cultures.* The Arts in Society Annual Conference, Lisbon, Portugal.

Nan, J. K. M., & Ho, R. T. H. (2014). Affect regulation and treatment for depression and anxiety through art: Theoretical ground and clinical issues. *Annals of Depression and Anxiety, 1*(2), 1–6.

Nan, J. K. M., & Ho, R. T. H. (2017). Effects of clay art therapy on adult outpatients with major depressive disorder: A randomized controlled trial. *Journal of Affective Disorders, 217,* 237–245.

Panksepp, J., & Watt, D. (2011). Why does depression hurt? Ancestral priMei-yee-process separation-distress (PANIC/GRIEF) and diminished brain reward (SEEKING) processes in the genesis of depressive affect. *Psychiatry: Interpersonal & Biological Processes, 74*(1), 5–13.

Schore, A. N. (2009). Right-brain affect regulation: An essential mechanism of development, trauma, dissociation, and psychotherapy. In D. Fosha, D. J. Siegal, & M. F. Solomon (Eds.), *The healing power of emotion: Affective neuroscience, development & clinical practice* (pp. 112–144). New York and London: W.W. Norton & Company.

Schutz, L. E. (2005). Broad-perspective perceptual disorder of the right hemisphere. *Neuropsychology Review, 15*(1), 11–27.

Sholt, M., & Gavron, T. (2006). Therapeutic qualities of clay-work in art therapy and psychotherapy: A review. *Art Therapy: Journal of the American Art Therapy Association, 23*(2), 66–72.

Stein, M. (1998). *Jung's map of the soul: An introduction.* Chicago and La Salle, Illinois: Open Court.

von Franz, M. L. (1980). *Alchemy: An introduction to the symbolism and the psychology.* Canada: Inner City Books.

Wilson, F. R. (1998). *The hand.* New York, NY: Vintage Books.

Winship, G., & Haigh, R. (1998). The formation of objects in the group matrix: Reflections on creative therapy with clay. *Group Analysis, 31,* 71–81.

4

Demystifying the Individualistic Approach to Self-Care

Sewing as a Metaphorical Process for Documenting Relational and Communal Care in Disability Culture

CHUN-SHAN (SANDIE) YI

Getting discount massages through Groupon is often one of my top choices for self-care. That is, if the first five minutes could go by without receiving comments about my physical disability. I call the first five minutes of massages "the anxious five." I lie face down on a massage table. A white sheet covers my body, and I am wearing nothing but underwear. I never know how the massage therapists are going to react as soon as they discover that I only have two fingers on each hand and two toes on each foot under the sheet.

Massage Therapist (MT):	"How is the pressure?"
Me:	"It's okay; I can take more though."

I continue to keep my eyes closed as I feel tension release from the increased pressure on my tight shoulders. The therapist then moves her hands from my shoulders to my arms and then to my wrists. It is no surprise that more questions follow:

MT:	"Did you have an accident?"
Me:	"Um . . . no. I was born like this."
MT:	"But you still function alright, right?"
Me:	"Uh . . . yeah, pretty much . . ." (I answer with sleepy eyes.)

A few moments later . . .

MT:	"So, what do you do now?"
Me:	". . . Um . . . I teach and I am working on a PhD in disability studies." (Am I being interviewed in the middle of a massage?)
MT:	"Oh, good for you! You made it this far, and you can help other people with disabilities!"

Some massage therapists might not ask about my impairments, but the way they touch, hold, and put pressure (or don't do any of the above at all) on my hands and feet reveals how they feel about my body. The purpose of receiving a massage is to be in a judgment-free space where one feels accepted, pampered, and well taken care of. The last thing that I want to think about is how I can help others when lying down on a massage table for some *me time*. So, I decided to join group yoga, where I would not be the only one seeking self-care. At the end of my first Kundalini yoga session in a new studio, the teacher approached me after class.

Yoga teacher (YT):	"It's wonderful that you came! I saw the way you move with your hands and feet—you can do a lot!"
Me:	"Um . . . I have practiced yoga before."
YT:	"Were you born like this? . . . What do you do now?" (asked with much enthusiasm)
Me:	"Yes . . . I was. I am an art therapist and I'm working on a PhD."
YT:	"Oh, that's very nice of you! You help disabled people . . . you must be so patient. . . . Now, you can give back to society. You can show others that nothing can stop people like you."

"People like me?" People like me, who were born with or acquired a disability, desire to pamper our bodies and minds when we are tired, frustrated, and defeated because we often experience microaggressions on a regular basis. We are turned into "inspiration porn," a term coined by late disability activist Stella Young (2014), meaning that we are considered to be doing something extraordinary when we are simply doing something mundane, such as going to school or work, shopping, or taking a yoga class. We are constantly expected to prove ourselves and show our productivity and worth as model citizens who can take care of ourselves so we don't become burdens to society. But when we try to relax and have fun after a long week of hard work, people remind us that we have the responsibility to inspire and help others "despite of" our disabilities. People like me, who realize that "nothing can stop people like you" is a false superhero tale.

Introduction

People who choose to become mental health care providers, as I have, often have the personality and innate ability to relate to others' pain and struggles. We are prone to compassion fatigue because we are ethically bound to support others who have experienced trauma, harm, and the unbearable (Hinz, 2019). We are seen as people with enough patience for working with "those" disabled people, whose needs are stigmatized as "special" and "hard to deal with." Society often prizes our work with the disability population as charity and us as saints and saviors. Does the same stigma and expectation apply to people like me who are both disabled and therapists? How do we, disabled and ill therapists, make sense of the stigma and deconstruct the savior syndrome, so we not only survive ableism but also thrive along with our disabled and ill clients/patients?

In the United States, independence and self-determination are the ideal attributes for a person's success. In other parts of the world, personal success depends on "saving face"—not shaming your family name and bringing prosperity to honor your ancestors. The individual's accomplishments reflect how well they meet the social expectations and take care—to recharge and maintain—their productivity in comparison to others. In other words, success depends on individuals' efforts to help themselves first.

The mentality of "pulling yourself up by the bootstraps" has deeply impacted the way we think about self-help and self-care in a capitalistic society (Gordon, 2018; Ward, 2015). The same "pulling yourself up by the bootstraps" mentality also impacts art therapists, who must present themselves as professional workers in front of clients/patients and colleagues with whom they work—especially when the field of art therapy strives to be recognized as an esteemed helping profession among other mental health care fields. It often requires art therapists to perform an authoritative presence and demonstrate "I've got it handled!" The individualistic norms shaped by neoliberalism have inevitably cultured art therapists to employ a capitalistic approach, focusing on individuals' responsibility for their own well-being (Gipson, 2017). As art therapists aim to serve clients/patients and keep up with the demanding capitalistic mental health care industry, art therapists don't always do a good job of asking for help when we are the helpers. How we handle stress, burnout, or countertransference through self-care often becomes an individualized responsibility that takes place behind closed doors.

The emphasis on individual efforts and ability to overcome challenges or setbacks without help has further cultivated a class-based, ableist culture where disability is considered an individual problem and a burden on the social welfare system. Professional mental health care providers inherit an interventionist model (Yi, 2019) when working with people who experience any sort of disability or illness. An interventionist approach is based on the medical model that disability resides within the individual person who does not fit the norm and cannot fully participate in society; therefore, such a person needs to be "normalized" or make adaptations by receiving clinical and mental health intervention from professional experts.

It is inevitable for art therapists who are disabled and/or ill themselves to internalize ableism, especially when disability culture community is absent in their lives. Some of us may choose "passing" as a survival skill and detach ourselves from disability. Those who can may "pass" by concealing their impairments and their need for help to avoid disability stigma. Those who can may also fall into an overachieving "supercrip"[1] narrative in which their accomplishments are seen as proofs for ridding their disability (Clare, 1991). They hold positive "can-do" attitudes and present themselves as overcomers to inspire non-disabled people without examining or addressing the existing systematic and environmental prejudice against disabled people. They may make attempts to be accepted as "normal" by blatantly denying or rejecting their disability identity and affiliation even if their disabilities are apparent.

I examine the role of disability culture in self-care through the lens of disability studies. I engage the theory of complex embodiment (Siebers, 2008) as I challenge existing self-care strategies: through retelling an earlier period of my practice, where I first shifted from making art about disability as a personal struggle to a shared cultural and political alliance with fellow disabled women artists, I reflect on the power that the metaphor of sewing and the act of repairing has on disability narratives. I argue that knowledge of disability culture is fundamental for art therapists' professional development. Later I will use examples of my artwork to illustrate a precursor of a collective care model for a sustainable self-care practice for art therapists, especially for art therapists who have experienced disability and/or illness. I hope to offer this chapter as a way to complicate the meaning and practice of self-care for the field of art therapy.

Self-Care: A Personal Disability History

In *Disability Theory* (2008), Siebers called attention to the complicated nature of disability by locating the bodymind in the social, cultural, economic, and political contexts the disabled bodymind inhabits. Instead of seeing "body" and "mind" as separate entities within white, Western culture (Clare, 2016), "bodymind" refers to how mental and physical states process lived experience as one unit (Price, 2014). Examining how disability is often seen as merely an individual's tragedy, loss, or defect, Siebers encouraged readers to recognize the multiple social realities and meanings that shape one's disability experience and identity. The theory of complex embodiment therefore leads us to engage in a conversation beyond the stereotypical rhetoric of disability. Complex embodiment often requires unpacking one's own internalized perspectives and stereotypes regarding disability and care. This was certainly a necessary part of my learning as an art therapy student.

Before the age of 25, I was estranged from the disability community and my disability identity. I was taught not to see my body as disability but only as "differences." People around me saw my passion and skills in art, and I proved to be evidence of how "disability did not hold her back." My ambivalent relationship to disability became further entangled when I took "Exceptional Child, Exceptional Art" (Henley, 1992), a special education class taught by an art therapist during college. I was able to connect class material to my own experience of being "different." I unconsciously avoided naming my experience as "disability" due to the stigma attached to disability and my internalized ableism, and I was applauded for my refusal to see myself as "broken." My interest in becoming an art educator in special education somehow rewarded me as a "warrior" who would model for and perhaps "make other disabled people's lives better."

I first learned about the concept of "self-care" in art therapy graduate school back in 2003. I learned about response art (Fish, 2019), and I was taught to "make art about it!" whenever I felt drained or defeated by the presenting issues, difficult feelings, or conflicts from working with clients. I was constantly challenged to use art to explore what I was learning during graduate school. Sometimes, I was frustrated by the "illustrative" nature of images created in the context of art therapy. I felt pressured by the expectation to master art for self-care because I felt I needed to show my readiness to compete with other mental health care providers. When not making art to process issues, I felt I was not working on my training! At times, I felt like a hypocrite when I found making art as self-care limiting, especially when I was exploring disability in an ableist dominated culture.

During an in-class presentation on self-care, I revealed that I was struggling with a personal memory, and I was not able to make art about it. What I had done was cut up my Taiwanese disability ID card with scissors the night before. It was an old ID card that had framed my very existence as an impaired person with an "untreatable" diagnosis from doctors and as a benefit taker by the social welfare system. I cried as I talked about the emotional process that cutting the ID card had been and my desire to be seen as "just a person." Cutting my disability ID card along with claiming my personhood was regarded as self-liberation and self-care. I received strong support and empathic responses from my art therapy community. I value and am grateful for the opportunity to engage in such a cathartic experience. However, my internalized oppression and understanding of disability remained unchallenged. It had never occurred to me or to the people around me that disability is a social construction that is continuously shaped by a neoliberal ideology. Self-care had been conceptualized as an individualized process without the integration of social, cultural, and political contexts.

Disability and Helping Relationships

The previous paragraphs show how I experienced internalized ableism. My understanding of disability was further challenged when I began working for charity-based institutions, which made me examine the existing dynamics within the helping relationship that many disabled people experience. The charity model positions disabled people as the helpees on the receiving end. Although the charity model is very well intentioned, it often represents disabled people as victims. The charity model seldom focuses on disabled people's self-determination and self-representation. In training, art therapy students are eager to learn skills to help clients/patients by asking, "What can I do?," "What's my job?," and "How do I serve?" It is a priority to train future therapists to examine their role in the helping relationship; the "I" in each question inevitably draws focus on the position and value of the helper. Helpers do not always recognize the power positions they take on as the givers, as the presumably "normative" people, and as those who have social capital. The savior syndrome instilled in the helpers often places emphasis on the virtue of helping. In *Bodies in Commotion: Disability and Performance*, Sandahl and Auslander (2005) pointed out that the relationship between the non-disabled helper and the disabled helpee is shaped and determined by helpers' internal "moral barometer" (p. 3): how good of a person they are depends on how much they help or save disabled individuals.

The notion that "I gain more than I give when I help disabled people" shows the rewarding experience of helping others. At the same time, it mirrors the individualistic mentality that neoliberal ideology constructs by rewarding people who are able to contribute to others in society. It daunted me that I had been in the position of the helpee as a disabled person in my life; now as I became an art therapist who assumed the power position of a mental health care professional, I asked, "Where do I position myself as a disabled art therapist of color? Why am I drawn to work with disabled clients/patients?" I realized I needed to sort out my own connections to disability as I entered a helping relationship with a fellow disabled person.

Sewing as Storytelling: The Meaning of Sewing and "Repairing"

Storytelling is a thread that connects people. In most cultures, the use of needlework has existed to portray and archive political movements, individual life events, marriages and family trees, life achievements, and social status (Baker, 2016; Boone, 2015). The embellishment of embroidery work shows wealth, taste, and style and reflects the political climate and social values that existed within the time depicted. The pictorial nature of embroidery and quilting composes narratives, such as the *arpilleras*[2] created by Chilean women during Pinochet's dictatorship and Hmong women's creation of story cloths.[3] Sewing provides a physical representation of lineage for people to trace back to their heritage and family of origin. Sewing physically ties human connections.

Sewing has been my way to tell stories. I have been drawn to sewing and craft making since I was a young child. Any kinds of crafting techniques that required fine motor skills—which doctors and occupation therapists worried that I would live without—always attracted me madly and dearly. Perhaps it was the watchful strangers, who nervously monitored the way I manipulated thread and needles, who trained me to be skillful at using my hands efficiently under time pressure. I remember myself as a child, with sharp focus and sweat on my hairline, determined to do well and to achieve perfection in arts and crafts with my hands. Looking back as an adult, I realized that my perfectionism had come from a desire to stop people from intervening and helping me before I even had a chance to try.

Repair is a verb that has torn me apart in different ways. Many of us who live with disabilities and/or illness often are told that we need to be fixed. *Repair* suggests that we are broken to begin with. In undergraduate school, I began exploring sewing as a process to trace and track the history of my bodymind, particularly through the surgical scars between my fingers. In the *Gloves for Two* series (Figures 4.1 & 4.2), I made three sets of gloves for my hands, indicating

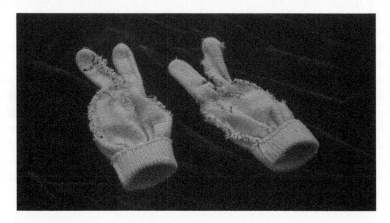

Figure 4.1 Gloves for 2, series 1 (studio documentation photographed in 2001), found object and thread

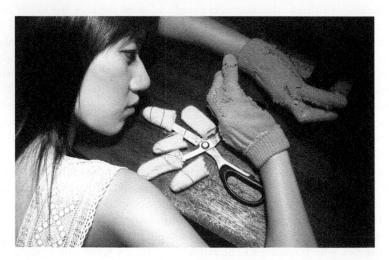

Figure 4.2 Gloves for 2, series 1, 2005, found objects and thread

Source: Photographer: Cheng-Chang Kuo

the three stages I went through as I learned about my experiences of receiving stares from others: rejection of the norm, self-contemplation, and celebration of being different (Yi, 2010). For the purpose of this chapter, I will only discuss the first pair of gloves. I cut the "extra" six digits off of a pair of store-bought gloves, leaving only four to match my two fingers on each hand. I repaired the now-two-fingered gloves with surgical thread, following the actual scars on my fingers. The scars recorded the stitches that I once had from reconstruction surgeries.

The *Gloves for Two* series was made as the result of my frustration with the lack of fashion accessories, including gloves, on the market for me. The process of repairing a pair of "perfect five-fingered gloves" was a defiant gesture against the normative measure of what qualifies as a "full" and "complete" human body. Sewing has become my way to investigate the mixed messages I've received, which are often overloaded with people's emotional responses to my body and to examine how ableism and sexism shape people's understanding about disability. *Repair* began taking another form after I came out as a disabled person. *Repair* now means pairing up with a fellow disabled person and creating disability culture narratives as a collective.

Are Art and Therapy for Self-Care Enough?

The power of "witnessing" in group work helps individuals get a sense of "I am being seen" or "I am not alone" through the energy of group dynamics (Block, Harris, & Laing, 2005). I made art alongside fellow graduate students during my training and with colleagues in professional supervision sessions after graduation. I saw therapists for individual therapy for self-care and terminated therapy after I achieved my treatment goals. My therapists were helpful, but the treatment-focused nature of our therapy sessions together meant that their presence was periodical. I felt that there was always something missing in my self-care routine. At that moment of my life, when I used art as self-care it felt like an individual lonely path, and I was fighting against bias and oppression all alone because my disability was talked about as a singular personal struggle, an adversary story. Later, when I discovered the disability activist community, I realized that what I had been missing was a community of people who share similar disability experiences and who talk about disability from a politicized perspective.

In 2006, I began working in Taiwan as an art therapist. I received a traveling artist grant for collecting stories about children and adults who shared my particular disabilities. I departed for the trip with the mindset of an art therapist who wanted to bring the healing power of art making to my interviewees. When I met them, I realized that they were not interested in making art. They took care of me during my visit. They wanted to know about my stories as someone who was born with an apparent disability, over tea or at the dinner table where homemade meals were served.

As I immersed myself in the disability activist community in Taiwan, I realized that I needed to set the institutional practice aspect of art therapy—contractual therapy relationships between a therapist and a client/patient—aside and relearn the meaning of "care" from my community. I learned that most people in the disability community considered art a luxury, a career path reserved only for people in middle and upper classes. I felt out of place when I made art about my feelings for self-care. This is not to say that art making no longer had value to me. Rather, the reality of Taiwanese culture made me realize that eating and sharing food with disabled people is also the art; strategizing demands and slogans for protests are the craft for creating relationships in disability community. Mending broken wheelchair seat cushions and sleeves torn by pushing manual wheelchairs, dreaming up and sewing sexy lingerie with disabled sisters, and cleaning and decorating mobile devices such as walkers or canes are what connect people.

In 2009, when I left Taiwan and landed in the San Francisco Bay Area to pursue an MFA degree, I began participating in local and national disability rights rallies through ADAPT, a grassroots disability rights organization. I was also involved with Sins Invalid, a disability justice-based performance project with a focus on the experiences of disabled artists who are people of color, queer, and/or trans. On the one hand, the disability rights movement opened my views about fighting for equality: I learned negotiation skills, lobbying strategies, and ways to build community at the frontlines. As single-issue activism, disabled people's independence is portrayed as "we can and we want to be productive members of the society." On the other hand, my participation as an artist-in-residence with Sins Invalid cultured me to see independence as interdependence because disability is not the only identity.

It was then that I began conversing with other disabled people who share mutual passions for arts, activism, and disability culture. A few fellow disabled sisters and I formed a bond through our shared disability and artist identities. I became increasingly interested in their experiences with coming out as disabled, their fashion choices, and how the medical procedures and rehabilitation interventions they had experienced shaped their lives. Self-care began taking place when we hung out with each other over snacks, coffee, or a stroll; we told our stories and found resonance. We were tired of people positioning us as "courageous" artists because of our impairments. We desired critical art critiques based on the merit of our concepts rather than its potential value to encourage others to feel good about their non-disabled status. We exchanged secrets for making ourselves feel pretty not despite our disabilities but because of them. Most importantly, we were seen as having fun in public. As disability studies scholar Petra Kuppers once said at a performance workshop, "[disabled people] having fun in the public is an activism" (Kuppers, 2013). We simply use the presence of our bodymind and state, "we exist, and we are living our lives."

Self-Care With and Within Disability Art Community

My Crip[4] artist sister Sunaura Taylor talked about her experience of getting braces to correct her L-shaped wrists. Her memories of the frustration and pain from the correctional therapy regime invited me to retell my story: the pain, fear, and also humor about getting correctional aids. We explored the connections of sensuality and impairment as we dreamt up fun ideas for prosthetic and assistive aids that would embody an individual's personality and styles. Another Crip artist sister Sadie Wilcox and I processed our experiences of coming out Crip and explored the way we balance our bodies when walking, standing, and sometimes (but rarely) running. As I listened to Sadie share about her burn experience and the surgical procedures that she went through, I was drawn to the suturing processes that she and I had both endured. Together, Sunaura, Sadie, and I accompanied each other and went down the memory lanes where disability culture and the sense of disability identity did not exist to support us when we needed them.

In response, I created *Em-brace*, a set of L-shaped, white plastic braces sculpted with organic contours and stitched with French knots on the top sleeve of the braces (Figures 4.3–4.6, Color Plate 5). The braces were made tailored to Sunaura's wrist curves and angles. Unlike the braces she had to wear as a child, Sunaura expressed how comfortable these braces are as they support her

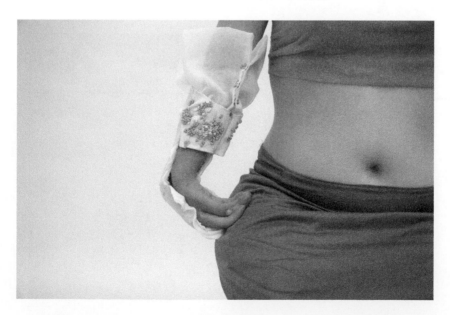

Figure 4.3 Em-Brace, 2011, plastic, embroidery thread, and fabric

Source: Photographer: Louisa Cabot DeLand

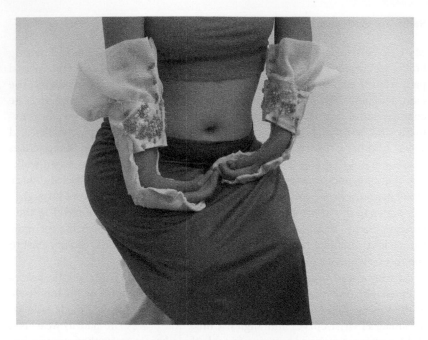

Figure 4.4 Em-Brace, 2011, plastic, embroidery thread, and fabric

Source: Photographer: Louisa Cabot DeLand

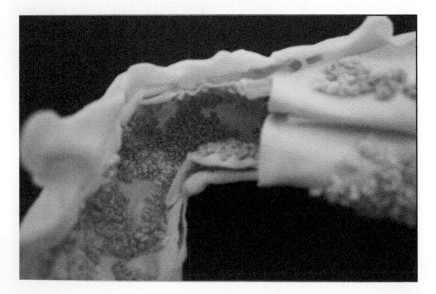

Figure 4.5 Em-Brace, 2011 (detail shot), plastic, embroidery thread, and fabric

Source: Photographer: Louisa Cabot DeLand

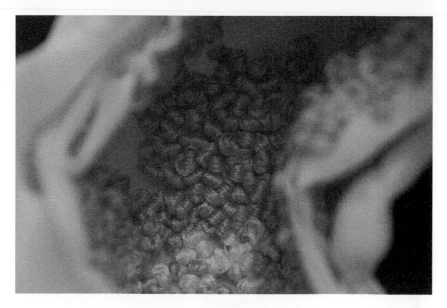

Figure 4.6 Em-Brace, 2011 (detail shot from the side), plastic, embroidery thread, and fabric

Source: Photographer: Louisa Cabot DeLand

in staying in her most natural physical state. People in society often demand to know "what's wrong with you?" when encountering a disabled person; the demand of full disclosure of disabled bodymind narratives shows the viewers' desire to assess the oddity, the disabled. When Sunaura wears the braces, viewers do not get to see the inner linings, which are embellished with French knots. The intricacy and the softness of the inner linings is reserved only for Sunaura. The silky and fine fabric decorated with embroidery holds Sunaura's wrists as if it is crowning disability on our own terms, as we reserve intimacy and joy only for us as Crips.

To create *Dermis Footwear*, I cast the scars on Sadie's legs with latex and created a pair of open-toed boots based on her stories of trauma and her formation of disability identity (Figures 4.7–4.9). I researched the surgical suturing techniques used by surgeons and imitated them as I stitched the latex scar pieces to form the walls of the boots. The boots flare out on the top like layers of flower petals blossoming, which speak to the formation of disability identity. When Sadie tried these boots on for the first time, she looked down and paused a moment, then commented on how the flaring petals look just like when her skin was peeling off during the fire. But this pair of boots now represents a new meaning about the burn experience for her.

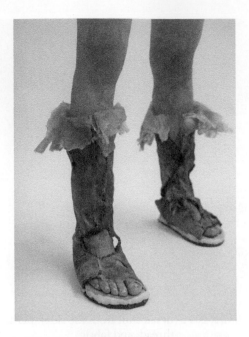

Figure 4.7 *Dermis-Footwear, 2011*, latex, plastic, cast human scar, and thread

Source: Photographer: Louisa Cabot DeLand

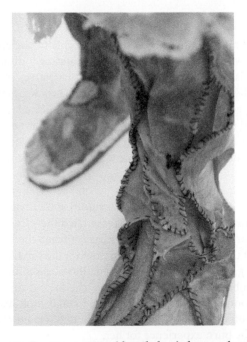

Figure 4.8 *Dermis-Footwear, 2011* (detail shot), latex, plastic, cast human scar, and thread

Source: Photographer: Louisa Cabot DeLand

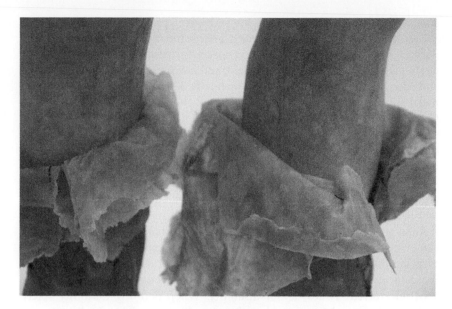

Figure 4.9 Dermis-Footwear, 2011 (detail shot), latex, plastic, cast human scar, and thread

Source: Photographer: Louisa Cabot DeLand

During the process of making these two couture pieces, Sunaura, Sadie, and I each maintained a studio practice as professional artists individually. My studio functioned like a couture shop where I took their measurements. I maintained an element of surprise and only revealed the final designs to them at the last fitting. Our disabled bodymind narratives jointly cultured a liberating and therapeutic experience, which made me feel alive and held by the co-existence of fellow Crips. These two pieces were a part of my MFA thesis exhibition in 2011. Since then, this project has become a pilot project for a Crip Couture manifesto, which I am currently working on for my PhD dissertation in fashion, intimacy, and disability heritage.

Reflection and Discussion

Throughout history, many craft practices have been deeply rooted in documenting domesticity, women's roles in society, and women's resistance (Robertson, 2011; Parker, 2012). Instead of documenting history with a pen or through typing, crafters use repetitive and time-consuming needlework to write and to create history. Crafters are instigators who explore and reveal hidden issues. As a disabled woman artist of color, I have used sewing as a way to trace, document, and create a shared disability family history. The slow stitches of care about disability narratives contrast the high-speed production that capitalistic society demands from all of us. I enacted the suturing process (emblematic of doctors in power) and created holding spaces/garments to house my Crip sisters' bodymind histories. I touched, held, and measured my Crip sisters' bodies and adorned them with art sewn by my hands. Their Crip bodyminds rejuvenated me and answered my desire to be seen and to be touched as well. This Crip haptic intimacy is something that I would not gain from massage or yoga.

What does the experience described earlier bring to my work as an art therapist? In writing about depression, Cvetkovich (2012) critically examined the way in which society positions depression under the domain of medical disease. Cvetkovich analyzed artists' and crafters' fiberwork and argued that mental illnesses, such as depression, should be seen as cultural and social phenomena. She stated: "The goal is to depathologize negative feelings so that they can be seen as a possible resource for political action rather than as its antithesis" (p. 3). Before I was exposed to disability culture and disability activism, self-care had meant a clinicians' skill. It helps increase insights about my clients/patients and counter-transference—my own unresolved "issues" about disability. When defining disability solely within pathological terms, such as "personality issues," "mal-adjustments" (in an ableist world), or "psychological problems," we see "disability" as symptoms, as the targets for elimination that require coping skills and treatments. When self-care is done in connection to disability culture, it reframed my relationship to disability and the meaning of self-care as an art therapist. Sewing, as a metaphor, turns surgical procedure from fixing to archiving our shared body and emotional experiences. Crafting about disability narratives is an action to document and envision disability as social, cultural, and political entities. Self-care is no longer about the individual self, it now means a collective living process, which has the potential to generate Crip coalitions and disability self-representations.

In *You Want to Be Well? Self-Care as a Black Feminist Intervention in Art Therapy*, Tillet and Tillet (2019) pointed to the limitation of feminist art therapy when race is left out of the discussion on gender. The authors discuss Black feminist self-care strategies as advocacy tools for raising critical consciousness, cultivating agents of change in young Black women, and creating community care. To further enrich feminist approaches to art therapy, I would argue that disability must be considered as an identity category alongside race and gender. In disability culture, Mad culture, and Deaf culture, people take on disability, self-claimed madness/psychiatric illness, and being Deaf as identity and pride (as in countering stigma and shame) and create a sense of communal belongingness and cultural affiliation.

Is disability shameful for art therapists to claim? Does the disclosure of disability or illness risk career opportunities for art therapists? As a disabled woman art therapist of color, I rarely encounter fellow art therapists who explore and integrate their own disability, Mad, or Deaf identities in professional practice, let alone how these identities intersect with their race and gender. The absences of these cultural identifications in art therapy are concerning. I once guest lectured on disability culture. A white student with a visual impairment said to me after class, "Disability means nothing," and suggested that his rejection of disability was what had led to his life achievements so far. A non-disabled woman student of color shared, "What if disabled clients end up not socializing and integrating with the rest of us [the non-disabled] because of disability culture?" Was the former comment a reflection of how the current dialogue, training philosophy, and curriculum of art therapy have not addressed art therapists' own intersectional disability experiences? Did the latter comment show the fear of losing control over disabled people as non-disabled therapists?

As art therapists and art therapy educators, we aim to provide "culturally appropriate" services to disabled and ill client/patients and students. When we do not recognize or educate ourselves about the complexity of disability, we often inappropriately see disability from a voyeuristic point of view while we claim to be the experts. Therapists' identity formation is essential to personal and professional development. The absence of disability studies and disability culture orphans disabled art therapists' experiences of learning and working in the field of art therapy. When therapists are disabled and/or ill, their Crip, Mad, and Deaf cultural identities are also critical for them to thrive professionally. When there is no support or care network for disabled art therapists to explore our disability identity and affiliations, the art therapy field not only reinforces the dichotomy and the power dynamics between "us" (non-disabled therapists) versus "them" (disabled patients), it also risks the readiness and quality of disabled art therapists' work. If there is no space for art therapists and graduate students with disabilities to "come out" and cultivate a sense of our own disability/Mad/Deaf belongingness, how can any art therapist be expected to exercise self-care and provide culturally and ethically appropriate support to disabled clients/patients in the future? If disability is only considered as a treatment target that is to be removed, intervened, and helped, doesn't the field of art therapy perpetuate a neoliberal, ableist practice with respect to disabled, ill, Mad, and Deaf art therapists?

The concept of self-care informed by a disability culture perspective can deepen the work both disabled and non-disabled therapists provide to clients. Self-care strategies must exist in relation to collective solidarity for sustainability. As we demystify self-care, we must remind ourselves that our work will be a crafting process: it is personal, communal, relational, and political. As artists, crafters, and art therapists, our job is to facilitate a sense of public intimacy by challenging existing values and boundaries. I recognize that it is not a one-person job to challenge the existing definitions and frameworks of disability in art therapy. I hope that the mission for advocating for fellow disabled art therapy students and practitioners will be a community care effort in the field of art therapy in the near future.

Notes

1. "Supercrip" is a term used by disability rights activists and disability studies scholars. It is defined as the representation of people with disability or illness who conquer their "limitations" by succeeding beyond the societal expectations. This representation is problematic because it focuses on the individual person's willpower to overcome difficulties without examining how the ableist society sets up a negative discourse around disability. Its use of positive language to portray disability, such as "overcoming their disability in spite of being a disabled person," fails to recognize the low societal expectations for disabled people. It also sets up a non-realistic expectation for all disabled people to attain the same level of success without considering each person's access to resources.
2. *Arpilleras* were used in Chile to represent pastoral scenes until Pinochet's regime, when they were then used to surreptitiously document the human rights violations of the regime. They are colorful patchwork cloth pictures depicting life hardship because of hunger, fear, and violence.
3. Hmong story cloths are often stitched with war and village life scenes. They can be seen in clothing and household decorations.
4. Crip, a self-reclaimed identity used by many politicized disabled people, came from the word *cripple*, which was once a derogatory term that non-disabled people gave to disabled people in the past. With knowledge of this piece of disability history, and the influence from fellow disabled artists in the San Francisco Bay Area, I began embracing my "Crip" identity as an artistic choice and style—art with a focus on Crip people's lived experience and narratives as design elements.

References

Baker, H. (2016, September 30). *Why English embroidery is storytelling with needle and thread.* Retrieved from www.ft.com/content/62c7a612-80cd-11e6-8e50-8ec15fb462f4

Block, D., Harris, T., & Laing, S. (2005). Open studio process as a model of social action: A program for at-risk youth. *Art Therapy: Journal of the American Art Therapy Association, 22*(1), 32–38. doi:10.1080/07421656.2005.10129459

Boone, A. (2015, July 5). *Embroidery: Storytelling and excess.* Retrieved from www.thistailoredlife.com/blog/2015/7/4/embroidery-storytelling-and-excess

Clare, E. (1991). The mountain. In *Exile and pride: Disability, queerness, and liberation* (pp. 1–13). Durham: Duke University Press.

Clare, E. (2016, January 19). *Writing a mosaic.* Retrieved from https://eliclare.com/book-news/writing-a-mosaic?

Cvetkovich, A. (2012). *Depression: A public feeling.* Durham, NC: Duke University Press.

Fish, B. J. (2019). Response art in art therapy: Historical and contemporary overview. *Art Therapy: Journal of the American Art Therapy Association, 36*(3), 122–132.

Gipson, L. (2017). Challenging neoliberalism and multicultural love in art therapy. *Art Therapy, 34*(3), 112–117. doi:10.1080/07421656.2017.1353326

Gordon, B. (2018, March 12). *Self-improvement and self-care: Survival tactics of late capitalism.* Retrieved August 19, 2019, from https://socialistrevolution.org/self-improvement-and-self-care-survival-tactics-of-late-capitalism

Henley, D. R. (1992). *Exceptional children, exceptional art: Teaching art to special needs.* Worcester, MA: Davis.

Hinz, L. D. (2019). Perils of the helping professions. In *Beyond self-care for helping professionals: The Expressive Therapies Continuum and the life enrichment model* (pp. 1–9). New York, NY: Routledge.

Kuppers, P. (2013, March). The olimpias: Heart athletes and disability culture presentation, followed by helping dance. *Access living and bodies of work's disability art and culture program.*

Talk presented at Access Living and Bodies of Work's Disability Art and Culture Program, Chicago, IL.

Parker, R. (2012). *The subversive stitch: Embroidery and the making of the feminine*. New York, NY: I. B. Tauris. (Original work published 1984).

Price, M. (2014). The bodymind problem and the possibilities of pain. *Hypatia, 30*(1), 268–284. doi:10.1111/hypa.12127

Robertson, K. (2011). Rebellious doilies and subversive stitches: Writing a craftivist history. In M. E. Buszek (Ed.), *Extra/ordinary: Craft and contemporary art* (pp. 186–203). Durham, NC: Duke University Press.

Sandahl, C., & Auslander, P. (2005). Introduction: Disability studies in commotion with performance studies. In C. Sandahl & P. Auslander (Eds.), *Bodies in commotion: Disability & performance* (pp. 1–12). Ann Arbor, MI: University of Michigan Press.

Siebers, T. (2008). *Disability theory*. Ann Arbor, MI: University of Michigan Press.

Tillet, S., & Tillet, S. (2019). "You want to be well?" Self-care as a black feminist intervention in art therapy. In S. Talwar (Ed.), *Art therapy for social justice: Radical intersections* (pp. 123–143). New York, NY: Routledge.

Ward, L. (2015). Caring for ourselves? Self-care and neoliberalism. In M. Barnes, T. Brannelly, L. Ward, & N. Ward (Eds.), *Ethics of care: Critical advances in international perspective* (pp. 45–56). Bristol, England: Policy Press.

Yi, C. S. (2010). From imperfect to I am perfect: Reclaiming the disabled body through making body adornments in art therapy. In C. H. Moon (Ed.), *Materials and media in art therapy: Critical understandings of diverse artistic vocabularies* (pp. 103–117). New York, NY: Routledge.

Yi, C. (2019). Res(crip)ting art therapy: Disability culture as a social justice intervention. In S. Talwar (Ed.), *Art therapy for social justice: Radical intersections* (pp. 161–177). New York, NY: Routledge.

Young, S. (2014, April). *Transcript of "I'm not your inspiration, thank you very much"*. Retrieved from www.ted.com/talks/stell_young_i_m_not_your_inspiration_thank_you_very_much/transcript?language=en

5

Emptying the Jar
Crochet to Unpack Toxic Racial Stress

MARILYN HOLMES

Introduction

I often joke about racism. Not in a "funny ha-ha" way but in the all too familiar "laughing to keep from crying" way. I find that one must have a sense of humor about the whole thing lest one drive oneself crazy. When I encounter what the literature terms as a "microaggression," an underhanded or even unintentional comment or action that often conveys a prejudiced attitude toward a marginalized person, I used to try to laugh and move on (Constantine, Smith, Redington, & Owens, 2008). I'd never forget, though. While microaggressions may be seen as an innocuous form of racism by some, for those on the receiving end working in higher education, they can lead to anxiety about success, exhaustion, and mistrust amongst colleagues (Cartwright, Washington, & McConnell, 2009). For Black graduate students it's not much better. Black graduate students are often left on shaky ground feeling distant from their peers and greater campus community (Cleveland, 2004; Green, 2016). As a Black student myself I can understand that sentiment.

"I'll just store it in a jar next to my heart and then, one day, I'll die."

I find myself saying that particular phrase, often with a smile and a silly laugh. It's a solid comeback—an explanation for my resistance to engaging in certain conversations. It's also kind of funny. The saying itself is a riff on a joke from John Mulaney's comedy special *The Comeback Kid* that I made my own (Mulaney & Thomas, 2015). "I'll keep all my emotions right here, and then one day, I'll die" (Mulaney & Thomas, 2015). It's a joke I've been making since I watched that special in 2015, but I noticed I began using it more often while studying in my graduate art therapy counseling program. It wasn't until I began doing some intense personal reflection that I understood why the joke doesn't quite land.

I've realized that it's not actually funny, is it? Holding pain so close to your heart. I've had my jar for a while now. Years actually. The lid is bedazzled with rhinestones and all cracks have been sealed with epoxy and duct tape. It's stuffed to the brim with more than a few negative experiences. After taking a detailed inventory, I've realized that most of the experiences are racially charged. Instances of microaggression and outright aggression have filled my jar leaving barely any room for anything else. Having to stay quiet around other—white—students because assertiveness paired with darker skin can be interpreted as aggression is something I've battled my entire academic career (Bryant et al., 2005).

Nevertheless, each new addition to my jar just makes it heavier. Developing a method of self-care that not only staunched the pain but successfully contained and externalized it became paramount to me not only continuing my education but ensuring the well-being of my mental health overall.

Racism in Counseling Education

Having been raised by a mother who worked in higher education, I was warned about the anti-Blackness inherent to academia. Even though I had been prepared, I still felt blindsided when confronted with unintentional racism from my peers and course materials. It wasn't as if I'd never encountered racism. I attended a predominantly white institution in Appalachia post-Trump's election. I'm *familiar* with racism. Encountering microaggressions (and sometimes out and proud aggression) has always been a norm. Fighting the battle not to internalize even unintentional prejudice has never been easy. Nevertheless, in a classroom where I'm exploring my own identity as both person and practitioner, the battle becomes even more difficult.

Part of the Black experience in academia is walking the line between hypervisibility and invisibility (Constantine et al., 2008). The hypervisibility provided by a perceivable difference in race can cause discomfort among other students and contribute to feelings of otherness in Black students (Gipson, 2015). There's an expectation of certain types of characteristics thought to be inherent to Black women: aggressiveness, dominance, extreme overachievement or underachievement, being overly friendly or not friendly at all (Cartwright et al., 2009). Understanding how to navigate predominantly white academic spaces is a skill that takes practice (Louis et al., 2016). Black art therapy students battle racism along several avenues including internships and in the classroom (Hiscox & Calisch, 1998). This method of navigation was a skill I used to have when I wasn't in a counseling program and didn't have to confront others or be confronted on issues of racism as an ethical necessity.

There's an emphasis in counseling education on congruence and genuineness (Jones, 1974; Kolden, Klein, Wang, & Austin, 2011). Being genuinely myself while maintaining my ability to exist safely within a predominantly white space does not always coincide. This raises questions about how much of myself I can share in educational spaces like classrooms and supervision. How much of myself do I share in those settings if I'm expected to be genuine? Is it always safe? Constantly negotiating space or, rather, whether I'm allowed to authentically take up space, is exhausting.

Process for Containing Racialized Stress

Containment Using Crochet

Learning about containers has been a fundamental part of my art therapy education. Symbolic containers, objects like boxes or vessels, can aid counselors by acting as a holding space for complex feelings (Thomas & Morris, 2017). Conversations about containment and compartmentalization have come up in nearly every class and supervision meeting, but I never really put the concept into practice in a healthy way until I had my first practicum experience. I was working with survivors of domestic violence seeking safety in a shelter. It was difficult work. I realized that if I wanted to be effective at my internship, I couldn't carry my own racial burden into my sessions and that tackling my own jar would also allow me to better address and combat my biases. A healthy form of containment became a must.

The question then became "what does containment look like for me?" I tried a number of strategies. I tried creating boxes (too impersonal) and journaling (too risky), but neither fully suited my needs. I tried affirmations and rituals, but it was difficult to find something that felt natural and authentic to me.

I found something that stuck when I learned how to crochet from a friend and mentor. I had always wanted to learn to crochet, and she promised me that dishcloths were easy. She patiently taught me how to make a dishcloth and lent me my first crochet hook until I could get my own set. That weekend, I stayed up all night deciphering a pattern for my first Amigurumi: a misshapen cactus with eyes and a smile. It wasn't pretty, but it was enough. I'd caught the bug. I'd learned to knit years before and had always found the process meditative, but crochet's build-ability appealed to me in an unforeseen way. My knitted work tended to be flat. Scarves and clothing pieces that could be laid out but rolled away so as not to take up space. My crocheted pieces could have a mass my knitted work never could.

Amigurumi are a type of crocheted and/or knitted craft that originated in Japan (Belton, 2006). They're stuffed animals (or zoomorphic items) that are known for their tiny size and sometimes embroidered faces. I fell in love with them because they were cute and compact, and I dreamed about lining my future office desk with them one day. I had no idea how important they would become to me. The most important thing about Amigurumi is that they are typically in one continuous piece rather than flat pieces that are sewn together at the end. Anything placed inside stays inside, insulated from the rest of the world. I carefully documented many new (and some old) negative experiences. My recollections. My feelings. What I wished I had or hadn't said. I wrote it all and carefully stuffed it inside one of my Amigurumi before I sealed it. There, all those thoughts and feelings are protected. Contained.

Jellyfish and Other Animal Symbolism

While watching nature documentaries on Netflix during a self-imposed self-care day, I learned about how toxic a jellyfish sting is. I wondered how something so tiny could potentially paralyze and kill. The conversations about toxicity and venom were always punctuated by one key fact: jellyfish apparently can't sting themselves. These creatures are able to contain venom that can kill a human being in a matter of minutes to hours, and yet they cannot use their own venom to harm themselves. If they could hold something so potentially poisonous, I imagined they could hold my toxins as well.

I found myself exploring other animal symbolism as well. An owl for a situation in which I wished I would have been wiser, slower to anger, and better picked my battles. A conch shell for an incident where I was feeling unheard, almost like I was talking to myself about my concerns, creating an endless echo. I choose animals that I feel connected to or that can teach me something. Sometimes I choose them just for comfort or strength.

Materials

The first jellyfish I created (Figure 5.1) was small enough to be held in one hand and constructed out of scraps of yarn from the art room of my first practicum site. I stuffed it with yarn clippings and polyfil before tucking my recollection of a negative experience inside it. I sealed it with a small chain loop so it could hang somewhere in my room. When it was finished, I squeezed it in my hands and lamented that it felt too light. The polyfil didn't feel protective enough. I felt that a container that would work best for me needed to be sturdy and hold its shape in the face of pressure.

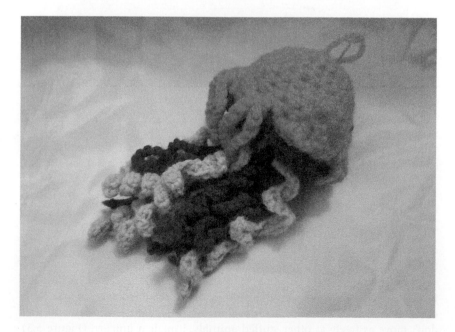

Figure 5.1 Jelly

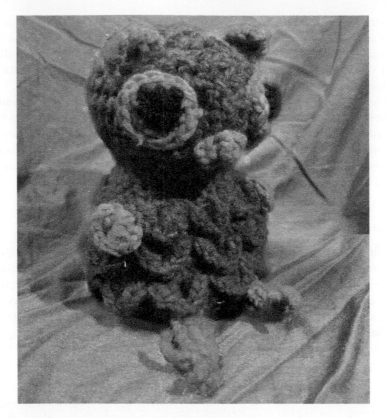

Figure 5.2 Oscar the Owl

After experimenting with other stuffing materials, I settled on 1" × 1" squares of denim cut from old pairs of jeans that I hadn't worn in years. When stuffed into an Amigurumi, the denim holds its shape. It's heavy—a physical weight even in my small projects. My owl (Figure 5.2, Color Plate 6) has been stuffed in boxes and smashed during moves between to two different apartments in six months, yet it has maintained its shape. The message inside has never been harmed. It's durable.

Process of Construction

This concept of durability led me to increase the size of my Amigurumi and construct them in more than one piece. An Amigurumi constructed in more than once piece can hold more than one recollection. Additionally, with more space for denim, it can become even more durable. The Amigurumi I make have the appearance of a standard stuffed animal, but when lifted one can note their excessive weight and stiffness. They become more like statues. Monuments that don't move as freely as other stuffed animals. I made a unicorn (Figure 5.3)

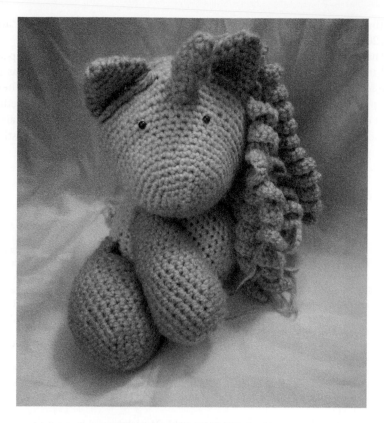

Figure 5.3 Tripod the Unicorn

from a cake of yarn I bought myself. It's made in soft neutrals that evoke a sense of calm in me. I didn't plan where the colors in the cake would land and let the yarn switch through tones organically. My unicorn is constructed in five separate pieces, each holding onto a toxic memory of a microaggression and my response to it. Right now he only has three legs. Even though I hope I never have to add a fourth, I know it's inevitable.

Conclusion

This process led me to develop a method of specified self-care in order to unpack my own issues regarding my responses to microaggressions. The facts are, as it stands right now, the world doesn't seem inclined to change. Racism is always going to be a fact of my life, and I have to find a way to deal with my experiences. In order to become the clinician that I want to be, self-care is a must. Developing good habits while still in school can only help me as I continue my journey from student to professional (Dorociak, Rupert, & Zahniser, 2017).

There are experiences I'm still trying to unpack. After all, my jar is deep and well-used (think Hermione's bag from Harry Potter), and if crochet was the cure to racism, I think someone would have found it well before me. There's still quite a bit to empty, but it's a comfort to know that I have one more method to set down the load if needed. There's a place where my pain can be contained but not forgotten. Respected but dampened. Where I don't have to keep stinging myself.

References

Belton, M., (2006). Zombies and robots and bears: Oh my! *Craft: Transforming Traditional Crafts*, *1*, 41–44.

Bryant, R. M., Coker, A. D., Durodoye, B. A., McCollum, V. J., Pack-Brown, S. P., Constantine, M. G., & O'Bryant, B. J. (2005). Having our say: African American women, diversity, and counseling. *Journal of Counseling & Development, 83*, 313–319.

Cartwright, B. Y., Washington, R. D., & McConnell, L. R. (2009). Examining racial microaggressions in rehabilitation counselor education. *Journal of Rehabilitation Education, 23*(2), 171–182.

Cleveland, D. (Ed.). (2004). *A long way to go: Conversations about race by African American faculty and graduate students*. New York, NY: Peter Lang Inc.

Constantine, M. G., Smith, L., Redington, R. M., & Owens, D. (2008). Racial microaggressions against black counseling and counseling psychology faculty: A central challenge in the multicultural counseling movement. *Journal of Counseling & Development, 86*(3), 348–355.

Dorociak, K. E., Rupert, P. A., & Zahniser, E. (2017). Work life, well-being, and self-care across the professional lifespan of psychologists. *Professional Psychology: Research and Practice, 48*(6), 429–437.

Gipson, L. R. (2015). Is cultural competence enough? Deepening social justice pedagogy in art therapy. *Art Therapy, 32*(3), 142–145. doi:10.1080/07421656.2015.1060835

Green, A. (2016). The cost of balancing academia and racism. *The Atlantic*. Retrieved from www.theatlantic.com/education/archive/2016/01/balancing-academia-racism/424887/

Hiscox, A., & Calisch, A. (Eds.). (1998). *Tapestry of cultural issues in art therapy* (1st ed.). Philadelphia, PA: Jessica Kingsley Publishers.

Jones, L. K. (1974). Toward more adequate selection criteria: Correlates of empathy, genuineness, and respect. *Counselor Education and Supervision, 14*(1), 13–21.

Kolden, G. G., Klein, M. H., Wang, C., & Austin, S. B. (2011). Congruence/genuineness. *Psychotherapy, 48*(1), 65–71. doi:10.1037/a0022064

Louis, D. A., Rawls, G. J., Jackson-Smith, D., Chambers, G. A., Phillips, L. L., & Louis, S. L. (2016). Listening to our voices: Experiences of black faculty at predominantly white research universities with microaggression. *Journal of Black Studies, 47*(5), 454–474.

Mulaney, J. (Writer), & Thomas, R. (Director). (2015). John Mulaney: The Comeback Kid [Netflix comedy special]. In *John Mulaney: The Comeback Kid*. Chicago, IL: Netflix.

Thomas, D., & Morris, M. (2017). Creative counselor self-care. *VISTAS Online*, Article 17. Retrieved from www.counseling.org/docs/default-source/vistas/creative-counselor-self-care.pdf

II
Craft as Culturally Resonant and Accessible

II

Craft as Culturally Resonant and Accessible

6

Embroidering Pieces of Place

ELIZA S. HOMER

Introduction

Some of my earliest memories of art making include needlecrafts. I recall the colorful embroidery sampler kits my grandmother gifted me each birthday and Christmas and our shared love of needlepoint. Years later, I intuitively incorporated hand sewing into my art therapy practice, knowing the rhythmic shared experience with a child abuse survivor would be soothing for her during a stressful period (Homer, 2015). The motivation for the study I describe in this chapter (Homer, 2019) began in 2005 when I was an exchange student in Morelia, Michoacán. My coursework immersed me in the culture of Mexico and provided me with a foundational understanding of the traditional stories and art of the region. I quickly became fascinated with the abundance of artistic expression. I learned that arts in Mexico have been a vehicle for the promotion of political and social causes, created for the masses, that the majority could understand (Vanina Celis, 2017). Whether illiterate or educated, Spanish-speakers or speakers of Indigenous languages, art became the platform for communicating revolutionary thought across cultures and socioeconomic status (Vanina Celis, 2017). However, despite the rich heritage of artistic communication within Mexican culture, this history does not seem to be reflected in the mental health services in Michoacán.

To explore current mental health concepts in Michoacán, I solicited support from Anayuli Torres Molina, a P'urhépecha psychologist trained in Western modalities (psychoanalysis) who works within the rural communities. When I asked if it had been difficult to combine her tools in psychoanalysis with the beliefs of the community, Torres Molina (personal communication, February 8, 2017) explained that the community accepted her by placing her within the construct of *curandero* (folk healer), specifically the *sukuami*, who heals both physical and emotional ailments and presides over ceremonies. She admitted that many of her clients ask for a ritual, such as taking water into the mouth and expelling it to remove a malady. She summarized, "'Ay, you are [a sukuami], ' . . . when are you going to remove the bad?'" When I suggested that art might serve as the ritual, a bridge between modernity and tradition, Torres Molina replied:

> That's something really interesting . . . and, at the same time, very noble, very beautiful, because to think about it [*artesenía*] in this way is another perspective that not only has to do with wanting to know but also wanting to know to be able to offer something.

Because creative expression has been used in many educational and therapeutic settings as a means to construct meaning and identity, prevent emotional and behavioral problems, increase self-esteem, and foster mutual respect, I began thinking about what Torres Molina expressed along with my own experiences, and I began to wonder about potential uses of traditional craft—*artesanía*—and if art making might support well-being. The art process, *tela bordada*, embroidered story cloths (see Figure 6.1, Color Plate 7), chosen for my study is but one of more than 30 types of traditional craft practiced by rural and Indigenous (known as P'urhépecha or Tarascan) artisans in the region surrounding Morelia, Michoacán. Specialized Tarascan handicrafts encompass a broad range of materials and techniques, including pottery, wood, textiles, toys and miniatures, metalwork, wax, plumage, leather, and glass, and each community produces a signature style that is recognizable by collectors. *Tela bordada*, which features embroidered scenes of daily life and ceremony in rural P'urhépecha communities, was selected for the study because of my own textile heritage and prior experience with utilizing needlecraft in treatment (Homer, 2015). Additionally, the scenes most directly present a narrative with materials that are easily accessible and portable (financially, materially, geographically, emotionally, and/or linguistically) and supported culturally responsive ethics through the inclusion of "traditions, rituals, ways of life, and customs" (Lahman, Geist, Rodriguez, Graglia, & DeRoche, 2010, p. 5).

Textiles: Stories Written in Thread

Throughout history and across cultures, fabric and needlework have been symbolic means to identify ethnic group and social status, as well as a vehicle for storytelling. During the late 18th and early 19th century, women in North America used needlework as historians and to have a voice; far more women were accustomed to using needles than pens to address values (Davis, 1998; Hunt-Hurst, 2004; Witzling, 2009). *Arpilleras*, story cloths, of Chile were smuggled out of the country to expose the atrocities under the dictatorship of Pinochet (Cohen, 2013; Garlock, 2016). Hmong story cloths depicted suffering and severe reprisals as a result of alliances during the Vietnam War; the cloths communicated a "social construct of memory" that "share[d] the intended affective mood" (Peterson, 1988, p. 14).

In Mexico, Zapatista women of Chiapas wove "a plurality of color organized as one beautiful tapestry" as a testament to the diversity of the region (Pellarolo, 2006, para. 35). In the Lake Patzcuaro Region of Michoacán, *tela bordada* originally drew on themes from ancient mythology and have evolved to depict events and rites of passage (Damon, 2016; Stein, 2015); the artisans of Santa Cruz shifted from replicating pre-Hispanic symbols to bringing folk traditions and rural experiences to life and in that process began to share with the world the importance of their work. As Berta Servin Barriga, a Santa Cruz master artisan, put it, "We must preserve and broadcast human values and support the diffusion and culture of folk art" (personal communication, January 12, 2017). As another artisan noted, "For many of the women, whose husbands went north to the States to find work, embroidery became 'a type of therapy'" (Fraser, n.d., Sanabria: embroidery, para. 2).

These histories suggest that the materials and techniques of *tela bordada* and other crafts are inextricably tied to the artisans' identities and traditions. However, in my research I found no evidence that narrative story cloths had been used in healing ceremonies for this population. I began to wonder if art making in this way could serve as a kind of ritual, a bridge between modernity and tradition. Could traditional story and artisan craft be used to build on familiar processes, much like a curandero or Indigenous healer uses ritual and traditional practices for physical healing? Could this create a link between *artesanía* and well-being, increasing cultural connection and creating a bridge between folk healing and Western mental health treatment, with the potential of increasing engagement in services?

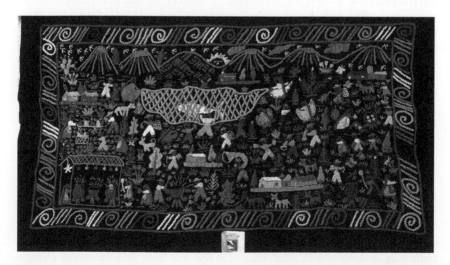

Figure 6.1 Tela bordada depicting community life by Berta Servín Barriga, approx. 29" × 17.5", embroidery on cotton

Until recently, scarce research had been compiled regarding the use of fiber arts in art therapy, and the majority of information published was not authored by art therapists but by others interested in the healing potential of these media (Cohen, 2013; Collier, 2012; Reynolds, 2004; Pellarolo, 2006; Pöllänen, 2015). Cohen (2013) and Garlock (2016) reported on their use of story cloths with female survivors of gender-based violence. They found that the graphic narratives created on fabric, embellished with simple embroidery and appliqué techniques, gave voice to traumas that had been difficult for the artists to verbalize. Processes that enriched the experiences of the participants were identified, including the social acceptability of coming together for art making as a stigma-reducing activity (Anderson & Gold, 1998). Rhythmic, repetitive motion (Cohen, 2013; Garlock, 2016; Homer, 2015) and bilateral stimulation to regulate hyperarousal (Garlock, 2016) are also integral to hand-sewing techniques.

Places in Time

To explore the potential of *tela bordada*, I conducted arts-based research, which focused on using narrative artwork within the context of place to interrogate the experience of place through engagement in traditional *tela bordada* among rural and urban university students in Michoacán (Homer, 2017, 2019). To ground myself in the technique, I personally engaged in the art making and interviewed local artisans to inform my experience with local ways of knowing (Homer, 2017). This allowed me to begin to form a framework for investigating the potential of using this technique by others (Homer, 2019) in relation to perceptions of identity, based on the concept that memories are formed in association with place and the notion that identity forms in relation to place, which has been called *place identity* (physical, social, and affective; Barwin, Shawande, Crighton, & Veronis, 2015).

Additionally, an exploration of the product and the process of embroidering highlighted a theme of time, specifically a slowing of time. Explaining a foundation for the contemplative practice of textile art making based on *Slow* Theory, Wellesley-Smith (2015) traced an underpinning of "sustainability, simplicity, reflection and multicultural textile traditions" (p. 6) and wrote of "a cultural revolution against the notion that faster is always better" (p. 12). Slow aims for quality over quantity and favors the journey over the destination, process over product—connection and reflection (Wellesley-Smith, 2015). Slow is not just about speed, it is about mindfully engaging in self-reflection, self-examination, self-monitoring, and shutting out external distractions to be alone in one's own thoughts with the aim of finding or creating meaning (Honoré, 2004). Slow embraces making use of what resources are available and promotes change (Lipson, 2012). Slow encourages looking at the how, what, why, and where of the work a person does, in relation to selves and others (Lipson, 2012).

As artist-researcher, I was slowed down by a cultural construct of time. This slowing-down process allowed me to be transported back in time through place memories. I felt hemmed in, constricted, by the leisurely rhythm of embroidering. This measured pace was simultaneously beneficial and detrimental. With each stitch, slow and deliberate, it was as if time itself slowed so that I had to sit with the images and recollections that were emerging, processing each detail as I pierced the cloth. Quieting the outside world, hours felt like they passed in an instant, yet the figures appeared on the scene at an unhurried pace; I found myself longing for them to move on. As a researcher and a therapist, I saw the potential for this technique to contribute to my sense of place and identity and overall sense of well-being. The lengthy progression of creating story scenes gave me time and forced me to sit with the images, contemplating what elements would be included, what elements needed to be voiced—the absence and the shadows amid idyllic landscapes.

Identity, Wellness, and Storytelling in Central Mexico

My interviews with local artisans and a mental health provider (Homer, 2017) provided insights on the role of *artesenía* in the community of Santa Cruz, Michoacán, with the aim of understanding, leading to the development of specific ways in which *artesenía* can potentially be used in art therapy to increase engagement in mental health services and to enhance psychotherapy goals in Mexico and communities with similar folk art traditions. Artisan Servín Barriga (personal communication, January 12, 2017) reported barriers to all health services with no community-based access in most rural areas, which underscored a benefit of utilizing local resources and materials. I identified six general themes from the interviews: well-being; identity; gender issues; expectations; Indigenous beliefs, fatalism, and the will of God; and the origins and role of folk art. In addition, themes of well-being, identity, gender issues, expectations, and experiences of place and time were also found within my phenomenological experience of art making and journaling. After completing my pieces (see Figures 6.2 and 6.3), I looked for overlaps, if any, between my experience and the themes expressed by the other participants and looked back to the literature. Through knowledge gleaned from my personal experience, I saw the potential for this technique, but would my experience be transferable? Would others have similar experiences?

The research design strove to honor place-based identities and traditions embedded in the culture. Professors Aguirre Ochoa and Barbosa Muñoz (2013) explored local sociocultural constructs and asserted, "In the case of Mexico and especially of Michoacán, a large cultural and historical tradition has existed based on the regulation of social relationships, social circumstances, and informal relations, which are not governed by law but by custom" (p. 557). Taking into consideration a concern about how to make my work accessible (financially, materially, geographically, emotionally, and linguistically) and how to empower the participants to honor their own intuition and knowledge, the design incorporated Indigenous theory that included storytelling, to honor the oral and artisanal traditions (Kovach, 2012; Wulff, 2010). I hoped to validate traditional folk art as a possible bridge between "modern" Western therapy practices and traditional healing, *curandismo*.

I searched literature on identity, wellness, views of illness, fiber arts, and storytelling, as these concepts relate to the population of Central Mexico. To provide context within the physical place where the research was conducted, the concepts of identity within rural populations of Michoacán, Mexico, were explored, which are in a state of flux due to economic pressures and modernization. Researchers White, Umaña-Taylor, Knight, and Zelders (2011) posited that identity strength was linked to academic achievement, self-esteem, and mental health among Mexican American youth. In Michoacán, a clash between modernity and tradition often results in identity crisis (Spears-Rico, 2015; A. Torres Molina, personal communication, February 8, 2017), and throughout Mexico, folk artists experience the contradiction of simultaneously being touted as national symbols while living in extreme poverty with poor quality of life (Novelo, 2002). Additionally, artisans in Michoacán create works to satisfy not their community but the retail public at large, such as tourists, relying on consumers who are not P'urhépecha to meet their economic needs (Garrido Izaguirre, 2015; B. Servín Barriga, personal communication, January 12, 2017).

In Mexico, *curandismo* encompasses treatment for maladies in domains of material, spiritual, and mental health (Garcia, 1998); suffering has cultural meaning (Garro, 2000); and physical health is tied to social ills (Rodriguez, 2012). Personal narratives become illness narratives related to somatic experiences in response to social or cultural tensions (Taggart, 2015). Other researchers have found that traditional societies such as those found in Mexico regard art as an element of life and do "not separate healing from art or religion" (Dufrene & Coleman, 1994, p. 145). Some of these researchers concluded that place (as in, regional, national, and/or geographical affiliation) provides context of culture in relation to self, others, and the environment and leads to identity formation (Barwin et al., 2015). Barwin et al. (2015) categorized three layers or modes of place: physical (location), social (locale, which comes with preconceptions of how it is used), and affective (sense-of-place subjective view that impacts how a person feels about or connects with a place).

Barkin and Barón (2005) recommended methods that strengthen and defend the traditions of rural Mexicans. Botha (2011) suggested mixing conventional qualitative methods with "uniquely indigenous ways of producing and holding knowledge, such as through alternative modes of consciousness, traditional relationships, and local practices" (p. 316). Stories shape how individuals react to life events. Individual, family, community, and national identities are shaped by stories, which through time become traditions (Mehl-Madrona, 2005).

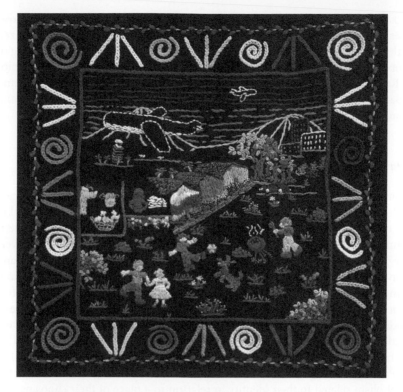

Figure 6.2 Eliza S. Homer, *California*, approx. 8 ½" × 8 ½", embroidery on cotton

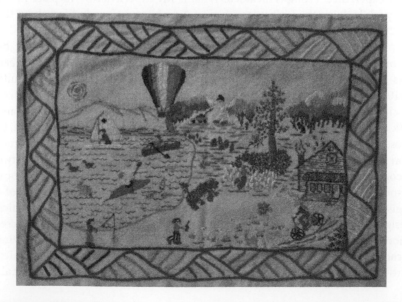

Figure 6.3 Eliza S. Homer, *Connecticut*, approx. 10" × 14", embroidery on cotton

Narrative therapy was built on the theory that individuals compose narratives about themselves and their experiences. These stories are contextualized within the perceptions of culture, which may lead to subconscious retelling of problematic or negative plots, causing the person to become "stuck" (Shapiro & Ross, 2002). Narrative therapy strives to assist individuals to identify and separate themselves from the problem, rename the issue, and externalize and re-author the story.

Tela Bordada as a Tool for Culturally Responsive Art Therapy

In order to explore the experience of engagement in *tela bordada* in Michoacán, with particular attention to what role, if any, the place of the scene depicted in the narratives has on associated memories and what meaningful way place is connected with identity formation, I recruited 13 participants from two university programs (Universidad Intercultural Indígena de Michoacán [UIIM] and Universidad Latina de América [UNLA]). UIIM is located in Pichátaro, a rural community in the P'urhépecha region of Michoacán and offers tuition-free education; UNLA is a private university located in the city of Morelia and has a student body from urban, affluent families. The eight UIIM participants were predominantly Indigenous (87.5%), and the majority (80%) of the five UNLA participants identified as Mestizo (mixed Indigenous and European decent).

Participants engaged in embroidering a narrative story cloth that depicted symbolism related to their identity in relation to a place of their choosing and wrote a reflection of their experience during and/or at the end of each of the 12 two-hour sessions in response to prompts to capture emotional expressions of their experience. Prompts included: What is my experience of the place in my story while doing this? What story/voice(s) do I hear? How do I feel about the process today?

Arts-based research includes data gathering through an art medium; by incorporating oral and folk art traditions, a symbiotic relationship between arts-based research and Indigenous theory is created (Kovach, 2012; Wulff, 2010). In this mutuality, "Respect is the foundation for all relationships" (Neel, as cited in Archibald, 2008, p. 23). Along these lines, I incorporated oral and folk art traditions by inviting Servín Barriga, an artisan and key informant, to present the history of the *tela bordada* technique and assist with art instruction during the first session. Selecting an instructor from one of the two recognized *tela bordada* collectives provided economic support, utilized local resources, honored the artisans, and minimized the risk of appropriation of a registered patrimonial craft by allowing the artisans to place limits on which design elements and techniques would be shared and by focusing on the creation of individual rather than community narratives. The choice of utilizing locally sourced materials and processes supported culturally responsive ethics, through inclusion of "traditions, rituals, ways of life, and customs" (Lahman et al.,

2010, p. 5). Additionally, instruction that used teachers who are part of the P'urhépecha community helped dispel the notion that traditional knowledge is of lesser value than so-called conventional learning (Vargas Garduño, Méndez Puga, Flores Manzano, & González Taipa, 2012). Data from participants' journals and artwork were analyzed through multiple processes to honor both Western and Indigenous ways of knowing. The final session included a debriefing of emerging themes and member checking to provide the opportunity for participants to rewrite any themes that did not harmonize with their experience.

Additionally, I engaged in artistic response before beginning data collection and during data analysis in addition to observational field notes, to explore personal processes and ways to disseminate the outcomes and/or empower the participants. I participated in two traditional backstrap weaving, *telar de cintura*, workshops to gain an understanding of ways of knowing in P'urhépecha artisan communities, which provided context for my observations during the sessions and metaphor for the process of data analysis. Weaving provided a lens by which I honored the storytelling process and traditional mores as guiding principles.

I chose a mixed-methods, arts-based, phenomenological approach for my study, using art making and reflective journaling, wherein art making was utilized during data collection (embroidered story cloths) and analysis (weaving) with the inclusion of a quantitative exploration of the possible role of ethnic identity using the Multigroup Ethnic Identity Measure (Esteban Guitart, 2010; Phinney & Ong, 2007). The organizing of individual threads and the act of weaving individual stories, interconnecting the warp (vertical threads) and weft (horizontal threads), metaphorically created a cloth with recurring patterns. Across groups, concepts related to affect regulation (e.g., becoming relaxed), connection to the group and social supports, increasing ego strength (e.g., expressions of accomplishment when gaining mastery with the technique), and meaning making through symbolism and color were evident. Another notion that emerged was the ability for reframing of the narratives from a negative to positive experience. Within the UNLA group, frustration tolerance and individual identity were prominent, whereas the UIIM group expressed an expanded sense of identity that included self, group, and community situated in place. Additionally, the UIIM group voiced their pleasure with the novel experience of creating space and time for self.

These expressions also appear to support the notion that engagement in *tela bordada* contributes to increased well-being. Based on the constructs of *well-being* in Mexico (e.g., Spears-Rico, 2015; Taggart, 2015)—namely happiness and social harmony—and *wellness* or health as holistic with components of physical, social/familial, and land connections, I looked for evidence in the spontaneous written reflections (in Spanish, one word, *bienestar*, translates as both wellness and well-being). Abundant data supported this theme, including declarations of physical sensations (e.g., relief from headache and stomach ache, increased relaxation and calmness, and stress reduction), affective-happiness experiences (e.g., laughter, hope, ability to understand and express feelings, freedom of expression, and resilience), social-familial experiences (e.g., connection with ancestors, family, group members, and community), and land connections (e.g., place-based memories, community stories, and agriculture).

Although all of the narratives and associated artwork depicted elements of place, the majority (77%) focused on an experience situated in place. For example, in the narratives the participants wrote of sensations of being transported in time and location to the associated memory. Almost half (46%) of the participants made explicit connections between identity and place. For the UIIM group, this was expressed in terms of gender roles within Indigenous communities, identification with place and gods of origin, and artisan traditions (see Figures 6.4 and 6.5), whereas the UNLA participants included symbolic representations of a place of personal growth (e.g., a river, personal space with favorite things, or a ropes course; see Figures 6.6–6.8). Although 61.5% named prior experience with needlework, none had worked with the specific technique of *tela bordada*, and they had previously only engaged in structured stitches (e.g., cross stitch) with designs originated by others. More than half (53%) of the participants had previously crafted using artisan techniques (e.g., feather work, textiles, embroidery, and clothing). An objective review of the narratives appeared to indicate that prior experience with embroidery did not have significant impact. Additionally, an exploration of symbolic elements evident in the researcher's narratives (see Figures 6.2 and 6.3) and the participants' artwork revealed cross-cultural commonalities and differences.

UIIM participants connected personal symbols directly to strong collective traditional identities. Francisco began with deities, Curicaueri the Sun and Nana Huare the Moon, creators of the Nahuatzen community (see Figure 6.5). Patricia depicted a central hummingbird icon reminiscent of the Mesoamerican god Huitzilopochtli (hummingbird of the left) often equated with the P'urépecha god Tzintzuuquixu (hummingbird of the south) who were credited with guiding their peoples to their homelands (see Figure 6.11). Rosa honored the significance of women in the community represented by feminine floral symbols (see Figure 6.4). In contrast with the communal identities expressed by the UIIM group, modern graphics were prominent expressions of individual identity for the UNLA participants. Alejandra's imagery lacked human and animal forms, instead featuring a basketball, a heart, and a river (see Figure 6.6). Margarita substituted a family system with a singular person and a stylized humanoid (see Figures 6.9 and 6.10). Veronica supplanted human connection with books and a pet (see Figure 6.7). The distinction between rural and urban, modernity and tradition, appeared juxtaposed in the narratives.

Consistent with my experience, issues related to place and time were evident with the participants. Three of the five UNLA participants and all of the UIIM participants situated their depicted memories in place, the context of which suggested affirmation of place as a key construct in identity development. Statements correlated to time included references to the present (e.g., time constraints for completing the project, the passing of time, etc.), the past (e.g., memories), and the future (e.g., plans to continue the practice of embroidery).

With a reported sense of being transported to the place and time of the memory, the participants and researcher alike evoked generational cross-cultural connections to needlecraft, reliving moments when mothers and grandmothers sat and stitched. The personal accounts recorded by the participants supported the benefits of intentionally making space for self-exploration and creating accessible places for that exploration. Some expressed that the project provided the first experience in which they had made time for self and had the ability "to tell *my* story" and to capture and embody their feelings.

Furthermore, although psychologist Torres Molina identified identity disorders as one of three major issues encountered in her private practice in rural Michoacán, the dysfunction stemmed from mixed identity anxiety. Mixed identity anxiety (dichotomy between racialized identities of Indio versus Mestizo) results from the struggle between past and present, tradition and modernization, rather than ethnicity itself, as P'urhépecha balance the drive to "preserv[e] their communities' intimacy and 'control' how they are perceived, consumed, and toured" (Spears-Rico, 2015, p. 1). Torres Molina, who identifies

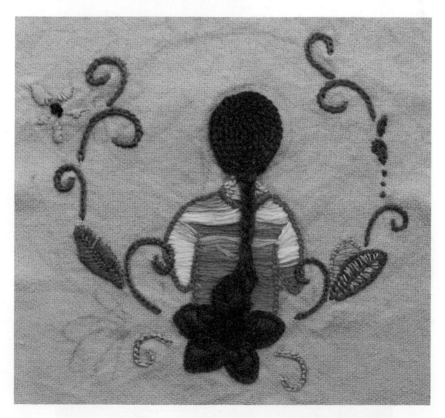

Figure 6.4 "Woman," Incomplete, approx. 10" × 10", embroidery on cotton

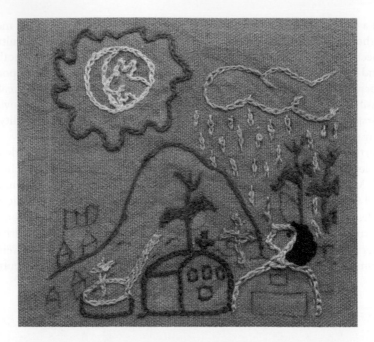

Figure 6.5 "The origin of the community Nahuatzen," Incomplete, approx. 10" × 10", embroidery on cotton

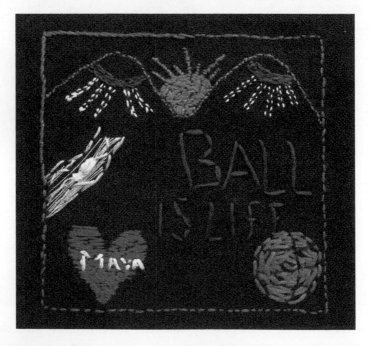

Figure 6.6 "The Essence of My Being," Final, approx. 10" × 10", embroidery on cotton

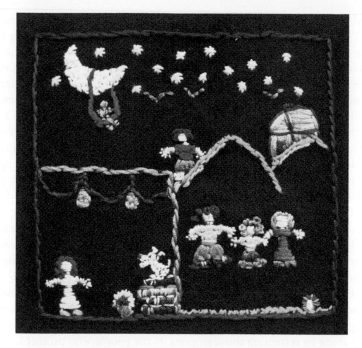

Figure 6.7 "Security and My Fears," Final, approx. 10" × 10", embroidery on cotton

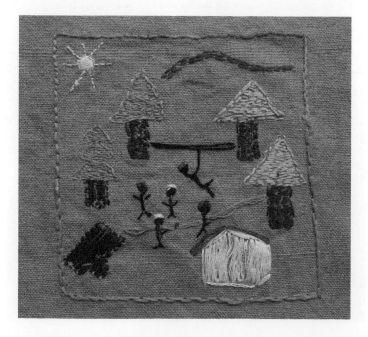

Figure 6.8 "Ropes Course," Final, approx. 10" × 10", embroidery on cotton

as P'urhépecha, explained the struggles with mixed identity, stating, "They say to me I'm not P'urhépecha. I'm neither here nor there and I suffer being in the middle of this, I don't know what it is. . . . It hurts me when they tell me 'you, yes, you are,' and it hurts me when they say 'you are not'" (personal communication, February 8, 2017). With the recognition that these identity crises are not based on U.S. criteria of ethnicity, a consideration of alternative measures of baseline indicators of psychological adjustment are warranted, such as ego strength or the House-Tree-Person elements instinctively portrayed by the participants, in conjunction with interpretation of the images by a mental health professional from the community. These measures might provide more appropriate indicators of an individual's level of adjustment associated with life stages and identity development, ranging from mixed-identity to bicultural identity (minority-traditional and mainstream-modern culture; Gfellner, 2016).

Narrative therapy strives to assist individuals to identify and separate themselves from the problem, rename the issue, and externalize and re-author the story. In the process of art making, evidence of identifying problems and re-authoring was implicitly and explicitly recorded by participants in my study. Patricia discovered her need to be in control. Francisco began with an externalized Indigenous story and identity, then embraced a new identity of "artisan" (see Figure 6.5). Veronica faced her initial personification of fears and made new meaning by reframing those persons as the people who protect her from

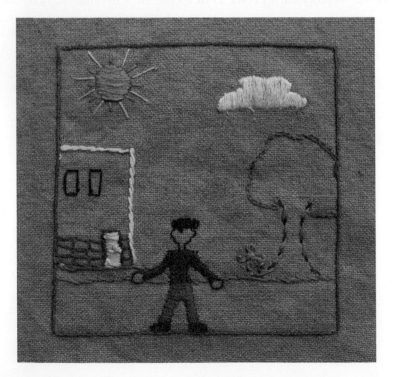

Figure 6.9 "A Future Spring," Final, approx. 10" × 10", embroidery on cotton

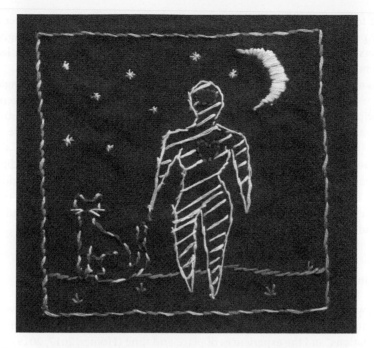

Figure 6.10 "Night Soul," Final, approx. 10" × 10", embroidery on cotton

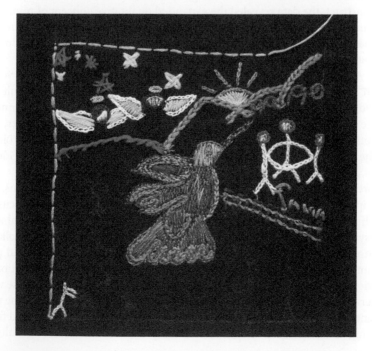

Figure 6.11 "Flying with life," Incomplete, approx. 10" × 10", embroidery on cotton

those fears (see Figure 6.7). Margarita found that her interpretations became more positive (see Figures 6.9 and 6.10). In each case, the narrative changed in process with the art making, rather than in isolation with the emotion-laden content of the stories.

As anticipated as the artist-researcher, a white woman from New England (Homer, 2017) and from the standpoint of the Mestizo-Campesino-Indigenous participants from Michoacán (Homer, 2019), a relationship with traditional craft materialized as a stimulus for memories, which implied that these processes can potentially be incorporated into art therapy practice in these communities in Central Mexico and in other communities with art traditions to enhance cultural connection and increase well-being. The textiles provided a means for colonized peoples to maintain Indigenous identities; the P'urhépecha artisans preserved pre-Hispanic symbolism through stories, dances, and folk art traditions.

Conclusion

Employing *tela bordada* in art narratives with Central Mexican university students surfaced key concepts—namely, well-being, identity, gender issues, expectations, and the experiences of place and time (Homer, 2017, 2019). Both the product and the process highlighted a theme of time, specifically a slowing of time. However, rather than limiting the meaning of "slow" to its quantitative construct, the data revealed the expanded qualitative concept of mindfully engaging in self-reflection, self-examination, self-monitoring, and shutting out external distractions to be alone in one's own thoughts with the aim of finding or creating meaning (Honoré, 2004).

As Aden et al. (2009) wrote, "Any single story/place holds multiple voices within it" (p. 316). The historical connection to needlecraft across cultures opened the way for culturally appropriate interactions, simultaneously connecting me and the participants in my study with ancestors, places, memories, and each other; the media became the vehicle to another time and place, embroidering the scene, weaving the cloth, transported in sensory imaginings (Gómez Flores, 2006).

Furthermore, although my research did not have a therapeutic focus, the participants articulated improved wellness and a novel experience with focusing on self to solicit emotional expression, which implies a potential for enhancing psychotherapeutic goals in Mexico and communities with similar folk art traditions. The commonality of experiences by myself as researcher and participants from urban and rural communities suggests that the incorporation of traditional crafts, such as needlework, crosses cultural boundaries for use with Western and non-Western populations. As noted in the experiences of the participants and myself, the memories and associated emotions that emerged from engaging in embroidery demonstrated the potential for increasing cultural connection by using a local craft—not as a didactic tool but as a pathway to self-expression and emotional content. Likewise, the participants endorsed the benefits of intentionally making space for self-exploration and the need for creating accessible places for that exploration. From this perspective, "slow" therapy using locally sourced materials and methods, such as artisan craft and emphasizing relationship, hope, and intention, may be a viable alternative to Western, formulaic, brief solution-focused approaches.

The specific locality of the art making and the limited number of participants may hinder generalization; however, building on the reported potential for healing through the combination of art and storytelling reported in the literature, there is support for using traditional craft, including *tela bordada*, as a culturally appropriate art therapy tool. It is my hope that other art therapists will be inspired by the potential of using traditional arts, whether *tela bordada* and other folk arts, dance, storytelling, or music, to open understanding of local, *natural* ways of knowing.

References

Aden, R. C., Han, M. W., Norander, S., Pfahl, M. E., Pollack, T. P., Jr., & Young, S. L. (2009). Re-collection: A proposal for refining the study of collective memory and its places. *Communication Theory, 19*(3), 311–336. doi:10.1111/j.1468-2885.2009.01345.x

Aguirre Ochoa, J. I., & Barbosa Muñoz, P. (2013). Violent subcultures and crime in Mexico. *Journal of Alternative Perspectives in the Social Sciences, 5*(3), 551–572.

Anderson, L., & Gold, K. (1998). Creative connections. *Women & Therapy, 21*(4), 15–36. doi:10.1300/J015v21n04_02

Archibald, J. (2008). *Indigenous storywork: Educating the mind, body, and spirit.* Vancouver, BC: UBC Press.

Barkin, D., & Barón, L. (2005). Constructing alternatives to globalisation: Strengthening tradition through innovation. *Development in Practice, 15*(2), 175–185.

Barwin, L., Shawande, M., Crighton, E., & Veronis, L. (2015). Methods-in-place: "Art voice" as a locally and culturally relevant method to study traditional medicine programs in Manitoulin Island, Ontario, Canada. *International Journal of Qualitative Methods, 14*(5), 1–11. doi:10.1177/1609406915611527

Botha, L. (2011). Mixing methods as a process towards Indigenous methodologies. *International Journal of Social Research Methodology, 14*(4), 313–325. https://doi.org/10.1080/13645579.2010.516644

Cohen, R. A. (2013). Common threads: A recovery programme for survivors of gender based violence. *Intervention 2013, 11*(2), 157–168.

Collier, A. F. (2012). *Using textile arts and handcrafts in therapy with women: Weaving lives back together.* Philadelphia, PA: Jessica Kingsley

Damon, A. (2016, March 29). *Mexican story cloths: Hand embroidery is still alive in Michoacán, Mexico.* Zinnia Folk Arts. Retrieved from http://zinniafolkarts.com/blogs/news/94798593 mexicanstoryclothshandembroideryisstillaliveinmichoacanmexico.

Davis, O. (1998). The rhetoric of quilts: Creating identity in African-American children's literature. *African American Review, 32*(1), 67.

Dufrene, P. M., & Coleman, V. D. (1994). Art and healing for Native American Indians. *Journal of Multicultural Counseling & Development, 22*(3), 145–152.

Esteban Guitart, M. (2010). Propiedades psicométricas y estructura factorial de la Escala de Identidad Étnica Multigrupo en español (MEIM) [Psychometric properties and factorial structure of the Spanish Multigroup Ethnic Identity Measure (MEIM)]. *Revista Latinoamericana de Psicología, 42*(3), 405–412. Retrieved October 16, 2017, from www.scielo.org.co/scielo. php?script=sci_arttext&pid=S0120-05342010000300005&lng=en&tlng=es.

Fraser, L. (n.d.). *Can a colonial crafts town survive modern Mexico?* [Web log post]. Retrieved from http://craftsmanship.net/can-a-colonial-crafts-town-survive-modern-mexico/

Garcia, C. C. (1998). *Diagnostic reasoning in traditional Mexican and Mexican-American folk medicine* (Master's thesis). Gonzaga University, Spokane, Washington. Available from ProQuest Dissertations and Theses Database. (UMI No. 304473702).

Garlock, L. R. (2016). Stories in the cloth: Art therapy and narrative textiles. *Art Therapy: Journal of the American Art Therapy Association, 33*(2), 58–66.

Garrido Izaguirre, E. M. (2015). *"Donde el diablo mete la cola": Estética indígena en un pueblo purepecha (México) ["Where the devil puts his tail": Indigenous aesthetic in a Purepecha village (Mexico)]* (Ph.D.). Universidad Complutense de Madrid, Madrid, Spain.

Garro, L. C. (2000). Cultural meaning, explanations of illness, and the development of comparative frameworks. *Ethnology, 39*(4), 305–334.

Gfellner, B. M. (2016). Ego strengths, racial/ethnic identity, and well-being among North American Indian/First Nations adolescents. *American Indian & Alaska Native Mental Health Research: The Journal of the National Center, 23*(3), 87–116. https://doi-org.ezproxyles.flo. org/10.5820/aian.2303.2016.87

Gómez Flores, C. J. (2006). *Bordados para ser contados* [Embroidered to be told]. Monterrey, Mexico: Mundo Sustenable A. C.

Homer, E. S. (2015). Piece work: Fabric collage as a neurodevelopmental approach to trauma treatment. *Art Therapy: Journal of the American Art Therapy Association, 32*(1), 20–26.

Homer, E. S. (2017). *Pieces of place: Finding meaning through the material and process of artisanal craft in Central Mexico* (Unpublished doctoral pilot study). Lesley University, Cambridge, MA.

Homer, E. S. (2019). *Pieces of place: Finding meaning through the material and process of artisanal craft in Central Mexico* (Doctoral dissertation). Lesley University, Cambridge, Massachusetts. Available from ProQuest Dissertations and Theses Database.

Honoré, C. (2004). *In praise of slowness: Challenging the cult of speed.* New York, NY: HarperOne.

Hunt-Hurst, P. (2004). Georgia history in pictures. *Georgia Historical Quarterly, 88*(4), 530–544.

Kovach, M. (2012). *Indigenous methodologies: Characteristics, conversations, and contexts.* Buffalo, NY: University of Toronto Press.

Lahman, M. K. E., Geist, M., Rodriguez, K. L., Graglia, P., & DeRoche, K. (2010). Culturally responsive relational reflexive ethics in research: The three Rs. *Quality and Quantity, OnlineFirst.* doi:10.1007/s11135-010-9347-3

Lipson, E. (2012). *The slow cloth manifesto: An alternative to the politics of production.* Textile Society of America Symposium Proceedings, 711. Retrieved from http://digitalcommons.unl. edu/tsaconf/711

Mehl-Madrona, L. (2005). *Coyote wisdom.* Rochester, VT: Bear & Company.

Novelo, V. (2002). Ser indio, artista y artesano en Mexico [To be indian, artist and artisan in Mexico]. *Espiral: Estudios sobre Estado y Sociadad, 9*(25), 165–178.

Pellarolo, S. (2006, March). *Zapatista women: A revolutionary process within a revolution.* Keynote speech presented at the International Women's Day event, California State University, Los Angeles, CA. Retrieved from www.inmotionmagazine.com/auto/sp_zw.html

Peterson, S. (1988). Translating experience and the reading of a story cloth. *The Journal of American Folklore, 101*(399), 6–22. doi:1. Retrieved from www.jstor.org/stable/540246

Phinney, J. S., & Ong, A. D. (2007). Conceptualization and measurement of ethnic identity: Current status and future directions. *Journal of Counseling Psychology, 54*(3), 271–281. doi:10.1037/0022–0167.54.3.271

Pöllänen, S. (2015). Elements of crafts that enhance well-being. *Journal of Leisure Research, 47*(1), 58–78.

Reynolds, F. (2004). Textile art promoting well-being in long-term illness: Some general and specific influences. *Journal of Occupational Science, 11*(2), 58–67.

Rodriguez, T. L. (2012). *Transnational quests for healing: Curanderismo in the South Texas Borderlands* (Publication No. 3525716) (Doctoral dissertation). The University of Wisconsin, Madison, Wisconsin. ProQuest Dissertations Publishing.

Shapiro, J., & Ross, V. (2002). Applications of narrative theory and therapy to the practice of family medicine. *Family Medicine, 34*(2), 96–100.

Spears-Rico, G. (2015). *Consuming the Native other: Mestiza/o melancholia and the performance of indigeneity in Michoacán* (Ph.D.). UC Berkeley, UC Berkeley Electronic Theses and Dissertations. Retrieved from http://escholarship.org/uc/item/16p2s3tn

Stein, P. (2015, April 10). *Embroidery from Lake Patzcuaro* [Web log post]. Retrieved from http://mexicobyhand.blogspot.com/2009/07/embroidery-from-lake-patzcuaro.html

Taggart, J. M. (2015). Native American oral narratives in Mexico and Guatemala. *Delaware Review of Latin American Studies, 15*(3). Retrieved from www.udel.edu/LAS/Vol15-3Taggart.html

Vanina Celis, S. (2017, September 11). El Taller de Gráfica Popular: 80 años de arte y revolucionario y popular en México [The people's graphic workshop: 80 years of revolutionary and popular art]. *Másdemx: Laboratorio de Conciencia Digital.* Retrieved from http://masdemx.com/2017/09/taller-de-grafica-popular-grabado-arte-revolucion-mexico-arte-revolucionario/

Vargas Garduño, M., Méndez Puga, A. M., Flores Manzano, N. D., & González Taipa, R. (2012). Training of P'urépecha elementary school teachers in interculturality. *Intercultural Communication Studies, 21*(1), 117–130.

Wellesley-Smith, C. (2015). *Slow stitch: Mindful and contemplative textile art.* London, England: Batsford.

White, R. M. B., Umaña-Taylor, A. J., Knight, G. P., & Zelders, K. H. (2011). Language measurement equivalence of the ethnic identity scale with Mexican American early adolescents. *Journal of Early Adolescence, 31*(6), 817–852. doi:10.1177/0272431610376246

Witzling, M. (2009). Quilt language: Towards a poetics of quilting. *Women's History Review, 18*(4), 619–637.

Wulff, D. (2010). Unquestioned answers: A review of research is ceremony: Indigenous research methods. *The Qualitative Report, 15*(5), 1290–1295.

7

Healing Roots of Indigenous Crafts
Adapting Traditions of India for Art Therapy Practice

KRUPA JHAVERI

Spirit and matter converse quietly
Ancestors whisper behind each gesture.
Hands, heart and body reassembling
Ancient patterns repeat alive with new eyes.
Movements carrying invisible codes
Breathing into visible awareness.

Identity and Perspective

The unusual circumstances of being born to Gujarati (North Indian) parents in the heart of North America paved the way for me to follow an unexpected path in life, both personally and professionally. Traditional art forms appeared sporadically throughout my upbringing, inciting curiosity through immersive rituals and experiences passed on from my mother and grandmothers. Facing confusion, discrimination, and acculturation in Colorado allowed me to question, consider, and later to be catapulted into a reconnection with my distanced Indian heritage. Beyond a career in the product-oriented world of graphic design, studying art therapy awakened a fascination with the innate cross-cultural phenomenon of creative processes developed in order to cope, express, and heal. In 2009, I followed an inner calling to return to my ethnic roots and survey potential applications of art therapy in Asia, eventually settling in Auroville, South India. As an international art therapist with a decade of grassroots experience in India, my multifaceted identity offers a unique viewpoint and context for the weaving together of ways of being and creating presented in the pages that follow.

The field of art therapy is currently experiencing growing pains in response to the calls for diverse voices to help decolonize the field internationally. One pathway to embody this change is by being open to ancient holistic wisdom such as the practical, positive, and universal approach of Indian psychology (Rao, Paranjpe, & Dalal, 2008). The prolific philosopher Sri Aurobindo Ghose, born in Calcutta and educated in England and India, synthesized Indian and Western thought at the turn of the 20th century to develop a spiritual path called Integral Yoga, unifying physical, mental, and emotional levels of awareness for a collective evolution (Ghose, 1999). He explained that "yoga is nothing but practical psychology" and has universal relevance in all aspects of living with awareness, impacting relationships from self into community and the world (Ghose, 1999, p. 44). By focusing on sensory and bodily experiences (physical), cognitive functioning and processing (mental), subjective sensitivity and responses (emotional), all as parts of a greater whole (spiritual), one can develop a culturally sensitive foundation for understanding and honoring ancient Indian art forms. This multidimensional yet interconnected framework of integral evaluation offers concrete direction on how to meaningfully bridge tradition into the modern context. Applying this framework within art therapy can serve to widen the access, relevance, and scope of global expressive and therapeutic work.

Craft is changing, along with ritual and tradition, all rapidly losing value in a modern globalized and technology-based world (Tyabji, 1999). In India, the core symbolism and metaphor within creative practices are being lost to commodification while maintaining a "stigma of inferiority and backwardness" (Tyabji, 1999, p. 115). Historian and philosopher of Indian art Coomaraswamy (1975) summarized that there are two major directions in Indian art, "the one inspired by the technical achievement of the modern West, the other by the spiritual idealism of the East" (para. 58). As craft is often valued superficially as functional and marketable product, it is judged for external, aesthetic, and technical beauty and therefore disconnected from the depth, story, and meaning it can also carry. Art therapy requires an initiation into accepting and honoring art as a process—sometimes chaotic, unfinished—and as a deeper reflection of our inner state, with the purpose of supporting our resilience (Malchiodi, 2020). As art is an ancient and underlying way of life in India, this cultural foundation has great potential to include common indigenous practices within art therapy, such as mehndi (natural temporary tattoos) and kolam (rice flour drawings). By understanding the cultural context of a traditional art form and studying the integral impact and essence of the practice through the physical, mental, emotional, and spiritual levels, traditional crafts can be sensitively adapted within art therapy practice to help restore relationships to our common, indigenous and healing roots.

Mehndi

Mehndi (also known as henna) is a plant that grows mostly in Asia, the Middle East, and Africa and has been used as a dye for hair, textiles, leather, and body decoration for centuries (Moazzam, 2014). The indigenous geography of the plant combined with historic isolation and exchange across cultures has led to varied mehndi traditions, uniting a wide range of religions including Christians, Jews, Muslims, and Hindus (Cartwright-Jones, 2006). Traditionally, the leaves are dried and ground into a paste and used to stain and adorn the hands and feet of a bride on the night before her marriage. Today festivals like Diwali, births, birthdays, and other rites of passage often include mehndi, with hired female artists adorning a circle of intergenerational women. Particularly in Asia, mehndi artists are often marginalized women otherwise restricted from independent work outside of their homes but are empowered by successful businesses through this niche art skill.

Upon asking such a mehndi artist what the patterns symbolize, she generally will not know but admits remaining loyal to specific designs she has copied and practiced to learn. There are visible connections to nature, to adornment and celebration of the feminine, as well as hidden images related to the union of husband and wife. When arranged marriages were more popular, it was an icebreaker game for the husband to find his name or initials in the mehndi designs on his wife's skin on their wedding night (Narayan, 2016). In the modern context, the symbolism within this tradition is lost to trendy global appropriation, even with common and dangerous allergic reactions resulting from hazardous chemicals added to darken the stain (Cartwright-Jones, 2006). Reconnecting to the essence of this practice by studying the integral impact of the art form (Table 7.1) informs the adaptation of it within therapeutic context.

When facilitating long-term group art therapy sessions with local youth in South India, one of my first considerations was to explore directives that reflected local cultural preferences, by attuning to the needs and capacities of my clients (Kristel, 2013). Initial interactions with this receptive mixed gender group helped establish the goal

Table 7.1 Integral Evaluation of Mehndi for Art Therapy

Physical Level	• natural medium from leaves of a plant
	• scent of eucalyptus and essential oils
	• cold, wet paste dries and stains skin
	• ingredients produce a cooling effect
	• design remains on body for up to two weeks
Mental Level	• concentration
	• fine motor skills
	• sense of mastery with new medium
	• imagination, symbolization
Emotional Level	• empowerment/sense of agency
	• grounding, calming effect while drawing
	• body awareness from sensations to memories
	• self-compassion and self-care
	• opportunity to transform/adorn scars and injuries
	• frustration tolerance and patience
	• non-attachment
Spiritual Level	• cross-cultural origin in a pre-wedding bridal ceremony
	• connected to rites of passage, celebration of body and spirit
	• communal experience of ancient body decoration ritual
	• deepened relationship to self, creativity, and nature

of original self-expression and empowerment in a non-judgmental space, differentiated from the usual copy-paste style of learning limited to stereotypic images. Trust in this cross-cultural therapeutic relationship was developed through rituals, including guided visualizations to reduce fear around art making and to discover a personally meaningful symbol to include within this adapted practice of mehndi. The youth first sketched these visualized images within hand tracings and later applied the designs with embellishments on themselves with natural mehndi cones in an atmosphere of noticeably silent concentration (Figure 7.1, Color Plate 8). Finally, the group chose partners and continued playful decoration on each other's bodies, building peer connection and empathy through the art to help address issues of bullying. Their sharing felt like a ceremonial celebration of diverse expressions unified by a group experience of drawing on their bodies together within a safe space. Encouraging the development and integration of personal symbols invited the youth to engage with the medium through a revitalized connection to their own culture.

In various cross-cultural and international settings over the last decade and through my personal practice and exploration of mehndi, I have found that this adapted process can serve as a tool for self-care for parents, teachers, helping professionals, in women's circles, and others looking to balance giving and receiving in their lives. It can support transition in the termination process by remaining for up to two weeks and is an opportunity to explore redefining scars and injuries on the body (Figure 7.2). There are layered benefits, considerations, and potential themes when working with mehndi, which, supported by an integral evaluation approach (Table 7.1), can be matched to appropriate and receptive populations according to their goals and needs.

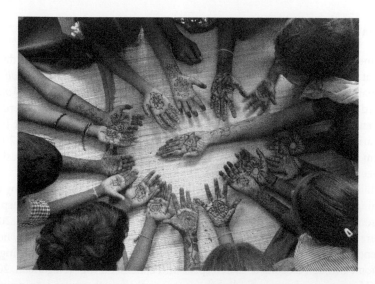

Figure 7.1 Mehndi art therapy process at Thamarai Center, Edyanchavadi Village, Tamil Nadu, India

Source: Photo: Krupa Jhaveri, 2012

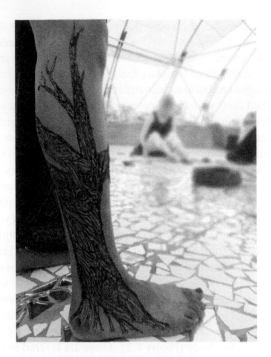

Figure 7.2 Mehndi art therapy process at Sankalpa Art Center, Auroville, Tamil Nadu, India

Source: Artwork, body and photo: Krupa Jhaveri, 2016

Kolam

Ground drawings are a traditional art form throughout India and Asia, dating back at least 2,000 years (Gode, 1947). In North India they are called *rangoli* and are mainly drawn for special occasions; in South India they are called *kolam*, a word that implies beauty, form, and play in the Tamil language, where the women practice every day (Nagarajan, 2005). Other names throughout India for variations of this tradition include *alpana* and *aripana* (Nagarajan, 2005). Kolam is an ancient Hindu ritual for creating sacred space at the threshold between home and the outside world (Nagarajan, 2019).

Millions of Indian women carry out this tradition daily before sunrise, by first cleaning and preparing the earth in front of their homes with water, sweeping, and sometimes also laying down a turmeric and cow dung base (Nagarajan, 2005) (Figure 7.3). This symbolic purification clears away the previous day and any negative energies, and the following ritual is a way to bring protection and blessings to the home through creating a "sacred space and ephemeral rug" (Nagarajan, 2005, p. 5). Many women begin by finding the center on their earth canvas, leaning into a kinesthetic balancing of mind and heart as the body becomes a pendulum (Figure 7.4) and then applying a series of dots and lines using a combination of rice flour and stone powder pinched and rolled through their fingers (Gitadelila, 2018).

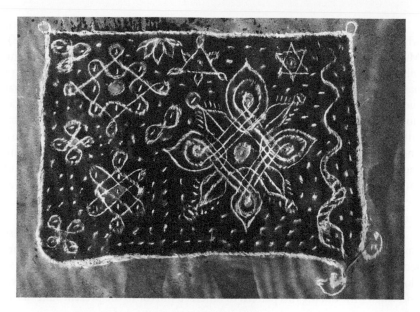

Figure 7.3 Kolam exploration on cow dung canvas with rice flour and turmeric, during Kolam Yoga training with Grace Gitadelila in Douceur, Auroville, India

Source: Photo: Krupa Jhaveri, 2016

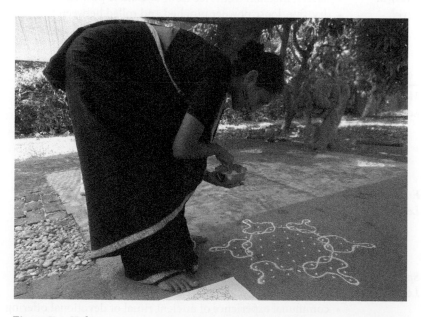

Figure 7.4 Kolam posture, in Kolam Yoga training with Grace Gitadelila in Douceur, Auroville, India

Source: Photo: Krupa Jhaveri, 2016

The knowledge of kolam is generally passed from mother to daughter, often when the daughter is between the ages of 6–12 years old (Gitadelila, 2018). Much of this metaphor, meaning, and symbolism is now lost, including the inherent wisdom of the designs, which hold a veritable syllabus for life. When I have asked various Indian women about the meaning of kolam, many reply that they simply do not know, yet express the tension of societal and family obligation with traditions, amongst feelings of pride, comparison, and competition with others. Today synthetic colors and shortcuts including stickers, stamps, and stencils speak to a growing disinterest and fewer young women learning the tradition (Nagarajan, 2005). By evaluating the integral levels of benefit and impact within this traditional art form, through individual and group experiences, I have explored the potential applications of this practice within art therapy (Table 7.2).

One example of the many layers of meaning and how the kolam process can function therapeutically is illustrated in Figure 7.5, which includes the varied process of creating the traditional *hridayam kamalam* kolam, translating as "lotus of the heart" (Gitadelila, 2018). In my experience creating this pattern and when introducing this pattern to others, a mirror to the present state of the

Table 7.2 Integral Evaluation of Kolam for Art Therapy

Physical Level	• natural medium from rice flour and stone powder • dry, fine, loose powder pinched and rolled between fingers • kinesthetic awareness of body as pendulum • drawing on the earth in front of home • grounding, balancing • ephemeral design on earth
Mental Level	• fine motor skills • concentration and memory • repetition and self-discipline • spatial, mathematic, and scientific learning • creativity and sense of mastery with new medium • imagination, symbolization
Emotional Level	• frustration tolerance and patience • empowerment/sense of agency • increased awareness of connection to body and earth • development of ritual, growth • clearing away negativity from the past, non-attachment
Spiritual Level	• protection and blessings for home • connection to cycles, shapes, elements of nature • communal experience of ancient ritual of devotional offering • acceptance and celebration of impermanence

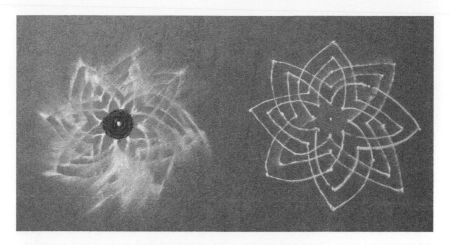

Figure 7.5 *Hridayam Kamalam* kolam, in Kolam Yoga training with Grace
Gitadelila in Douceur, Auroville, India

Source: Photo: Krupa Jhaveri, 2017

artist creating the design can be revealed through several facets: the patience to
lay out this design at any scale, the impulse to fix or change, the spaces and balance between the dots and lines, the dance of a surprisingly asymmetrical code
which reveals a symmetrically open design, the weaving across at all angles,
and the unconscious mistakes and slips of the hand. Every day the same pattern will appear differently when created by the same person, reflecting some
new insights through the details of the intuitive process. The rich, layered, and
deep reflection allows a space for self-awareness and growth on multiple levels
(Figure 7.5).

With the globalizing post-colonial complexity of Indian culture turning
toward consumerism, traditions like kolam are taken for granted and slowly
disappearing. In a community-based effort to revive and restore the significance of traditional art forms while supporting cross-cultural learning, a group
of graduate students from the School of Visual Arts (NYC) visited and collaborated with my organization Sankalpa in Auroville in 2015 for an intensive
credit course on multicultural issues within art therapy. Local Tamil women
were paired with the students to teach and share their traditional art practices
including mendhi, kolam, creating flower garlands, embroidery, and mandalas with flowers and seeds. The students engaged with curiosity and empathy,
empowering the women by reflecting the value in the rich "strengths and skills"
of their culture (Philip, 2015). The exchange prompted open discussion of
themes including hierarchy, power, privilege, poverty, disability, agency, biases,
and how to work in an adaptive culturally sensitive manner. Extensive thought
and preparation preceded the choices to focus on the needs and goals of the

local women practicing these traditions, including the seat of power remaining within the hands of the women holding these traditions within their culture, instead of the cross-cultural norm of visiting trainees imposing directives on locals. The context and application of each art form needs thoughtful consideration, as explored in more detail later.

Cultural Considerations

The implications of cultural appropriation, appreciation, and adaptation are part of a range of ethical considerations in any form of indigenous and/or cross-cultural art therapy practice, which requires research on the origin of each art form included. With little discussion on the topic of cultural appropriation in the field of art therapy, there is a widespread issue of stealing concepts (e.g. the mandala) from colonized cultures for commodified recipes and oversimplified use without context, reference, or credit to the true origin and ancient philosophy embodied in the art form. Many traditional crafts such as mehndi and kolam are under-documented beyond the designs involved, living mainly in oral and lived history by individuals and communities and requiring initial diligent research into the roots and essence of each tradition to respectfully avoid superficial exploitation, exoticization, or appropriation. When incorporating culturally referenced art forms into directives, there is a responsibility for the art therapist to both thoughtfully introduce the context, history, and background of a tradition and carefully consider the application and relevance of a traditional craft for a particular individual or group and their needs.

For those curious to try mehndi or kolam within sessions, knowing why and how this could be appropriate depends on the cultural identity of the therapist, the client(s), and the context of the therapeutic work. Whether these media are incorporated into art therapy sessions or not, the first step is a thorough personal exploration and research of the medium, fostering informed choices based on therapeutic goals and intentions instead of a superficial interest. Ideally, it is important for an art therapist to have direct contact with an individual practicing the art form in the context of its cultural origin to advise, give permission, and be credited for the respectful use of the tool. To avoid blatant appropriation, the historical and cultural background must be included with use of a culture-specific art form. In order to choose the media needed to meet the goals of a client or group, it's essential to know the language of "expression and containment, destruction and creation, control and spontaneity" in the materials (Moon, 2002, p. 60). To remain informed and sensitive, art therapists can engage in personal research, experience, and evaluation into the physical, mental, emotional, and spiritual impacts of the craft and how this can inform relevant, ethical applications and adaptations from a space of cultural appreciation. Art therapist and yogi Michael Franklin (2001) has explored thoroughly how yogic mindfulness is inseparable from the path of embodying these principles as an artist and art therapist, linking the mysterious ways to "verbalize the sacred" between all of these worlds (p. 103). As a therapist, the challenge and responsibility is authentic embodiment—staying aware of body, mind, heart and spirit within ourselves in order to offer balanced and all-encompassing spaces in which our clients can grow.

My own reconnection to the deep history, significance, and potential of each tradition is the basis for the ongoing cross-cultural work I dare to do internationally in an effort to revive, restore, and remember this disappearing knowledge through cultural adaptation of craft within art therapy. A unifying reverence for life in India involves adorning the body, marking the threshold of the home, and expressing oneself multidimensionally with intention, symbolism, and awareness that informs the culturally sensitive practice of art therapy here. My hope is that inspired art therapists will globally join this effort to responsibly and carefully look back into the marginalized, undervalued, and misunderstood traditions within the communities in which we work in order to inform a more equitable, restorative, and harmonious future for our field and the exponential benefit of all.

Restoring Meaning and Integration

Ethologist Dissanayake (1988) asserted that art, play, and ritual are individual and social functions of "making special" or an elaboration of the functional into aesthetic enjoyment, which promotes well-being and belonging. Traditional art forms like mehndi and kolam illustrate the interconnectedness of human and devotional relationships, reflecting an ancient indigenous philosophy, which can be consciously adapted and updated to be understood in our current shared reality. "The traditions of the past are very great in their own place, in the past, but I do not see why we should merely repeat them and go no farther," wrote Ghose (1999, p. 323). By studying the context and history of a tradition, we can begin to fathom the holistic benefits it offered as creative coping skills amidst the adversity of daily life. By understanding what each medium evokes within us individually, collectively, and universally, we can approach ways to adapt tradition into the context of contemporary therapeutic work.

On the physical and mental levels, crafts with an ancient tradition are refined skills and require practice to cross the perceived limits of capacity into meaning. Through the repetition of these practices, a deeper encounter allows an emotional exploration of metaphor, ritual, personal and collective symbolism, possibilities for greater self-awareness, and transformation of patterns both in the art and behaviors in life. In the examples of mehndi and kolam, a guided meditation and time to explore the patterns on paper in preparation often help to ease anxiety and support the transition in learning a new medium. Spiritually, the return to meditative skills allows us to integrate the cumulative physical, mental, and emotional benefits of these crafts, as a self-soothing relationship to our own art, to our communities, and to nature in a holistic and balanced way.

As part of a colonized system of thought, the handmade and imperfect quality of many crafts results in them being classified as primitive and therefore inferior (Dascal, 2009). These diminished crafts are in fact infinitely valuable as an honest and visible spiritual practice, mirroring both inner and outer nature. Ancient practices in many indigenous cultures employed materials creatively and thoughtfully sourced from nature, helping practitioners to stay grounded, humble, and aware of and in harmony with a wider wisdom. Through the use of nature-based materials, the movement of eco-art therapy similarly reconnects us to ritual for both individual and social balance through interconnection to our communities and the world (Speert, 2016). Within our current man-made ecological crisis, nature-based expressive arts therapy also returns us to an eco-centric perspective informed by and effectively reviving traditional indigenous practices around the world (Atkins & Snyder, 2018). As we contemplate the future of humanity and knowing where we come from, what we are part of, and how we are living out of balance with the natural world surrounding us, it seems imperative that we return to these roots for collective healing. Psychology—meaning "study of the soul"—somehow largely misses the vastness of health and well-being in relationship to nature as 40,000 years of indigenous people have researched, lived, and created based on this knowing (Farrelly-Hansen, 2001).

Kalmanowitz, Potash, and Chan (2012) clarified that "Eastern traditions point to holistic health by reminding us that separation is contrived and that all aspects of life influence each other" (p. 40). A revolution in neuroscience and trauma-informed care is revealing the limitations of contemporary psychology and medicine, as growing research demonstrates the inseparable links between mind, body, and health (van der Kolk, 2015). With the support of the integral approach for adapting traditional Indian art forms into art therapy, unlocking the four levels of awareness helps reassemble a more holistic image of self, in which art making is the key to our visible and externalized consciousness in nature. With consideration of the past, present, and potential future of these traditional art forms, I offer these experiments in embodying conscious and creative therapeutic tools that retain their deeper holistic significance to the field. The question now is, how can others sensitively adapt such traditions for use within art therapy? As art therapists motivated with integrity, can researching and reconnecting to our own personal creative lineages empower us, and can we in turn also access and provide similar possibilities for our clients? How we can collaborate to further explore examples of decolonizing art therapy through the power of craft around the world?

A beloved teacher, mentor, and collaborator in the realm of combining art therapy and yoga, Hari Kirin Khalsa (personal communication, June 20, 2019) shared in an interview, "ritual is a doorway to noticing that you are in sacred space." Many crafts throughout time and cultures carry this access to the sacred, the imaginal, the universal, the spiritual, and to a deeper understanding as part of a more holistic sense of well-being. Further research and bridging of these traditional crafts into art therapy in my cross-cultural work also includes affirmation dolls, embroidery, individual and group mandalas, mask-making, and basketry, among others.

Coomaraswamy (1975) suggested, "every real pattern has a long ancestry and a story to tell. For those that can read its language, even the most strictly decorative art has complex and symbolical associations that enhance a thousandfold the significance of its expression" (para. 46). As art therapists, I trust we can move beyond rigid colonized perspectives to retrieve the underrepresented creative traditions traced within our own lineages and the lineages of our clients and their communities. My current work includes documenting how indigenous art forms can reveal the links between ritual and resilience, allowing us to fathom, externalize, and heal intergenerational trauma. If we understand our holistic identities beyond this lifetime through the arts carried in our heritage, we can be empowered to adapt these crafts into tools and pathways to support our individual, collective, and universal growth and healing.

References

Atkins, S. S., & Snyder, M. A. (2018). *Nature-based expressive arts therapy: Integrating the expressive arts and ecotherapy*. London, England: Jessica Kingsley.

Cartwright-Jones, C. (2006). *Developing guidelines on henna: A geographical approach* (Master's thesis, Kent State University). Henna Page Publications, Stow, OH.

Coomaraswamy, A. K. (1975). The aims of Indian art in studies in comparative religion. *World Wisdom, Inc, 9*(1). Retrieved from www.studiesincomparativereligion.com/public/ articles/ The_Aims_of_Indian_Art.aspx

Dascal, M. (2009). Colonizing and decolonizing minds. In I. Kuçuradi (Ed.), *Papers of the 2007 world philosophy day* (pp. 308–332). Ankara, TU: Philosophical Society of Turkey.

Dissanayake, E. (1988). *What is art for?* Seattle, WA: University of Washington Press.

Farrelly-Hansen, M. (2001). *Spirituality and art therapy: Living the connection*. London, England: Jessica Kingsley.

Franklin, M. (2001). The yoga of art and the creative process: Listening to the divine. In M. Farrelly-Hansen (Ed.), *Spirituality and art therapy: Living the connection* (pp. 97–114). London, England: Jessica Kingsley.

Ghose, S. A. (1999). *The complete works of Sri Aurobindo*. Pondicherry, India: Sri Aurobindo Ashram Trust.

Gitadelila, G. (2018). *Kolam Yoga* training (verbal and unpublished materials) taught in regular sessions between 2016–2018 at Douceur, Auroville, India.

Gode, P. (1947). History of the Rangavalli (Rangoli) art. *Annals of the Bhandarkar Oriental Research Institute, 28*(3/4), 226–246. Retrieved from www.jstor.org/stable/44028067

Kalmanowitz, D., Potash, J. S., & Chan, S. M. (2012). *Art therapy in Asia: To the bone or wrapped in silk*. London, England: Jessica Kingsley.

Kristel, J. (2013). The process of attunement between therapist and client. In P. Howie, S. Prasad, & J. Kristel (Eds.), *Using art therapy with diverse populations: Crossing cultures and abilities* (pp. 85–94). London, England: Jessica Kingsley.

Malchiodi, C. A. (2020). *Trauma and expressive arts therapy: Brain, body, and imagination in the healing process*. New York, NY: The Guilford Press.

Moazzam, I. (2014, August 4). A brief history of henna. *The Express Tribune*. Retrieved June 20, 2019, from https://tribune.com.pk/story/741476/a-brief-history-of-henna/

Moon, C. H. (2002). *Studio art therapy: Cultivating the artist identity in the art therapist*. London, England: Jessica Kingsley.

Nagarajan, V. (2005). *Kolam: The traditional floor drawing*. Auroville, India: Ilaignarkal Education Center, Sri Aurobindo International Institute of Educational Research.

Nagarajan, V. (2019). *Feeding a thousand souls: Women, ritual, and ecology in India: An exploration of the kolam*. New York, NY: Oxford University Press.

Narayan, S. (2016, February 17). A quest to master the art of Henna. *Smithsonian Journeys Quarterly*. Retrieved May 15, 2019, from www.smithsonianmag.com/travel/henna-wedding-india-tradition-art-craft-180958087/

Philip, A. (2015, September 24). Of art and building bridges between cultures. The Hindu. Retrieved from www.thehindu.com/news/cities/puducherry/of-art-and-building-bridges-between-cultures/article7683870.ece

Rao, K. R., Paranjpe, A. C., & Dalal, A. K. (Eds.). (2008). *Handbook of Indian psychology*. New Delhi, India: Cambridge University Press India and Foundation Books.

Speert, E. (2016, October 27). *Eco-art therapy: Deepening connections with the natural world*. Retrieved from https://arttherapy.org/eco-art-therapy-deepening-connections-natural-world/

Tyabji, L. (1999). The story behind the stitches: Indian women, Indian embroideries. In *Maker and meaning: Craft and society: Proceedings of the seminar January 1999*. Chennai, Tamil Nadu, India: Madras Craft Foundation.

van der Kolk, B. (2015). *The body keeps the score: Brain, mind, and body in the healing of trauma*. New York, NY: Penguin.

8

Integrating Traditional Crafts Within Clinical Practice
A Cross-Cultural Group Case Study

MAHESH IYER

As a young Indian adult, son, art therapist, and human being, I have often been inclined to make sense of the world by plummeting into the creative arts. Through my exposure to multicultural populations in India and then the Middle East, I quickly recognized the capacity of art to unfold personal and collective experiences. This pursuit to "make meaning" creatively led me to the field of art therapy. As I trained to become an art therapist, I became more aware of my artistic process and experienced a strong urge to rewind time and seek out the roots of my creativity, culture, and influence (Manthe & Carolan, 2018). This led me to excavate my earliest sketchbooks covered with an energetic repetition of geometric patterns only to replicate a perfect symmetrical design laid down by my grandmother on the first page. This revealed a reservoir of interwoven reminiscences that spun around the Indian craft of kolam, an abstract symmetrical maze-like design joined on a grid of dots made using rice flour (Laine, 2009) and its adapted regional version rangoli made using various colored powder composed of basic patterns harmonized with symbol motifs (Steinmann, 1989).

An (In)visible Craft

Since ancient Indian times, art has carried a complexity between culture and traditional crafts to the extent that the line of delineation between the two is often blurred, highlighting the interweaving nature of both worlds. Historically, the British colonial officers disregarded kolam and its regional versions in their renumerations of Indian art and craft traditions (Sengupta, 1997), yet the Nobel laureate Rabindranath Tagore defined folk arts and village craft as "the best repositories of tradition" (Thakurta, 1992, p. 202) and viewed kolam as a "pure and unspoilt tradition" (Laine, 2009, p. 7). Anthropologist Anna Laine (2009) identified that there are no historical references to its cultivation as a craft form, however India's vast visual culture has always included kolam in its ongoing dialogue between photography, cinema, commercials, fine art, and religious festivals (Pinney, 2001).

The knowledge of this craft has strikingly survived solely through oral and visual histories transferred amongst generations. Kolam serves a purpose within a ritualistic and domestic setting, where women still engage in this craft every day as a meditative process to layer meanings, invoke deity, ward off evil, symbolize wellness, and create a sacred space (Tadvalkar, 2015). Given its undeniable presence in visual and traditional culture, on what account was the traditional craft of kolam and rangoli disregarded within a historical, artistic, and scholarly perspective? Laine (2009) recognized that the aim of her anthropological study is *not* to objectify a final product as art or craft but to give it voice and consider why it is used. She believed that perspectives that exclude everyday art or craft are wholly informed by ideas of aesthetic judgment.

Similarly, within the field of art therapy, we as practitioners regardless of our gender or theoretical orientation seek to help clients reclaim their voice through diverse methods of artistic expression. The arts have always served as a means to understand and amplify the client's perspective (Kapitan, 2015; Gilroy, 2006). From this establishment, it is in our nature to view traditional crafts forms for more than their customary use of religious or decorative purposes and find ways to integrate them into clinical practice. As a foreign student, I enrolled in a Masters in art therapy program in Singapore and learned about its multicultural context through critical observations, dialogues with local peers, and experiential training. I then integrated the traditional craft of rangoli in my clinical placement for older adults and found that the group garnered a range of therapeutic benefits. The following sections illustrate this process of integration through the use of a group case study in Singapore.

Population and Setting

St. Vincent's Home was established by The Catholic Welfare Services who act as an action arm for the Catholic Church in Singapore. They provide shelter with basic amenities for ambulant older adults who are 60 years or older and have no immediate family or financial sustainability to depend upon. As the shelter hosted elders from different walks of life they observed sporadic conflicts between residents with differing opinions. Therefore, art therapy services were initiated to build connections, increase engagement, and essentially improve quality of life and well-being for the residents (Bennington, Backos, Harrison, Reader, & Carolan, 2016; Stephenson, 2013).

At the time of the art therapy program's conception, the shelter hosted 14 residents consisting of 11 men and 3 women The group ranged between the ages of 66 and 95. All members came from a low socioeconomic background and solely depended on minimal monthly expenses allocated by the shelter. The group's ethnicity was predominantly Chinese Singaporean except for two men from Indian Singaporean and Eurasian Singaporean backgrounds. Prior to commencing group art therapy sessions, I conducted an initial observation of the group to gain familiarity with the residents. I then interviewed the senior social worker to understand the group's underlying attribute, which was identified to be a strong presence of predominant cultural, local, and national identities. Both these processes were consolidated within clinical supervision, and the goal of integrating culture-specific craft traditions was formulated. The rationale behind the program was to instill a sense of unity by inviting collective cultural themes through traditional crafts for residents to re-connect with their personal and collective identities (Prasad, 2013). All the artworks produced during the sessions were perceived through Stephenson's (2013) framework to understand successful aging in older adults. Stephenson's research outlined four art therapy program goals: "foster artistic identity; activate a sense of purpose and motivation; use art as a bridge to connect with others; and, support movement towards the attainment of gerotranscendence" (Stephenson, 2013, p. 151). The framework was implemented after considering the prominent parallels of group art therapy objectives, context, and population. Furthermore, by observing the artwork created within the group art therapy sessions through a culturally informed lens (Kapitan, 2018), two additional themes of *cultural integration* and *personal and culture-specific expressions* were identified.

Given Singapore's multifaceted global landscape, the city is home to diverse ethnic groups comprised mainly of Chinese, Malay, and Indian along with their respective belief systems (Statistics Singapore, 2017). The cultural values stemming from these systems inevitably influence the identity of individuals and groups (Essame, 2012). To attempt to mimic Singapore's inclusive identity within group art therapy sessions, a diverse range of culture-specific crafts closely associated with four nationally celebrated cultural festivals were introduced. Rangoli, associated with the Indian festival of Deepavali, was one of these crafts. The following section will detail how this traditional craft was adapted and integrated for the residents. The consolidation of data was conceived by perceiving the group as a single entity and identifying emergence of themes modeled by Stephenson's (2013) framework. All members are assigned pseudonyms to maintain confidentiality as per international research guidelines.

Integrating Rangoli

Rangolis are usually created on the floor; however, to effectively adapt the traditional craft for the residents, yoga mats were elevated on tables to symbolize the grounding nature of the craft for the residents. Traditional colored powder was substituted with tactile materials such as feathers, varied colored pebbles, and shells for easier use to maintain residents' autonomy. Rangoli was introduced to the group in two successive sessions so that members could gain familiarity and build the skillset to express themselves freely. The distributed experience allowed members to move beyond creating a conventional form of rangoli to expressing a personalized design with intent and meaning. Members commenced their first rangoli by independently drawing their own outlines using pre-drawn guiding dots (Figure 8.1).

A simple diamond shape was strategically adopted to form a linking point between each member's rangoli (Figure 8.2). The rationale behind this idea was to allow residents to explore the idea of boundaries, share a dot, and

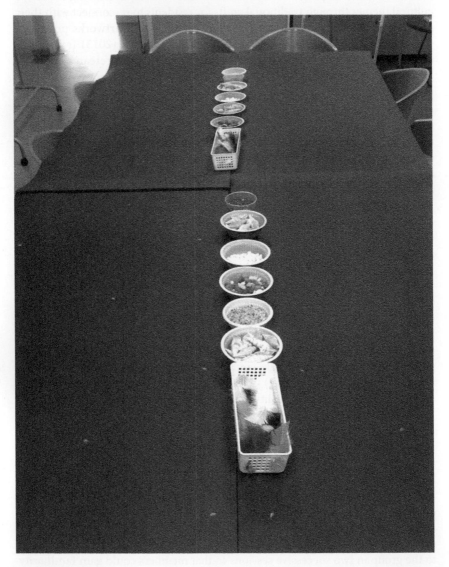

Figure 8.1 Mahesh Iyer, *Guiding dots*, session eight, chalk on yoga mats

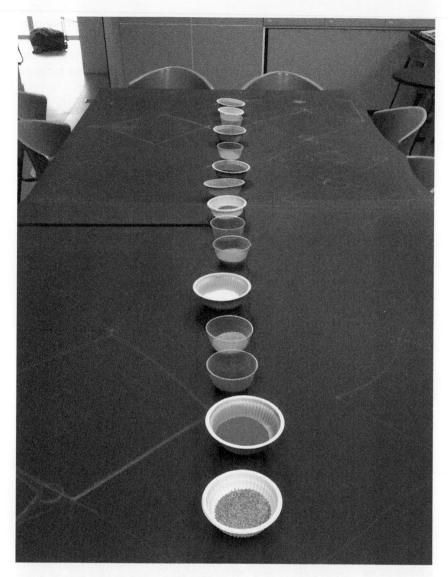

Figure 8.2 Group members, *Self-drawn boundary*, session eight, chalk on yoga mats

simply become aware of their neighbor. Our most recently admitted resident, Mr. Kong, was observed to be getting acclimated and building trust within the group art therapy sessions. He only verbalized in Chinese, minimally, and he refrained from creating any artwork. However, due to the demanding nature of rangoli in terms of space, the session settled Mr. Kong next to Mr. Goh, an older resident suspected of developing symptomatic criteria for dementia and typically observed to be internally engaged with ongoing narratives in Chinese. Within all previous art therapy sessions, Mr. Kong and Mr. Goh were never observed to socialize with one another, however, during this session, the group witnessed an emerging relationship in their rangolis (Figure 8.3).

Both group members used pebbles that playfully surpassed self-drawn boundaries. Their affect levels were positive; they laughed, gestured, and collaborated intentionally. The intersections in their process marked a new-born friendship as two incomplete pieces gradually became one coherent artwork. This was Mr. Kong's first initiative to use art as a way to connect with others (Stephenson, 2013).

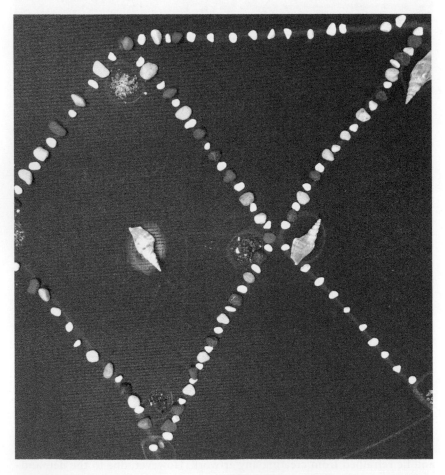

Figure 8.3 Mr. Goh and Mr. Kong, *Untitled*, session eight, pebbles, shells and chalk on yoga mat

In contrast to the above collaboration, Mrs. Xin and Mrs. Yi Ling have always encouraged and influenced each other's creative expression in the group art therapy sessions. During the first rangoli making session, both members presented similar styles with mutually revised ideas (Figure 8.4 and Figure 8.5). However, in the second rangoli making session, Mrs. Xin carefully illustrated the engagement ring on her finger and proudly exhibited it to the group (Figure 8.6). Although it is common to see personal expression appear in art therapy (Lusebrink, 2004), it is important to note that Mrs. Xin, who comes from a Chinese ethnic background, was able to identify with an Indian culture-specific artform and symbolically represent her marriage in her artistic expression.

Meanwhile Ms. Yi Ling developed her artistic identity and developed a deeper relationship in her process (Bennington et al., 2016). Her second rangoli

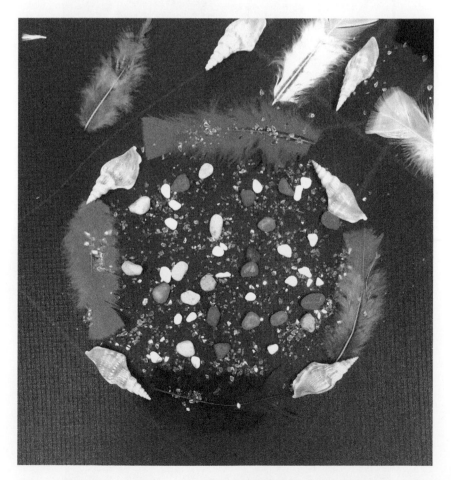

Figure 8.4 Ms. Xin, *Untitled*, session eight, pebbles, shells and feathers on yoga mat

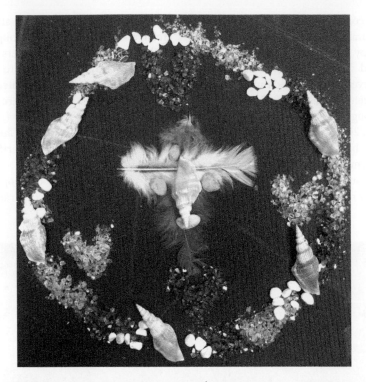

Figure 8.5 Ms. Yi Ling, *Untitled*, session eight, pebbles, shells and feathers on yoga mat

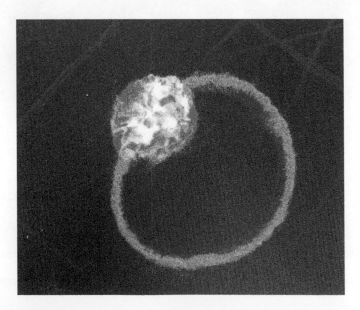

Figure 8.6 Ms. Xin, *Wedding ring*, session nine, colored powder on yoga mat

work presented an appealing blend of colors. The purposeful alternation of shells complimented by a defined border using the colored powder showcased on overall holistic thought of composition (Figure 8.7). Mrs. Xin demonstrated a significant level of personal and symbolic expression while Mrs. Yi Ling developed her unique style and artistic identity (Stephenson, 2013).

Mr. Koh is the oldest member of the group, embracing life each day at age 95. During group art therapy sessions, he was instrumental in the quality of the program translating Chinese to English and vice-versa. Compared to Mr. Koh's first rangoli (Figure 8.8), his second attempt showcased a deliberate thought

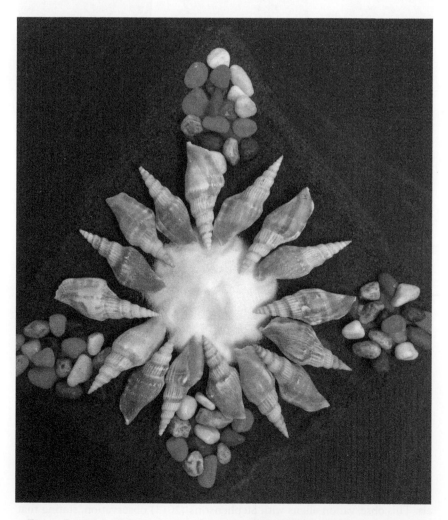

Figure 8.7 Mrs. Yi Ling, *Untitled*, session nine, pebbles, shells, and colored powder on yoga mat

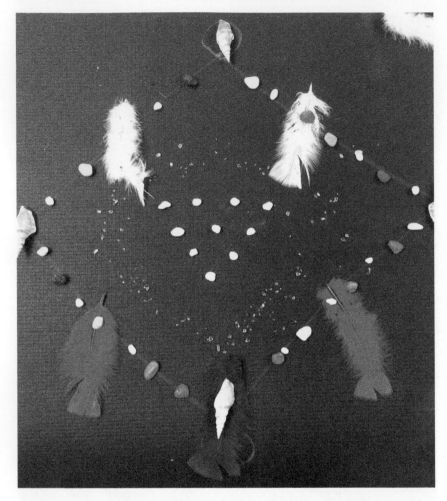

Figure 8.8 Mr. Koh, *Untitled*, session eight, pebbles, shells, and feathers on yoga mat

about composition—the red outer boundary complimented by an inner circle within which laid a hand drawn six-point star (Figure 8.9). Furthermore, accurately creating forms by hand is an acquired skill in rangoli, however Mr. Koh was strongly motivated to do so. While some residents requested unconventional tools such as brushes or thick paper to assist their process, Mr. Koh overcame these challenges by carefully handling and maneuvering the materials. This observation aligns with Stephenson's (2013) observation, stating that experimentation in artmaking fosters motivation and fuels a sense of purpose. Mr. Koh also shaped four anchoring symbols on the vertices of the diamond by

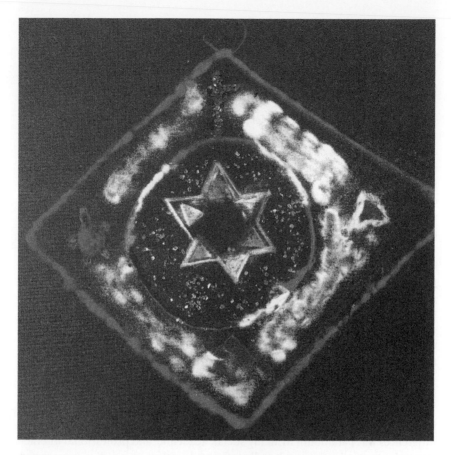

Figure 8.9 Mr. Koh, *Untitled,* session nine, pebbles, colored powder, and chalk on yoga mat

hand: the Christian Cross studded with purple stones on top, a purple triangle or pyramid outlined with yellow on the right, a purple square below, and a turtle with a red shell on the left, popularly known as a symbol of longevity in Chinese culture (Turtle in Chinese culture, n.d.). Apart from the two geometric shapes, the rangoli reflects an emergence of significant personal and religious symbols. Rangoli makers often incorporate the divine presence through symbols of God (Laine, 2009; Dohmen, 2001). By including the Christian Cross and the six-pointed star referenced to represent the Creator's Star in Christianity (Six-Point Star, 2017) as well as the turtle iconic to a long life such as his own, it may be that Mr. Koh had created his own sacred space in the rangoli, drawing on the cultural roots of the craft.

Carolan and Stafford (2018) recognize that "art has the capacity to facilitate a multiplicity of experiences of knowing in ways that cognitive linear processes do not" (p. 23). Keeping this in mind, whether conscious or unconscious, Mr. Koh was able to personalize the art form and generate free expression. His work indicated a strong artistic identity, an activated sense of purpose in technique, and emergence of personal and cultural expressions. Towards the end of the second and final session of rangoli making, residents were provided with a polaroid camera to photograph their work due to its impermanent nature. Mr. Koh personally shared his deep engagement with the craft's philosophy and its ties with Buddhism. Stephenson (2013) conceptualized gerotranscendence as an arrival to an age where self-esteem, wisdom, and the little things in life are embraced. As I reflect upon my conversations with Mr. Koh, I realize that they always revolved around his everyday routines that made him feel contented. Through the analytical lens of viewing the group as a single entity, several observations were seen to align with Stephenson's (2013) four goals of art therapy with older adults.

Additionally, incorporating traditional crafts as strategic interventions evoked a theme of cultural integration represented with several examples of personal and culture-specific symbolism. Conclusively, it was found that the group members garnered a range of therapeutic benefits from the group art therapy program. This case study demonstrates one possible way of enabling clinical art therapy practice with traditional crafts to thrive within multicultural contexts. The processes of integration demonstrate an important focus for future research in the field of art therapy. I encourage art therapists to persevere a deeper understanding of their own cultural expressions and gain the required skillsets to integrate them within their art therapy practice.

In my personal lived experience, I have been fortunate to be exposed to several multicultural populations. Understanding the interplay of cultural differences was paramount in all my social, academic, and professional interactions. However, adopting a culturally informed art therapy practice encouraged me to become self-reflexive of my own cultural background and mindful of appropriately integrating its elements in my clinical practice. This in turn helped me prioritize the integrity and dignity of individuals from other diverse cultural contexts and clear generalizations from my perceptions as an art therapist. I believe that as the art therapy profession develops, it is only natural that cultural and traditional crafts are integrated purposefully within therapeutic practice. In doing so, we invite multicultural inclusiveness, promote relevancy, and contribute to the international use of art therapy.

References

Bennington, R., Backos, A., Harrison, J., Reader, A. E., & Carolan, R. (2016). Art therapy in art museums: Promoting social connectedness and psychological well-being of older adults. *The Arts in Psychotherapy, 49*, 34–43.

Carolan, R., & Stafford, K. (2018). Theory and art therapy. In R. Carolan & A. Backos (Eds.), *Emerging perspectives in art therapy: Trends, movements, and developments* (pp. 17–32). New York, NY: Routledge.

Dohmen, R. (2001). Happy homes and the Indian nation: Women's design in post-colonial Tamil nadu. *Journal of Design History, 14*(2), 129–139.

Essame, C. (2012). Collective versus individual societies and the impact of Asian values on art therapy in Singapore. In D. Kalmanowitz, J. S. Potash, & S. M. Chan (Eds.), *Art therapy in asia: To the bone or wrapped in silk* (pp. 91–101). London, UK: Jessica Kingsley.

Gilroy, A. (2006). *Art therapy, research and evidence-based practice.* London, England: Sage Publications.

Kapitan, L. (2015). Social action in practice: Shifting the ethnocentric lens in cross cultural art therapy encounters. *Art Therapy: Journal of the American Art Therapy Association, 32*(3), 104–111.

Kapitan, L. (2018). *Introduction to art therapy research.* New York, NY: Routledge.

Laine, A. (2009). *In conversation with the Kolam practice: Auspiciousness and artistic experiences among women in Tamilnadu, South India.* Gothenburg, Sweden: School of Global Studies, Social Anthropology and Institutionen för globala studier, socialantropologi.

Lusebrink, V. B. (2004). Art therapy and the brain: An attempt to understand the underlying processes of art expression in therapy. *Art Therapy: Journal of the American Art Therapy Association, 21*(3), 125–135.

Manthe, L., & Carolan, R. (2018). Ethics in art therapy. In R. Carolan & A. Backos (Eds.), *Emerging perspectives in art therapy: Trends, movements, and developments* (pp. 93–104). New York, NY: Routledge.

Pinney, C. (2001). *Public, popular, and other cultures.* Oxford: Oxford University Press.

Prasad, S. (2013). The impact of culture and the setting on the use and choice of materials. In P. Howie, S. Prasad, & J. Kristel (Eds.), *Using art therapy with diverse populations: Crossing cultures and abilities* (pp. 76–84). London: Jessica Kingsley.

Sengupta, S. (1997). *Highlights and halftones: The Rajview of Indian Art, 1850–1905.* Delhi, India: Asia Pacific Research Information.

Six-Point Star (Hexagram; Star of David). (2017, January 19). Retrieved April 2, 2018, from www.religionfacts.com/six-point-star

Statistics Singapore. (2017). *Population trends.* Retrieved from www.singstat.gov.sg/publications/publications-and-papers/population-and-population-structure/population-trends

Steinmann, R. (1989). Kolam: Form, technique, and application of a changing ritual folk art of Tamil Nadu. In A. L. Dallapiccola (Ed.), *Shastric Traditions in Indian Arts* (Vol. 1, pp. 475–491). Stuttgart: Steiner.

Stephenson, R. C. (2013). Promoting well-being and gerotranscendence in an art therapy program for older adults. *Art Therapy: Journal of the American Art Therapy Association, 30*(4), 151–158.

Tadvalkar, N. (2015). A language of symbols: Rangoli art of india. In S. Garg (Ed.), *Traditional knowledge and traditional cultural expressions of South Asia* (pp. 173–186). Colombo: SAARC Cultural Centre.

Thakurta, T. G. (1992). The ideology of the 'aesthetic': The purging of visual tastes and the campaign for a new Indian art in late nineteenth/early twentieth century Bengal. *Studies in History, 8*(2), 237–281.

Turtle in Chinese Culture. (n.d.). Retrieved April 2, 2018, from http://chinesehoroscop-e.com/astrology/turtle-in-feng-shui.php

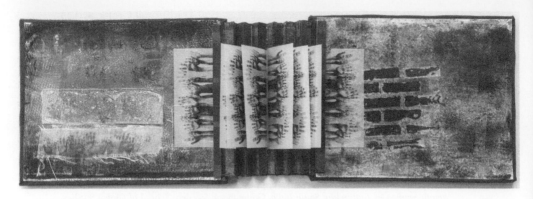

Color Plate 1 La Frontera/Wall

Source: Lynn Kapitan (Chapter 1)

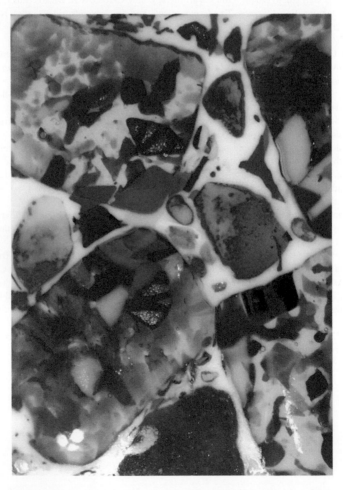

Color Plate 2 Rejoinder (after of repurposed broken pieces)

Source: Jessica Woolhiser Stallings (Chapter 2)

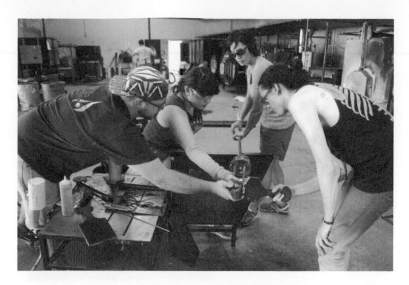

Color Plate 3 Three glassblowing instructors helping youth shape molten glass (Chapter 2)

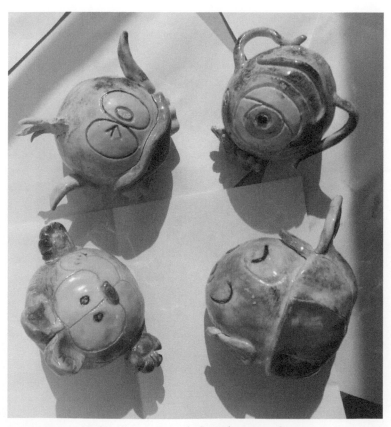

Color Plate 4 Four ladies playing mahjong

Source: created by pottery studio participants (Chapter 3)

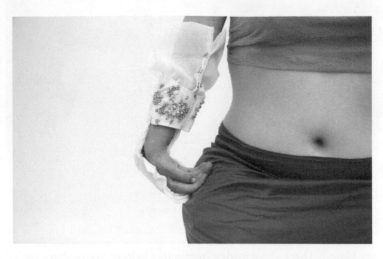

Color Plate 5 Em-Brace, Chun-shan (Sandie) Yi, 2011, plastic, embroidery thread, and fabric (Chapter 4)

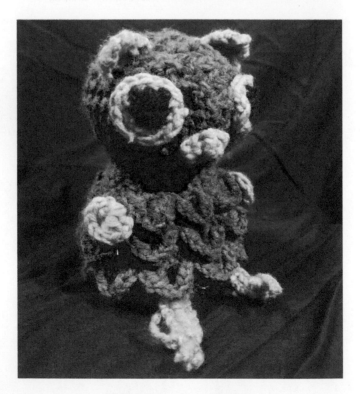

Color Plate 6 Oscar the Owl

Source: Marilyn Holmes (Chapter 5)

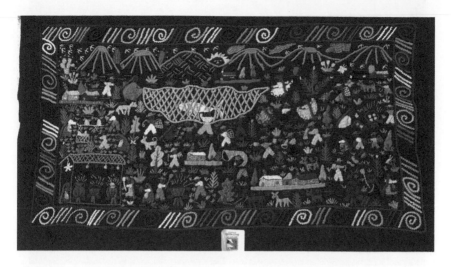

Color Plate 7 *Tela bordada* depicting community life by Berta Servín Barriga, approx. 29" × 17.5", embroidery on cotton, (Chapter 6)

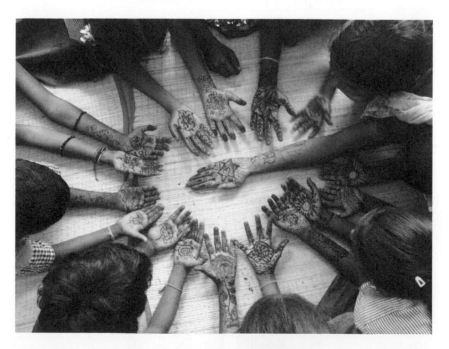

Color Plate 8 Mehndi art therapy process at Thamarai Center, Edyanchavadi Village, Tamil Nadu, India

Source: Photo: Krupa Jhaveri, 2012 (Chapter 7)

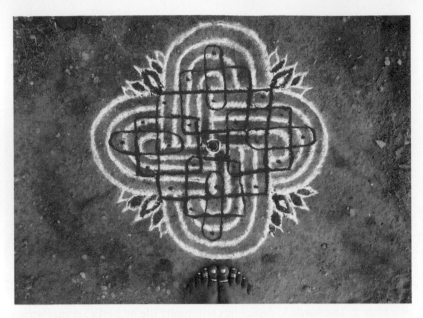

Color Plate 9 Kolam collaboration on the theme of cultural integration, between Mahesh Iyer (gray lines) and Krupa Jhaveri (background image)

Source: Artwork by Mahesh Iyer & Krupa Jhaveri, 2019

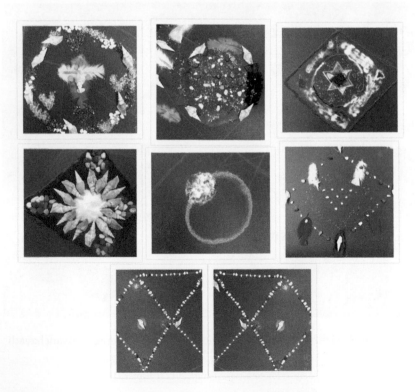

Color Plate 10 Group members, *Examples of rangoli*, sessions eight and nine, mixed media on yoga mats, (Chapter 8)

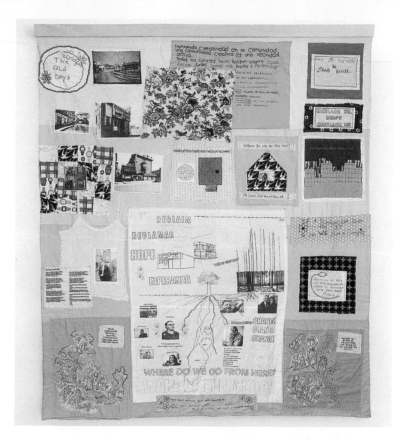

Color Plate 11 Wake Up Everybody Collaborative Quilt, Crafting Change group (Chapter 10)

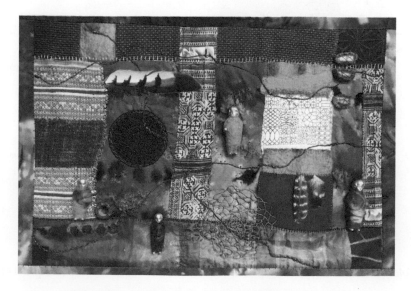

Color Plate 12 Separation I: Immigration Series, 2018

Source: Lisa Raye Garlock (Chapter 12)

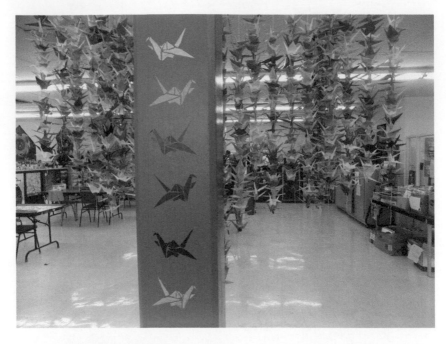

Color Plate 13 An installation of 1,000 paper cranes on display in the art studio following a workshop taught by a resident mentor (Chapter 13)

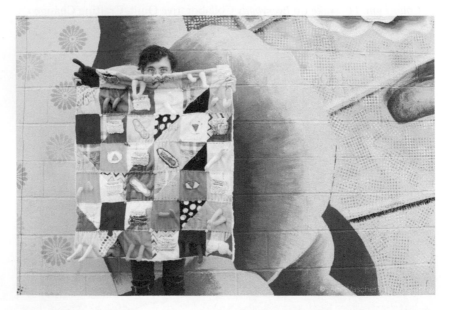

Color Plate 14 Mikey Anderson, *Queer Quilt*—mix media fiber crafts (Chapter 14)

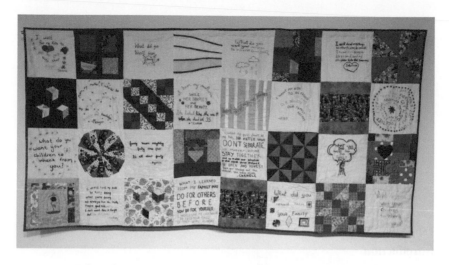

Color Plate 15 Envisioning Justice show quilt (Chapter 15)

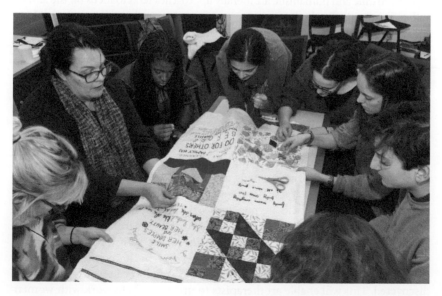

Color Plate 16 Quilting Circle (Chapter 15)

9
Using Crafts in Art Therapy Through an Intersectional Feminist Empowerment Lens
The Case of Bedouin Embroidery in Israel

MICHAL KATOSHEVSKI AND EPHRAT HUSS

Introduction

Crafts in the Western art world since the Renaissance have been considered a lesser form of art compared to so-called fine arts including poetry, architecture, and sculpture (Parker & Pollock, 2013). Industrialization further reduced the need for craftspeople. Even with the renewed interest in craft practices in Western countries, crafts are often associated with working class people, often from racial and ethnic minorities. Craft is not usually associated with creativity or with social arts (Berger, 2005; Kaimal et al., 2017; Lippard, 1995; Timm-Bottos, 2011).

This marginalization of craft practices can also be found in art therapy discourses: Psychodynamic and humanistic art therapy approaches tend to focus on the aim of authentic individualized self-expression and on process rather than product (Huss, 2015; Kaimal et al., 2017; Rubin, 1999). When the field was first forming, art therapists were at pains to be differentiated from occupational therapists, who used crafts to work on motor skills. In more current art therapy theories, crafts have been conceptualized as a calming, mindful activity that helps to self-regulate emotions and improve mood, as in the case of drawing mandalas as a form of meditation. Crafts have also been understood as a way to support problem solving, perseverance, and other skills often lost in neurological impairment (Collier, 2011; Dalebroux et al., 2008). Crafts are often not considered "creative" in terms of authentic self-expression, therapeutic in terms of providing a way to reach the unconscious, or socially communicative in terms of social art aiming to shift society.

We seek to challenge these assumptions, claiming that because crafts are associated with women who are poor or working class and/or people of color, they lend themselves to socially contextualized analyses from an intersectional feminist perspective. This may enable art therapists to use crafts to explore working class women's cultural forms of expression. In this context, craft's levels of therapeutic gain, empowerment, and social action can be unpacked and discovered. This will enable art therapists to utilize crafts to work with women within their social realities (Leone, 2018; Moon, 2010; Timm-Bottos, 2011).

If crafts are an art form associated with poor women, often from marginalized ethnic groups, then by definition they can become a site to address and empower the marginalization and voicelessness that these women often experience within Western societies as poor women in minority groups. Third World poor women's voices are often silenced and are not heard by the dominant culture and maybe not by art therapists. Crafts could be a way to change this (Mohanty, 2003; Motzafi-Heller, 2000; Talwar, 2003; Spivak, 1987). How can crafts used in an art therapy context become a medium to create "effective" speech acts that enable a woman both to "encounter her own voice" and to be "heard" by the dominant culture (Spivak, 1987)?

Hocoy (2002) argued that art as self-expression is a deeply Western construct, not necessarily suited to people from different cultures. Hudson (1960) described the process of learning depth perception in Africans observing Western art, demonstrating that art perceptions are cultural rather than universal skills. Acton (2001) warned against being a "color blind" art therapist and ignoring the cultural differences and approaches to healing of different peoples. Bhabha (1994) claimed that multiculturalism, a concept widely used in art therapy training, assumes that all cultures are interchangeable. He stated that the "vocabularies" of each culture cannot be automatically translated into other languages, as they have different comments and connotations in their specific contexts.

Cole (1996) stressed the importance of artifacts as something simultaneously ideal and physical and thus serving as a reservoir of cultural meanings. Crafts are thus "culturally-embedded aesthetics." As Mahon (2000) wrote, crafts are inseparable from "broader social contexts . . . and struggle over cultural meanings" (p. 470). On the other hand, although the conception of art as Westernized individualized self-expression is limited, viewing the crafts of people from non-Western cultures as a static expression of culture is also limiting and "archeologizes" crafts activities into a static past, when in fact they are constantly evolving and often hybrid expressions that react to cultural transitions in different ways. As Lippard (1995) stated:

> Notions of authenticity imposed from the outside that lead to stereotypes and false representations, freeze non-Western cultures in an anthropological present or an archeological past that denies their heirs a modern identity or a political reality on an equal basis with Euro-Americans.
>
> (p. 12)

Within current global culture, individuals can belong to multiple and transitional cultural contexts simultaneously, which they can embrace and resist, in different ways. Thus, crafts are not anthropological static forms of expression but may be an arena within which to integrate, challenge, and express these multiple identities. In terms of class and culture, women's crafts groups are utilized as a way to enable women to earn money in a culturally sanctioned way (Abu-Rabia-Queder, 2007). For example, crafts making enables women to embroider at home while looking after children and remaining within socially designated female spaces. In terms of feminist empowerment, the shared-reality group of the embroidery collective can be understood as an empowering and thus therapeutic space, enabling women to gain social support and information as well as to define their identity as related to a sociocultural shared group reality and thus raise social consciousness (Saulnier, 1996).

Crafts have a variety of uses that can allow individuals to integrate cultural identity and to gain power from their traditional cultures, while at the same time resisting and expanding it. Using crafts as a way of gaining knowledge and financial power enables power in the patriarchal and hegemonic community. We have experienced this social theory of crafts in action in a group of Bedouin women in southern Israel who use embroidery as a tool of empowerment and in doing so have transformed the different ecological circles of individual, group, and community. As the full case studies of these women have been previously published (Huss, 2009, 2012, 2015), our aim here is to focus on the ways that crafts groups with Third World impoverished women can become an art therapy practice that is connected to social theories. We hope that this will be of use with other groups who are similarly marginalized.

Embroidery in the Context of Traditional Bedouin Culture

The individuals described herein are Bedouin women living in townships in the south desert of Israel. Although the Bedouin are Muslim, they have integrated early pre-Islamic customs into Islam, specifically ones related to survival in the desert, that define them as indigenous people (Meir, 1997). They originate in different groups: the "Sum Ran," considered to be the original Bedouin tribes; the "El-Abed," who are black Sudanese Bedouin; and the "Hum Ran," who are Arab *fellah* (farmers) who joined the Bedouin tribes (Barakat, 1993; Meir, 1997).

Traditional Bedouin society, similar to many collective non-Western cultures, is defined as "high context" according to Barakat (1993), emphasizing the collective over the individual, a slow pace of societal change, and a sense of social stability as a value. The values of generosity, hospitality, reciprocity, pride, valor, and strength are manifested through societal codes of indirect communication, conflict avoidance, and the use of mediators (Cole, 1996; Joseph, 1999; Tal, 1995). Collectivist culture can be described as "the production of selves with fluid boundaries organized for gendered and aged domination" (Joseph, 1999, p. 12).

It is helpful to draw on Cole's (1996) definition of context to grasp the terms "context" and "collective." According to Cole, context is not the "surroundings" external to the individual but rather the "connected whole that gives coherence to its parts" (p. 135). These cultural norms are made visible in the Bedouin embroidery in which the collective pattern gives coherence to each shape and color. The aesthetic language is one that stresses the importance of balance, measure, and spacing and that challenges the eye with puzzles and provides a mystical sense of infinity (Irving, 1997). Thus, art's role within Arab culture is to stimulate an intellectual challenge and to convey respect for order that pleases the viewer (Nasr, 2002). From this perspective embroidery is itself an "art therapy," in that it "embroiders" women back into the values that they believe in and that create a coherent cultural support system for them.

Power for Arab women is relative to other Arab women, rather than being compared to the male public arena. Women from non-Western collective traditional minority cultures in general and Bedouin women as well tend to express themselves indirectly through networks of kinship and friendship that can have consequences for men in their community (Joseph, 1999; Tal, 1995; Yamini, 1996). This hierarchical social organization is also apparent in embroidery aesthetics. In this context of power, embroidery is a way of decorating the home, camels, and women themselves—helping to protect against the evil eye and therefore powerful. The embroidered dress also conveys information about status, number of children, hierarchy as a wife, and life transitions such as mourning to people in and outside of the tribe. Skill in embroidery also creates social networks of help and competition, and it symbolizes group pride in that different tribes use different patterns of embroidery. The power is expressed visually, in a silent, non-confrontational way (that is "silent" verbally but "loud" in terms of color). This reflects the indirect use of power described earlier and parallels Third World feminist practices and claims that words are constructed to express male experience while women often express themselves in non-verbal and indirect ways. Thus, embroidery becomes a gendered act of empowerment, of self-expression, and of social interaction (Mohanty, 2003; Motzafi-Heller, 2000).

Bedouin Embroidery in the Context of Cultural Transition

The previous description of the role of embroidery within Bedouin culture is, however, static and anthropological. Similar to other indigenous groups throughout the world, under the influence of the dominant Israeli culture Bedouin society is undergoing change from a collective to an individualistic culture and from a nomadic lifestyle to one fixed in permanent settlements (Meir, 1997). This has resulted in a dramatic change in the social organization of the Bedouin community.

The well-being of Bedouin women depends upon the well-being of their male relatives and their reactions to the aforementioned societal changes. As a result, unemployment and child benefit supports from the state have become the central sources of income for impoverished Bedouins in the townships (Bar Tzvi, 1986; Meir, 1997; Tal, 1995). According to Brownwell (1997), Arab-Palestinian women are oppressed doubly, both by men and by the Israeli political regime. According to Tal (1995), Bedouin men perceive the possibility of work and free movement outside the tribe as a threat to the traditional roles of women. As a result, women are increasingly under men's control. Due to the forces of modernization, women are no longer busy with agricultural work; rather, all are in the house together for many hours, intensifying the age-old mother-in-law/new bride conflict. Polygamy has risen due to modernization as men desire a more educated wife or wish to enhance their declining sense of power (Al-Ataana, 1993; Cohen, 1999; Gilboa-Negari et al., 2017). Simultaneously, due to the limitations on hunting and a nomadic lifestyle, men have taken over roles that were previously under women's control in the home, such as overseeing the educating of children. The externalization of social responsibilities to state authorities, who invest limited resources and often lack cultural relevance for the community, has resulted in the decline of collective family support and funds (Kapri et al., 2002; Lewando-Hundt, 1978).

Bedouin women do not live according to their tribal culture anymore but rather are caught between the values of Western "modern" culture and collective culture, and this increases the marginalization of impoverished women (as compared to middle-class women who are able to mobilize resources to shift to the hegemonic Westernized culture through, for example, studies and financial ability). Shifting embroidery trends embody these cultural transitions. Due to increased mobility and variety of available materials, strong primary colors are now rendered in varying shades, and there are more types and styles of embroidery. Bedouin crafts are on the decline because Islamic movements disapprove of time spent on embroidery, embroidery can be machine made, and embroidered clothes are worn less by younger generations (Tal, 1995). Dresses are now made with one fewer panels, and embroidery has been dwindling (Fugel, 2002).

Due to these shifts, a dynamic and multi-faceted definition of culture may be especially suitable for people undergoing rapid cultural change: culture can no longer be seen as static but rather involves a hybridization of various, at times conflicting, cultural norms within any given person at any given time. Women often are defined as the "carriers" of traditional culture and are expected to pass it on to their children, whereas men are allowed to enter the modern culture. However, this may or may not be what they want. This means that rather than defining what crafts these women should do, based on anthropological notions of what is "authentic" for them, a phenomenological participatory approach could help women define for themselves what interests them and what is relevant to them, from both their traditional and current cultures. Crafts can be an excellent place to integrate different art discourses and to negotiate the transition from homeostasis to change in a visual way that is less directly challenging (Avruch, 1998; Huss, 2009, 2012).

The following examples show how embroidery crafts were used by a group of Bedouin women living in poverty during the cultural transition described earlier. This group of 12 women asked to learn crafts, rather than do art therapy. They met once a week for 12 weeks in the social services welfare offices of their township. All research subjects signed an agreement to allow their crafts to be described but not photographed within the context of the research. The university ethics committee approved the project (Huss, 2012).

As stated previously, the aim of the following vignettes is not to present the full case study but rather to illustrate how crafts are used in art therapy through an empowerment lens. This includes three levels: (a) on the individual level, to gain a coherent voice by integrating hybrid cultural identities; (b) on the group level, to create a support system within which to co-produce knowledge and provide support; and (c) on the community level, through negotiating Bedouin community and Israeli culture in terms of gaining knowledge and money that increase social, symbolic, and financial power in relation to the external culture and in relation to the Bedouin patriarchal culture.

Individual Level: Integrating Hybrid Cultural Identities

The women in the group decided what crafts they wanted to use: some wanted to create traditional Bedouin embroidery while others wanted to learn to paint with fabric colors to make "modern" jewelry crafts that they could sell and wear—both options were provided. Some women integrated older techniques with more contemporary crafts designs. These hybrid products were then sold at a crafts fair and were very popular. The process of deciding on both types of crafts and the integration of both of them enabled a creative safe space in which to practice integrating both tradition and modernity in new ways. One woman stated: "Silk painting is the opposite of embroidery in that you make abstract droplets of color that you have no control over, while embroidery you have to plan in advance . . . it's nice to combine them." A young woman embroidered a square according to accepted norms but added a heart shape to it. She stated that she wanted to get married but also wanted love, and she thought marriage was the "end" of freedom. She explained, "After marriage, you stay home and do not get to see anything, anymore." All the women concurred, laughing and nodding their heads in agreement. Another young woman wore jeans and a tight top, but embroidered traditionally, learning from the older women in the group. She thus integrated dual cultural sources—one in her modern clothes and one in her traditional embroidery—about the role of women and about love and marriage, as well as dual cultural messages in her dress and her embroidery.

These examples resonate with the previously mentioned literature about how crafts can provide a space to integrate hybrid identities, rather than "anthropologizing" women into traditional cultural modes, as men tend to situate them or forcing them to use expressive modes that are not inherent to their culture, as sometimes happens in art therapy (Hogan, 2003; Kaplan, 2000). In these examples, crafts became innovative and original integrations of old and new crafts aesthetics.

This type of innovation and integration can be understood as an aesthetic stand, as expressed by Arnheim (1996), who stated, "All problem solving has to cope with an overcoming of the fossilized shape . . . the discovery that squares are only one kind of shape among infinitely many" (p. 43). By selling jewelry, the women gained financial power and also shifted stands of what is traditional cultural expression in the larger Bedouin community. In this sense, this act was subversive.

It is important to note the group leader also brought crafts books for the group to look at, which enabled the women to see new ways of using embroidery including stitching words rather than abstract designs. One woman prepared an embroidery template that included the words "beware of bad people." She explained that she was scared of the "bad" youth in her neighborhood and felt that many dangers existed outside her home. She wanted to warn her children and have an embroidered message like this at the entrance to her home. Due to poverty and social marginalization, there is much crime and drug use among impoverished Bedouin youth. The original aim of embroidery on clothes is to provide information about the Bedouin women. This use of crafts as a didactic tool is a central aim of arts discourses throughout history, as shown in religious art, in the past and present, and also in areas such as Western advertising (Huss, 2012). As stated previously, embroidery is also used as an amulet against the evil eye in Bedouin culture. Embroidering this message helped to provide the magic protective powers of embroidery as an amulet, as well as to provide information, with words that warn about the dangers of modern culture. The integration of magic and didactic uses of crafts served to justify the ability of the mother to look after her children.

Group Level: Creating a System Within Which to Co-Produce Knowledge and Provide Support

Feminist therapy defines women as experts on their situations: a central method is to utilize the shared-reality group space to explore issues together, problem solve, and situate personal experience within social contexts (Huss, 2015). Modernization often disrupts the collective element of women's spaces and power in indigenous cultures. By creating an embroidery group, this power was returned to the women. The use of traditional embroidery enabled a culturally sanctioned space that was not perceived by men as subversive and therefore was not viewed as a threat.

One woman in the group stated: "I learnt lots of things in this group, new ideas, some of them I use at home, I take the good ideas and use them at home." Others shared that it gave them a chance to leave home and meet people outside the tribe and extended family, to create new friendships. The women also started meeting up together in the evening, outside of group sessions. At the end of each group session the women showed and explained what they had made that day; this enabled a space for building group coherence. Often, the crafts object held the Bedouin culture, while the discussion around it challenged or disrupted the traditional culture or provided suggestions of how to deal with marginalization effectively.

In one session, a woman made a small traditional embroidered amulet to protect children and shared: "This is the main joy of the women—to have children." Another woman reflected, "But when they are older, it is hard. For instance, I have problems with my daughter who wants to be with her father, and to leave me alone." A third woman suggested, "You should let your daughter go with her father, because for her it is important." The second woman responded, "But she leaves me all alone. She goes with his new wife and his children, and I am left all alone." The third replied, "Still, you must think of her. . . . We will help you—we are your friends. We know it's hard for you, but it will be okay—you can come to visit us in those times, or come here to embroider and make some money."

In this example, we see how the craft object, which holds deep cultural power, sanctioned the ability of a mother to protect her children and to be a good mother. This in turn may have enabled a discussion of the difficulties of being a good mother in a society where mothers may be replaced by new wives. The women within the group space provided both practical solutions and emotional support for this problem. This type of discussion also became subversive to the patriarchal society, showing how women negotiate power indirectly.

As part of the combination of crafts and art that the women asked for, the women wanted to make embroidered dolls for their children, as they could not afford to buy them toys. The women made any character that they wished. One woman made embroidered dolls of a sheik and his wife. She separated the dolls, explaining that the woman was in the women's part of the tent, "She is saying, 'yes, yes,' but not doing what he says." The woman ignoring the sheik "encountered" her own power or resistance and shared it in the group of women. This example, through humor and irony, showed the other women that they (as a group) had power over their various oppressors. Thus, the sheik is the comic "fool" of the story, not knowing that he is being disobeyed. All of the women laughed. This example reveals the indirect ways that the women resist the power of men in their culture (Abu-Lughod, 1995; Huss, 2015).

The use of crafts as a focus for a group process enabled renegotiation of power within the group itself between women from different Bedouin ethnic hierarchies. For example, a Black Bedouin woman in the group (the lower "caste" within Bedouin culture and thus the lowest status group in the crafts group) worked carefully on a silk brooch that was embellished with embroidery on a painted background. She wanted to use gold paint as a base but hesitated. Finally she reached over, took the bottle of expensive paint, and made her background gold—constantly looking at the other women and at the group leader. The woman had shifted her status within the group through using the most expensive paint; she had claimed power within the group zone. This was not verbal, but occurred within the craft making process and dynamics of the women.

Community Level: Negotiating Bedouin Community and Israeli Culture

Finally, the crafting group also enabled individuals to gain knowledge that is power, to earn money that enabled them to engage in the external world, and to more directly challenge patriarchal hierarchies. For example, one woman described her pride in her new skills that she could show to the community as a whole. At the end of the sessions, she spoke of the pride she felt in her embroidered brooch and how she wanted to wear it to a wedding the following day where she would tell everyone that she had made it. She said, "it is not the cost of the brooch that I am proud of, but that I made it and that everyone at the wedding will acknowledge my skill."

Another example of secondary gains around the embroidery group that are empowering is the new information and knowledge that women received in the group. The financial gains of the crafts group as an NGO enabled the group to pay for lecturers on issues that the women were interested in, such as women's reproduction health and women's rights. These lectures provided knowledge about hegemonic culture and enabled the women to "enter modernity" in a way that does not challenge men because it occurred in a traditional crafts space where the women were seemingly compliant to their traditional tribal roles. The women could embroider and listen to a lecture at the same time. One woman stated:

> We sit and talk and embroider, then we sometimes have a lecture, and we talk about it, and then we take our money . . . and go home . . . we can continue embroidering at home if we need more money, and we learn important things.

Another explained, "We need lots of things—emotional help, and support, and to have fun, but first of all, we need to earn money, because that gives us real power in the home." The women discussed how having money enabled them to negotiate power with their husbands in the real world. For example, one woman remarked, "My husband wants my sons to work and earn money, but I told them they have to study, and now I have money to pay for their studies."

Another community-level benefit was that embroidery helped to maintain traditional roles while creating new ones. One woman explained:

> I wanted to learn to drive and my husband said "no," and the other women in the tribe laughed at me that I want to be a man, but also I was embroidering, I am a women, and also, I earned my own money, so I bought a driving theory book and I learnt it, and then when my husband said he won't pay for my lessons, I told him, that's ok, I have my own money.

Summary

In sum, these specific examples demonstrate how to "read" craft as a form of art therapy based in feminist empowerment theories. In the group of Bedouin women, crafts were used to integrate their cultural identity on the personal level and to gain power from traditional culture, while at the same time resisting and expanding it. As Lippard (1990) stated:

> Hybrid and emotionally complex stories derived from both tradition and experience, old-new stories, challenge the pervasive "master narratives"

that would contain them. . . . It has become clear that the hybrid is one of the most authentic creative expressions in United States.

(p. 57)

This hybrid expanded from the individual to the group to the community. It included craft processes, skills, products, and the conversations and knowledge gained while co-creating a shared reality group space. It expanded to the financial gain that was sanctioned by the cultural norms. Thus, the different ecological circles of individual, group, and community were all transformed through the crafts. Additionally, this chapter suggested a new way to "listen" to crafts as voices of the "other". As Fine (1994) in her book *Working the Hyphens* noted: "Rather than trying to study the 'other' or to give voice to the other, researchers are called to listen, instead, to the plural voices of those 'othered' as constructers and agents of knowledge" (p. 76). This conception of crafts can be understood as an effort to "listen" to how our clients use crafts within their social contexts.

References

Abu-Lughod, L. (1993). *Writing women's worlds: Bedouin stories.* Berkeley, CA: University of California Press.

Abu-Lughod, L. (1995). The objects of soap opera: Egyptian television and the cultural politics of modernity. In D. Miller (ed), *Worlds apart: Modernity through the prism of the local,* 190–210. London, UK: Routledge.

Abu-Rabia-Queder, S. (2007). The activism of Bedouin women: Social and political resistance. *HAGAR: Studies in Culture, Polity & Identities, 7*(2), 67–84.

Acton, D. (2001). The "color blind" therapist. *Art Therapy, 18*(2), 109–112.

Al-Ataana, M. (1993). Connection between marital status of Bedouin woman and her self image and psychological well being. (Master's thesis) Bar-Ilan University, Tel Aviv, Israel.

Arnheim, R. (1996). *The split and the structure: Twenty-eight essays.* Berkeley, CA: University of California Press.

Avruch, K. (1998). *Culture and conflict resolution.* Washington, DC: United States Institute of Peace.

Barakat, H. (1993). *The Arab world, society, culture and state.* Los Angeles, CA: University of California Press.

Bar Tzvi, S. (1986). Traditions and ancient custom of the Negev Bedouin. *Notes on the Bedouin, 17,* 15–20.

Berger, M. A. (2005). *Sight unseen: Whiteness and American visual culture.* Berkeley, CA: University of California Press.

Bhabha, H. (1994). *The location of culture.* London, England: Routledge.

Brownwell, P. (1997). Multicultural practice and domestic violence. In E. P. Congress (Ed.), *Multicultural perspectives in working with families* (pp. 217–236). New York, NY: Springer.

Cohen, M. (1999). The status of the Bedouin women in Israel economic and social changes. *Maof Vemeaseh, 5,* 229–237. (In Hebrew).

Cole, M. (1996). *Cultural psychology: A once and future discipline.* Boston, MA: Harvard University Press.

Collier, A. F. (2011). The well-being of women who create with textiles: Implications for art therapy. *Art Therapy: Journal of the American Art Therapy Association, 28*(3), 104–112.

Dalebroux, A., Goldstein, T. R., & Winner, E. (2008). Short-term mood repair through art-making: Positive emotion is more effective than venting. *Motivation and Emotion, 32*(4), 288–295. http://dx.doi.org/10.1007/s11031-008-9105-1

Fine, M. (1994). Working the hyphens. In *Handbook of qualitative research.* Thousand Oaks, CA: Sage.

Fugel, T. (2002). The language of the dress of the Negev Bedouin women. *Notes on the Bedouin*, *34*, 217–223.

Gilboa-Negari, Z., Abu-Kaf, S., Huss, E., Hain, G., & Moser, A. (2017). A cross-cultural perspective of medical clowning: Comparison of its effectiveness in reducing anxiety and pain among hospitalized Bedouin and Jewish Israeli children. *Journal of Pain Research*, *10*, 1545–1552.

Hocoy, D. (2002). Cross-cultural issues in art therapy. *Art Therapy*, *19*(4), 141–145.

Hogan, S. (Ed.). (2003). *Gender issues in art therapy*. London, England: Jessica Kingsley.

Hudson, W. (1960). Pictorial depth perception in sub-cultural groups in Africa. *The Journal of Social Psychology*, *52*(2), 183–208.

Huss, E. (2009). A case study of Bedouin women's art in social work: A model of social arts intervention with "traditional" women negotiating Western cultures. *Journal of Social Work Education*, *28*(6), 598–616.

Huss, E. (2012). *What we see and what we say: Using images in research, therapy, empowerment, and social change*. London, UK: Routledge.

Huss, E. (2015). *A theory-based approach to art therapy: Implications for teaching, research, and practice*. London, UK: Routledge.

Irving, R. (1997). *Islamic art in context*. New York, NY: Abrams Press.

Joseph, S. (1999). *Intimate selving in Arab families: Gender, self, and identity*. Syracuse, NY: Syracuse Press.

Kaimal, G., Gonzaga, A. M. L., & Schwachter, V. (2017). Crafting, health and wellbeing: Findings from the survey of public participation in the arts and considerations for art therapists. *Arts & Health*, *9*(1), 81–90. doi:10.1080/17533015.2016.1185447

Kaplan, F. (2000). Now and future ethno-cultural issues. *Art Therapy: Journal of the American Art Therapy Association*, *19*(2), 65–79.

Kapri, H., Roznik, R., & Budekat, B. (2002). *Welfare services in the unrecognized settlements*. Jerusalem: Israeli Ministry of Welfare. Study Project. (Hebrew).

Leone, L. (2018). *Crafting change: Craft activism and community-based art therapy* (Doctoral Dissertation). Mount Mary University, Milwaukee, WI.

Lewando-Hundt, G. (1978). *Women's power and settlement: The effect of settlement on the positions of Negev Bedouin women*. (Doctoral thesis). University of Edinburgh, Edinburgh, UK.

Lippard, L. (1990). *Mixed blessings: Art in a multicultural America*. New York, NY: Pantheon.

Lippard, L. (1995). *The pink glass swan: Selected feminist essays on art*. New York, NY: New Press.

Mahon, M. (2000). The visible evidence of cultural producers. *Annual Review of Anthropology*, *29*(1), 467–492.

Meir, A. (1997). *As nomadism ends: The Israeli Bedouin of the Negev*. Boulder, CO: Westview Press.

Mohanty, C. T. (2003). Under Western Eyes: Feminist scholarship and colonial discourses. In R. Lewis & S. Mills (Eds.), *Feminist postcolonial theory: A reader*. Edinburgh, Scotland: Edinburgh University Press.

Moon, C. H. (Ed.). (2010). *Materials and media in art therapy: Critical understandings of diverse artistic vocabularies*. New York, NY: Routledge. Motzafi-Heller, P. (2000). Reading Arab feminist discourses. *Hagar: International Social Science Review*, *1*(2), 63–91.

Nasr, S. H. (2002). *The heart of Islam*. San Francisco, CA: Harpers.

Parker, R., & Pollock, G. (2013 [1981]). *Old mistresses: Women, art and ideology*. New York, NY: I.B. Tauris & Co, Ltd.

Rubin, J. (1999). *Art therapy, an introduction*. Philadelphia, PA: Bruner and Mazel.

Saulnier, C. (1996). *Feminist theories and social work*. New York, NY: Haworth Press.

Spivak, G. C. (1987). *In other worlds: Essays in cultural politics*. New York, NY: Methuen.

Tal, S. (1995). *The Bedouin women in the Negev in time of changes*. HaNegev, Israel: Joe Alon Center for Bedouin Culture. (Hebrew).

Talwar, S. K. (2003). Decolonization: Third world women and conflicts. In S. Hogan (Ed.), *Gender issues in art therapy* (pp. 185–193). London, UK: Jessica Kingsley.

Timm-Bottos, J. (2011). Endangered threads: Socially committed community art action. *Art Therapy: Journal of the American Art Therapy Association*, *28*(2), 57–63. doi:10.1080/07421656.2011.578234

Yamini, M. (1996). *Feminism and Islam*. London, UK: Garnet Publishers.

III
Craft as Empowerment and Activism

10

Finding Our Way Together
Exploring the Therapeutic Benefits of Collaborative Craft Activism

LAUREN LEONE

For the past 3 months we've put our hearts, heads, and our hands together to create a quilt that expresses a cause. . . . Art is a light that never gets dull or old. This art is called craftivism, which is a social process of collective empowerment, action, expression, and negotiation. Hopefully our quilt will jump-start a movement that makes sure that we as a community are included, not excluded, from the process of change.
—Excerpted text from the *Wake Up Everybody* quilt presentations, written by Brenda, member of the Crafting Change group

Throughout history, people have used craft to express themselves, to build community, and even to resist social and political oppression. As an art therapist with emancipatory aims for my work and a long history of using fiber art in my own art making, I wanted to more concretely explore the benefits of craft—both its individual therapeutic impact and its community-building potential—particularly when it is used to support art therapy participants in being change agents. With this goal in mind, I designed a collaborative craft activism project with members of an art therapy sewing group at a community health center in the Boston area (Leone, 2018, 2019). Together we created a quilt that aimed to raise community awareness around the gentrification and displacement impacting the local neighborhood. Almost three years after our first project wrapped up we still continue to meet to work on new projects. This experience has demonstrated that in a community model of art therapy, collaborative craft activism builds individuals' capacity to address issues that affect their communities and that developing these skills serves a therapeutic function.

Craft Activism

There is a historic precedent for the use of craft as a form of activism. Examples include abolitionist quilts created before and during the U.S. Civil War, some of which even contained explicit opposition to slavery via poems and images (Lufkin, 2019); British suffragists' strategic use of the stereotypical association of embroidery with femininity to create the banners that were essential to their political action (Wheeler, 2012); Gandhi's call for Indians to spin their own cotton as a form of non-violent protest of British textile laws during the Indian independence movement (Sharma & Bhaduri, 2019); and *arpilleras*, or story cloths, created by women during Augusto Pinochet's dictatorship in Chile, to document the incarceration, torture, and death of tens of thousands of people (Agosín, 2008).

This use of craft as activism is currently known as *craftivism*, a term to describe the use of craft for activist purposes that emerged at the beginning of the 21st century (Greer, 2011). Craftivism can be traced to several social and political movements, including third-wave feminism, environmentalism, anti-capitalism, anti-sweatshop organizing, and antiwar politics (Robertson, 2011). Commonalities among different craftivism projects are that they have a participatory element, employ a democratic process of decision-making and creation, use cross-disciplinary mediums, and advocate for an ongoing mission related to political engagement. Craftivists rely on a mixture of technology, public spaces, and nontraditional art spaces to share their skills and information (Black & Burisch, 2011).

One of the most often-cited forms of art activism, the *AIDS Memorial Quilt*, can be seen as a precursor to the craftivism projects that emerged two decades later. The project brought national recognition to a critical issue that many people were trying to avoid or overlook, and the use of the quilt served to bring another dimension to AIDS activism by focusing on mourning and remembrance (Reed, 2005). Conceived by Cleve Jones, a gay rights activist living in San Francisco, the project began in the mid-1980s with the creation, by friends and partners, of individual 3' × 6' quilt panels that each represented a person lost to the disease. The project quickly gained momentum and national attention in the United States. The quilt was first displayed on the National Mall in Washington, DC, during the second National March on Washington for Lesbian and Gay Rights in 1987 where, according to the NAMES Project Foundation, almost 2,000 panels were displayed; an estimated half a million people saw the quilt over the course of the weekend. Today the number of panels has grown to almost 50,000 (The AIDS Memorial Quilt, n.d.).

A powerful contemporary example of how quilts can be used as activism can be seen in the work of the Social Justice Sewing Academy (SJSA). SJSA, founded by quilter, educator, and activist Sara Trail in 2017, is a "youth education program that bridges artistic expression with activism to advocate for social justice" (SJSA, n.d.). SJSA conducts workshops in schools, prisons, and community centers where adult volunteer mentors teach youth "to use textile art as a vehicle for personal transformation and community cohesion and become agents of social change" (SJSA, n.d.). Youth create quilt blocks illustrating the social justice issues important to them, and then these squares are sent to volunteers who embellish and embroider them. The embellished blocks are then sewn together to create quilts that are exhibited in museums, galleries, and quilt shows. The foundation of the SJSA process is to center the voices of marginalized youth and encourage intergenerational and intercultural dialogue that results in "a truly collective vision—both hopeful and critical—for social justice" (Schmidt, 2019, p. 304).

Another powerful example of how the quilt form can serve as a site for activism is an arts-based community project created by Michelle Napoli and Michaela Kirby (2019), which I had a chance to participate in. Their project began with the intention to create a space for open dialogue about healthy sexuality. They invited community members to create images of vulvas using a dry-wool felting technique with the purpose of facilitating "a process where one can recognize a part of our body that is often hidden, denied, disowned, or pathologized, to critically question what has been made taboo by society" (p. 284). These images were then assembled onto a quilt titled the *Vulva Quilt*, which also featured anatomical and slang words as "another step in breaking the silence and taboo" (p. 286).

Despite the therapeutic and transformational potential evident in these examples, the practice of craftivism is currently facing justified criticism, as individuals illustrate how craftivism has fallen short of its inclusive aims and has even resulted in silencing marginalized voices (e.g., Feliz, 2017; Ivey, 2019; Schmidt, 2019) and/or erasing or appropriating historic uses of craft and craft activism (Han Sifuentes, 2017; Ivey, 2019). Another important critique of craftivism is that the crafts that many people in the Global North have historically engaged in as leisure activities constitute poorly paid or unpaid labor for poor and working class people and people of color throughout the world (Han Sifuentes, 2017; Portwood-Stacer, 2007; Robertson & Vinebaum, 2016).

Some scholars have also questioned whether craftivism is in fact as feminist in practice as proclaimed. Communication and gender studies scholar Laura Portwood-Stacer (2007) challenged the craftivist belief that simply choosing to make something imbues the creative act and product with feminist activism. She asserted that "for feminist praxis to be truly effective, it must transcend the individual and recuperate a social politics that takes broad, radical change as its ultimate goal" (p. 17). Curator Ele Carpenter (2010) noted that as certain forms of crafting became associated with the "retro feminine fashion" of the mid-20th century, they inadvertently reinforced gender stereotypes about women's roles as homemakers, which has detracted from the valuable history of craft employed as activism. She argued that the commodification of the DIY/craft movement served as a "cutesy approach to selling craft back to women as a form of artificial liberation" (Carpenter, 2010, para. 17) and warned that this commercialization can co-opt the political aims of activist craft. I agree that the commercialization of the DIY/craft movement has capitalized on concepts of empowerment and liberation and can reflect a consumerist culture (Dawkins, 2011; Ouellette & Hay, 2008; Solomon, 2013), although I think it is important to note that despite having similar roots, craftivism is not synonymous with the DIY craft community. All of these critiques raise important considerations for art therapists interested in incorporating craft activism into their practice.

There is evidence in the craftivism projects described earlier of a potential to contribute to genuine empowerment and liberation for participants. My hope is that the Crafting Change group can serve as an example for how culturally relevant craft techniques, such as quilting for African American women, can be used in a way that strengthens cultural pride rather than being appropriative or tokenizing. I also hope it provides one model for how craft activism can be employed in an equitable and socially just art therapy practice that results in marginalized voices being centered and amplified, not erased, left out, or disregarded.

The Crafting Change Group

The Crafting Change group assembled as part of my doctoral research in September 2017. In total, there have been eight of us in the group—three members from a preexisting art therapy sewing group (one of whom had just joined the group the day this project started), two sisters of one of the members of the sewing group, the health center's director of behavioral health, and a mental health counselor who provided occasional translation services. All of us identify as women, and we range in age from 34 to 75, with five of the members being seniors. Our group is also culturally and racially diverse, made up of African Americans, Afro-Latinas, an Asian Filipina, and one white person (me). One group member's first language is Spanish, and she has been in the process of learning English while our group has been meeting.

We meet at a community health center in the Roxbury neighborhood of Boston, and most group members live in Roxbury or nearby. About 65% of Roxbury's population is made up of African Americans and immigrants from Africa, with people of Hispanic or Latinx roots accounting for 25% and white people representing about 10% of the population (Roxbury Historical Society, n.d.). Roxbury has the second-highest rate of mental health hospitalizations among Boston's neighborhoods and struggles with community violence, leading to high rates of posttraumatic stress disorder (Whittier Street Annual Reports, 2016). Despite these and other challenges, Roxbury has a rich history of arts and culture, including jazz clubs and public art, as well as grassroots activism (Roxbury Historical Society, n.d.).

The core of the Crafting Change group, as well as the original research project that it grew out of (Leone, 2018), is the practice of participatory action research (PAR): a process that results in co-researchers developing critical consciousness (Freire, 1970), which in turn results in capacity building and agency through knowledge generation. This iterative process involves collaboratively creating plans, taking action on them, reflecting on the action, and making our subsequent decisions in response to our experience so far. Craft practices—particularly those that lend themselves to collective practice, such as knitting circles and open shop time—complement the PAR process, as they can promote community building, storytelling, and appropriate pacing for exploration, action, and reflection, all of which are integral to the PAR process. The Crafting Change group established this technique as our foundation when we first began meeting, and we continue to use this process today. The project described here unfolded in three stages based on this participatory action process: (a) naming the issue and planning the project, (b) reflecting and taking action through creating, and (c) exhibiting our creation and sharing our message.

Naming the Issue and Planning the Project

We dedicated our first two meetings to identifying the issue we wanted to address and to plan the project. I provided examples of historical uses of craft activism and contemporary craftivism projects, and we collaborated as a group to identify an issue in the community that group members wanted to address. Initially, we were interested in creating a quilt to commemorate the many jazz clubs in the neighborhood that have closed over the past few decades, seeking to highlight that the neighborhood, which is often associated with crime and poverty, in fact has a rich cultural history.

As we continued to explore this issue, however, the group concluded that the real reason the jazz clubs were no longer active was the gentrification and displacement taking place in the neighborhood. Participants were concerned that the community wasn't paying close enough attention or didn't feel empowered to intervene in the changes happening in the neighborhood. We perceived that a lack of community cohesion might be part of what allowed these processes to happen, and so we decided to focus our project on calling attention to gentrification and displacement in the hopes of motivating viewers into action.

I taught the group about a range of possible craft methods, including knitting, crochet, embroidery, appliqué, and quilting. We decided that a quilt would be the right format for our project, given that many group members felt a cultural connection to the strong tradition of African American quilting and had memories from their youth of family members quilting. The quilt itself, with its traditional symbolism of caring, comfort, and association to the domestic sphere, seemed like a subversive way to call attention to issues of gentrification and displacement, as people who are no longer able to stay in neighborhoods they have called home for decades are having their safety and comfort compromised. We also decided to use embroidery and appliquéd photo transfers to illustrate images of historical community spaces that no longer exist, alongside historical local and national leaders who had fought for justice and equity. We titled the quilt *Wake Up Everybody* to reflect our desire to call attention to issues related to gentrification and displacement and to encourage the greater community to take notice and take action.

Reflecting and Taking Action Through Creating

Over the next three months we shared knowledge and skills as we created the quilt. I provided the group with a range of craft materials, including solid and patterned fabric; embroidery floss; notions (e.g., buttons, ribbons, and zippers); and tools such as fabric glue, scissors, and rotary cutters. We had two sewing machines and tools for hand sewing. I provided books about craftivism, African American quilting traditions, and technical instructions on quilting and embroidery.

We used my laptop in each session to research the history of the neighborhood and community leaders, including downloading images to include in the quilt, which we printed onto inkjet fabric sheets. Although some crafting and art-making materials are quite expensive, quilting supplies can be inexpensive and are therefore fairly financially accessible; most of the fabric for our quilt came from donations or old sheets. Some individuals even brought in fabric that had personal meaning to them, such as family members' clothing.

Each of us decided on a theme for a square we wanted to create for the quilt, and as we worked on these individual pieces we collectively reflected on the problems of gentrification and displacement through discussion, storytelling, and the art-making process itself. One issue we discussed at length was how displacement specifically affects seniors. We also talked about former local and national community leaders who had inspired group members in their sense of social justice. Ideas and direct quotes from our discussions often made their way directly into the images and words that individuals included on their quilt squares (Figure 10.1, 10.2, 10.3).

As we crafted together over the course of several weeks, we began to notice themes emerging both from the crafting process and from the quilt we were creating. The stitching action served as a metaphor for the issues being addressed, as described by one group member: "The stitches . . . it's stitching things together like we're trying to stitch ourselves back together and our city back together because of gentrification." Participants also reported that the stitching process was "relaxing," "therapeutic," and "intimate." Also, because sewing by hand can be a slow process, some group members took the squares they were working on home between our sessions, creating a transitional object that they reported made them feel connected to our group and our mission between meetings. And because of the slow process of hand stitching, we spent longer in conversation with each other than we anticipated, which supported us in developing mutually respectful, trusting relationships with each other.

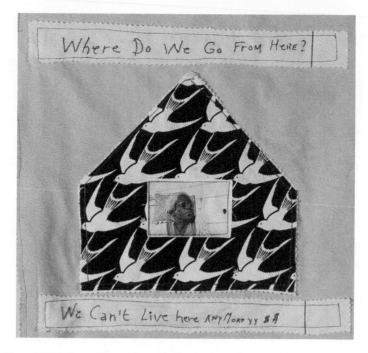

Figure 10.1 Brenda's square, *Wake Up Everybody* Collaborative Quilt

Source: Photo by Sarah Trahan

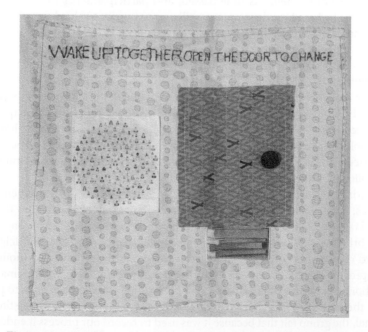

Figure 10.2 Sarah's square, *Wake Up Everybody* Collaborative Quilt

Source: Photo by Sarah Trahan

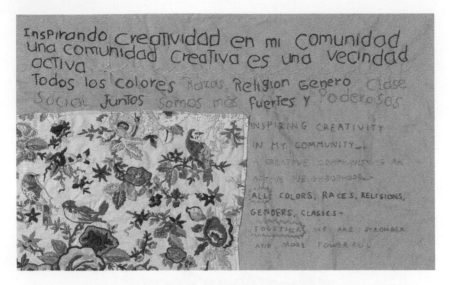

Figure 10.3 Francisca's square, *Wake Up Everybody* Collaborative Quilt

Source: Photo by Sarah Trahan

The quilt project took longer than we had initially planned for, but participants felt it was important to continue working, as the mission of the project was important to them. As time passed, and participants began to take over specific tasks based on their unique skills, everyone was valued for what they individually brought to the collective. This engagement in community building allowed for people's strengths to be recognized and named as we came to rely on each individual for different needs, rather than feeling that we each had to do a little bit of everything.

Our quilt became an object that held individual stories and perspectives while also housing a collective message. The symbolic function of the quilt as an object where many different pieces create a unified message parallels how we were able to each contribute to the group based on our tacit skills and personal histories with crafting and activism and while also learning from and building the collective knowledge of the group.

During this first project I created a "stitched journal" to document the themes, images, and phrases that came up during our meetings (Figure 10.4). I would take notes while we met and then embroider and appliqué between meetings, bringing the journal back to the group each week to show participants and to confirm that I was accurately documenting our process and thoughts. This process eventually took on a sort of "secretarial" function, but it remained collaborative: participants decided how to finish it and eventually even to place it on the quilt. Even though that wasn't my original intention for the stitched journal, the group felt that because it was used to record our process it ended up embodying the intentions of our quilt; thus, it should be a part of the quilt itself.

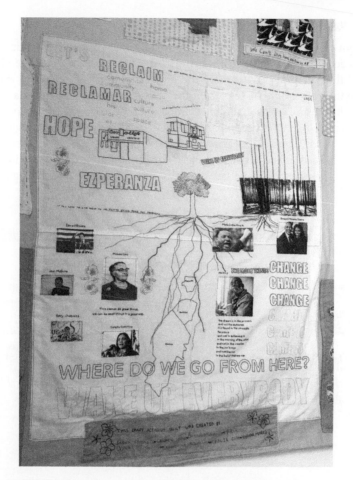

Figure 10.4 Lauren's stitched journal

This stitched journal also served as a form of arts-based inquiry and allowed for an important self-reflexive process, as I used the time I worked on it between group sessions as a way of examining the role my identities and social location as a white, cisgender, heterosexual, able-bodied woman with class and citizenship privilege played with respect to privilege, assumptions, and biases and how those identities and social location might impact the research process and the group as whole (Talwar, 2010). Relationships are dynamic; thus, so are identities and positions within groups. Throughout the time our group has been meeting, I have found myself fluctuating between holding the roles of researcher, facilitator, collaborator, advocate, and listener/witness. It's essential that I examine my power due to these varying responsibilities and roles (Ottemiller & Awais, 2016). Additionally, as I am still an outsider to this community, I was and continue to be deliberate about negotiating power with and transferring control to the community as the group continues to meet and our projects unfold (Kapitan, 2018).

Exhibiting the Quilt and Sharing Our Message

As we got closer to completing the quilt, we began to plan and strategize about what to do with the quilt once it was finished (Figure 10.5, Color Plate 11). We decided that the best way to share the knowledge we had generated through creating the quilt would be to present the quilt in a range of settings via a "travelling exhibit" and engage audiences in conversation about the rationale for why we created it. One group participant wrote a script for the presentation, which we edited together and translated into Spanish for one of our Afro-Latina members to read in her native language. The presentation would also include a reading of the poem "Still, I Rise" by Maya Angelou—also in both English and

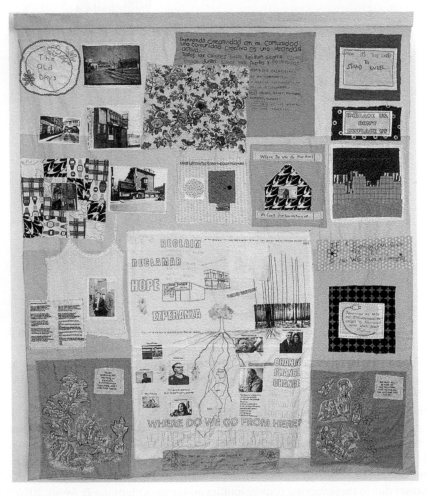

Figure 10.5 Wake Up Everybody Collaborative Quilt

Source: Photo by Sarah Trahan

Spanish—as the group felt it embodied the spirit of our project and the conviction we wanted to imbue in our audience.

We scheduled our first presentation at the community health center where we had been meeting, and shortly after were invited to give another presentation about our project at the center's senior holiday lunch. We strategized about who to invite to the presentations based on who we felt would benefit from hearing our call to action, as well as who had the institutional power to potentially ally with us to effect policy about development in the neighborhood.

The presentations were very well-received, which reinforced our group's sense of the project's importance and our motivation to continue to share our work with the community. We have since taken several additional opportunities to present the quilt—some by invitation and some by application, some within Roxbury and some in other neighborhoods and cities—in a juried gallery show themed around the concept of "sanctuary," at a craft museum's "Make a Difference Day," for a university art therapy class, for a senior group at a local YMCA, at the Museum of the National Center of Afro-American Artists (located in Roxbury), and at a housing justice forum focused on the Boston housing crisis, inequality, and diversity.

Crafting Change Now

Perhaps the strongest testament to the value of the craftivism experience for participants is that our group continues to meet over two years after the conclusion of our first project. Throughout this time we have continued to develop community and build trust. Since we completed *Wake Up Everybody*, we have worked on two other large projects. The first project involved creating a book of photographs entitled *Crafting Change: Finding Our Way Together* (Franklin et al., 2018).[1] The book allowed each co-researcher of the Crafting Change group to have a tangible record of our collaborative process and a product to show friends and family. It also served as a quiet and approachable way to disseminate our research findings alongside our public exhibitions and presentations, which involved a lot of coordination and effort from participants. The book also allowed us to make the message of the quilt even more portable than the quilt itself. Because the quilt itself is quite large and embroidery and appliqué are best seen close up, the book contains zoomed-in detail photos to represent all of the elements of the quilt in addition to wide shots of the whole quilt. The group also decided to include photos and brief bios of all co-researchers in order to provide more context for the project. The book's title was inspired by the following description: "Action research is a process rather than a product, and as such, our invitation is one of finding our way together rather than getting to a predetermined end" (Herr & Anderson, 2015, p. 155). This phrase exemplifies the process of conceiving this project, carrying it out, and presenting it to the community—and our group's ongoing focus on collaboration and consensus decision-making as we continue to navigate new projects together.

Our second major project, currently underway, is a new quilt that combines group members' personal experiences with our exploration of craft activism.

The project began as one participant's idea to create a quilt for Mother's Day that focused on women who have been mentors or have been inspiring for group members in our own efforts to have a positive impact on our communities, but it has since expanded to include direct reference to craft activism we had previously discussed in the group.

At the beginning of our first project I showed photographs of Judy Chicago's *The Dinner Party* while discussing the feminist art movement of the 1970s. I noted that some feminists took issue with the fact that only one Black woman, Sojourner Truth, is represented in the art piece (Walker, 1983) and also that, although the work was regarded as collaborative, Chicago was criticized for taking full credit for the conception and creation of the piece and inadequately recognizing other contributors (Jones, 2005).

Our new quilt combines these ideas and aims to pay homage to women of color who have inspired group members through arts, sports, politics, social justice, and/or community organizing. These individuals have made significant contributions to history but many remain under-appreciated, which has inspired the working title for our new quilt: *The Hidden Figures Dinner Party*.

This project has served an educational purpose for the group as we teach each other about the historical accomplishments of people we weren't all initially familiar with. The quilt is taking the form of a collection of embroidered portraits of 25 individuals, ranging in chronology from Ida B. Wells to Aretha Franklin, and will also include a list of about 100 additional embroidered names of individuals we want to honor and bring viewers' attention to (Figure 10.6).

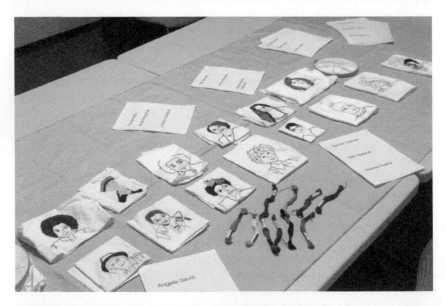

Figure 10.6 Embroidered portraits for *The Hidden Figures Dinner Party* Collaborative Quilt

Our plan is to finish this quilt in time to exhibit it for International Women's Day 2021, and we are currently reaching out to partner with organizations where we feel exhibiting the quilt will provide educational and activist impacts. We are also planning a photo book of this new quilt, which will feature educational material about each of the individuals represented on it.

Reflecting on Our Experience

In preparation for writing this chapter and in maintaining the collaborative and power-sharing practices we have established, I facilitated the group in a critical dialogue circle so we could reflect on how things have shifted since the official research project ended in December 2017. I wanted to be sure each group member's perspective and voice was accurately portrayed as I wrote about our work together.

The most prominent theme to come from our most recent discussion was the importance of community and a sense of belonging. One participant stated, "The main point I would like emphasized is how the group has come together as a family," continuing, "I don't think that would have been possible without the art therapy piece, but [art therapy] is only a piece of what goes on here." Another participant responded to this statement by saying, "True, we help each other." A third said, "It makes me feel like I'm a part of something, and I really enjoy and I hope it never ends." A fourth participant stated, "I thank God that we're still here, as a group, as a family. And I appreciate that, because over the last 4 to 5 months, there have been a lot of changes [at the community health center]." She summarized: "I appreciate that we're still together."

A second important theme that came up through this discussion was how the Crafting Change group provided something that felt like it transcended the day-to-day and provided participants with support. One individual shared, "It gives me something to do, it gives me something to look forward to, it gets me out of the house and keeps me kind of busy. It helps me focus. And I depend on art therapy because it keeps me kind of calm and settled." Another stated, "I think we each like [the group] for different reasons, but I think the break [from] doing what you do every day is a blessing, and also you're getting something out of it." A third stated, "Art therapy has got me over a lot of hurdles."

Perhaps one of the most important results for me personally has been the frank intercultural discussion the group has been able to have about race and class, on societal and very personal levels. One participant in particular commented on this, sharing directly to me that she initially would have chosen to not come to the group "specifically because you are white," as she has historically been "steadfast on not allowing people to use [her or her people] for upward mobility" but that the focus on craft attracted her in spite of this, and that the way we worked together allowed her to build a relationship with me.

As we continue to develop trusting relationships the mutual support between group members has become even more prominent. A few weeks ago a participant entered the group and said she was doing well, but other participants perceived sadness in her affect and pressed her on this. In response, she shared some family stress she was managing and others offered support, advice and reminded her to reach out to them when she is having a hard time. One member stated, "When [she] walked in, you can tell she's hurting, and it's like, 'Let's stop and acknowledge that.' That's beautiful to me." Another responded, "You can call me anytime—I'm always around. If I don't want to talk to you, I'll call you [back] later, but I will always answer." She added, "You never know where you're gonna get help from. It doesn't have to be in the doctor's office—there's many doctors in this community that have no degree."

This anecdote is indicative of the strongest theme to come out of the discussion, which was the idea that helping others is not only the right thing to do but feeds the helper as well. One participant described this as follows: "It doesn't cost me anything to lift people up. Not only does it not cost you, but it *gives* you. I think that is what stood out to me before, and stands out to me now." This statement also reflects the sense of empowerment that group members have built to meet their own and each other's needs, rather than relying solely on larger systems.

Therapeutic Benefits of Collaborative Craft Activism

The Crafting Change group demonstrates that collaborative craft focused on activism and practiced in a community-based art therapy context can support individuals in empowering themselves and being change agents. Our group supports members in (a) expressing social realities, (b) building community, (c) accessing art and social action, (d) pacing social interaction and reflection, (e) crossing boundaries, (f) being subversive, (g) being awakened and awakening others, and (h) creating a forum for speaking and being heard.

Expressing Social Realities

Early views on craft in art therapy denied its expressive value because of its historical association with the creation of functional objects (Kramer, 1975; Ulman, Kramer, & Kwiatkowska, 1977). But the Crafting Change group directly challenges these beliefs. We have used culturally resonant practices to create artworks that are functional objects but also symbolic and expressive. Craft can indeed be used to engage in creative, expressive work, whether focused on activism or not. We have even found meaningful fiber-specific symbolism in our stitching process, which arose in our group's internal conversation and in the phrasing of the messages included on our first quilt that we wanted our audience to see. The unique contributory format of quilting has allowed us to retain our individual voices while multiplying them into a collective voice—we created an artwork that communicated the group's shared message in addition to all the participants' individual messages. And we've watched at our exhibitions as attendees approached the quilt, first looking from afar but then drawing near to see the details of the stitching and the embroidery, creating a sense of intimacy.

Building Community

When group therapy participants craft together, individuals' experiences are validated in an atmosphere of mutual support (see, e.g., Garlock, 2016; Huss, 2010; Moxley, Feen-Calligan, Washington, & Garriott, 2011; Reynolds, 2000). When art therapy is placed in a social justice context, as is the case for our group's work, validation and support take on increased importance and support participants' self-empowerment and capacity for action. People who feel supported are better equipped to speak their truth and confront power imbalances. This has been evidenced in our group when individuals advocated for themselves when interacting with administrators at the community health center where we meet and during presentations of the quilt. We have also identified mutual trust and support within the group as attributes that serve us individually, and we have also shared the insights and knowledge from our work with our friends and families, as well as our larger community.

Although storytelling is a common feature of crafting groups (Garlock, 2016; Moxley et al., 2011; Reynolds, 2004), it may be of more critical importance in groups focused on emancipatory practice. In our group's experience, in a social justice context, storytelling has provided group members with a way of sharing knowledge with each other and has conveyed information and advocacy to community leaders. We have used collaborative craft as a form of activism to direct attention to cultural landmarks that no longer exist in the neighborhood, employing storytelling to share important history and community knowledge. Art therapists and community artists can honor individuals' cultural and historical knowledge by employing collaborative craft practices to support dialogue. When extending this premise to social justice, the idea that everyone has important contributions to make supports ordinary people in instigating the change needed in their communities, rather than feeling the need for outside experts (Kapitan, Litell, & Torres, 2011; Timm-Bottos, 2017; Timm-Bottos & Reilly, 2015). Additionally, our group has found that a shared sense of purpose toward our activist goals creates community, and, reciprocally, the sense of community we built lends itself to this shared mission.

Accessing Art and Activism

In an art therapy context, fiber craft can accommodate a range of skill levels. Individuals can contribute to the knowledge-creation process based on their own unique strengths, skills, and experience, and can be valued for those contributions. In our case, each participant's unique skills have helped to build a collaborative atmosphere that, over time, has led to greater sharing of skills and knowledge, which suggests capacity building and mastery. Group members use the collaborative crafting process to identify and reflect on issues in the community that we seek to change and in the process rebuild a sense of community that we have identified as lacking. Group members also have taken control of how to share our new learning with the community so that the impacts are multiplied.

Pacing Social Interaction and Reflection

Within literature on both therapeutic craft (e.g., Reynolds, 1999) and craftivism (e.g., Corbett, 2017), the slow process of crafting has been proposed as a way for individuals to take time to reflect on issues they are seeking to address. Art therapy's roots in Western psychology, as well as the U.S. cultural value of individualism, emphasize the benefits of individual reflection; however, in community practice, individual reflection is only one part of the benefit of craft. One of the ways collaborative crafting builds community is that it encourages participants to become closer and more familiar with one another. The extended time for collective reflection supports the complexity of engaging in critical examination of social issues. Meanwhile, community support allows the responsibility for change to shift from the individual to the collective, which moves away from the neoliberal idea that "healing" is an individual responsibility (Gipson, 2017; Talwar, 2019).

Crossing Boundaries

Art therapists have observed that artworks created in sessions may serve as transitional objects that can be carried outside the session to maintain a sense of connection (e.g., Homer, 2015; McCulloguh, 2009; Morris & Willis-Rauch, 2014). The transportability of many fiber crafts may serve a similar purpose, as seen with Crafting Change group members who bring their quilt squares home to work on them, thereby maintaining a sense of connection with the group between meetings. The individual quilt squares also represent the social justice focus being carried into individuals' lives between meetings, which facilitates a multiplier effect whereby the larger community learns from those engaged in knowledge construction in smaller community settings. Additionally, the portability of the final products we create means that we can bring our quilts into different settings and communities, thus exposing a wider range of audiences to our work. If we created something site-specific, such as a mural, this wouldn't be possible. And the book we created about our first project makes this process of sharing our learning even more feasible.

Being Subversive

There is a long history of individuals and groups using craft subversively. In our work, we exploit the connotation of quilts as comforting, nurturing, and related to the home. The *Wake Up Everybody* quilt—a symbol of shelter and protection—confronts gentrification and displacement, two forces that directly challenge peoples' comfort, well-being, and safety. We also subvert popular opinion of crafting as a benign hobby for older women—something that is harmless, even time-killing busywork (Chansky, 2010; Greer, 2019). Instead, we have found that craft takes on a new meaning when the very individuals who are routinely considered "benign" and powerless subvert societal expectations and create a strong and powerful call for social justice. Clearly, collaborative craft activism holds material and symbolic potential that individuals can strategically employ to ensure impact.

Being Awakened and Awakening Others

Although the Crafting Change group identified an initial intent of "waking up" the community with our first project, several participants reported that through the process, they effectively woke *themselves* up as well. They have recognized that they have something important to say and feel an increased personal drive and motivation to contribute more to their community, coupled with the agency to actually do so. Depending on their personal histories, they defined this either as a first awakening or as a reawakening of a dormant part of themselves: by focusing on the process of sharing a call to action with their community, participants have found an increased sense of empowerment and feel compelled and motivated into action as well.

Creating a Forum for Speaking and Being Heard

Arundhati Roy, an Indian writer and activist, stressed that "it is not so much that communities and their members are voiceless, but that others have intentionally turned a deaf ear to their well-being and concerns" (as cited in Watkins & Shulman, 2008, p. 276). Using craft in an effort to foster self-empowerment, build community, examine social realities, and effect change can create a forum for speaking and being heard by one's community—whether literally—as in the case of the Crafting Change group—or figuratively. Several art therapists have noted the potential catalytic effects that occur when art therapy participants share their artwork with their community (Andrus, 2017; Block, Harris, & Laing, 2005; Houpt, Balkin, Broom, Roth, & Selma, 2016; Morris & Willis-Rauch, 2014; Thompson, 2009), including social power. When people who have been marginalized gain visibility in the larger culture by sharing art about their experience, "power flows from that visibility with an insistence on mutual respect, equality, and support for self-determination" (Kapitan, 2014, p. 3). By creating and presenting the quilt, group members have found an audience for their voices and an ability to make an impact. The process has also resulted in group members gaining access to power brokers and spaces where marginalized voices are not always welcomed; in this way the group has been able to engage the community in dialogue about the issues we feel need to be addressed.

Conclusion

Incorporating craft activism into art therapy practice offers a powerful and effective way to incorporate a social justice model into community practice and functions as praxis. Craft activism can build individuals' capacity to address the issues that affect them and their communities, and developing these skills serves a therapeutic function. Building on the powerful history of people who have used craft to claim power and resist against social and political oppression, craft activism can be a way for contemporary art therapy practitioners and participants to envision and craft the change that is needed in their communities.

Note

1. To see the Crafting Change: Finding Our Way Together book visit crafting-change.laurenleone. com

References

Agosín, M. (2008). *Tapestries of hope, threads of love: The* arpillera *movement in Chile* (2nd ed.). Lanham, MD: Rowman & Littlefield.

The AIDS Memorial Quilt. (n.d.). *About.* Retrieved from www.aidsquilt.org/about/the-aids-memorial-quilt

Andrus, M. (2017). *Private to public: Therapeutic impact and ethics of sharing artwork in trauma resolution* (Unpublished doctoral dissertation). Mount Mary University, Milwaukee, WI.

Black, A., & Burisch, N. (2011). Craft hard, die free: Radical curatorial strategies for craftivism in unruly contexts. In M. A. Buszek (Ed.), *Extra/ordinary: Craft and contemporary art* (pp. 204–221). Durham, NC: Duke University Press.

Block, D., Harris, T., & Laing, S. (2005). Open studio process as a model of social action: A program for at-risk youth. *Art Therapy: Journal of the American Art Therapy Association, 22*(1), 32–38. doi:10.1080/07421656.2005.10129459

Carpenter, E. (2010). Activist tendencies in craft. In G. Cox, N. Haq, & T. Trevor (Eds.), *Concept store #3: Art, activism and recuperation* (pp. 86–91). Bristol, England: Arnolfini. Retrieved from https://research.gold.ac.uk/3109/1/Activist_Tendencies_in_Craft_EC.pdf

Chansky, R. A. (2010). A stitch in time: Third-wave feminist reclamation of needled imagery. *Journal of Popular Culture, 43*(4), 681–700. doi:10.1111/j.15405931.2010.00765.x PMID:20645475

Corbett, S. (2017). *How to be a craftivist: The art of gentle protest.* London, England: Unbound.

Dawkins, N. (2011). Do it yourself: The precarious work and postfeminist politics of handmaking (in) detroit. *Utopian Studies, 22,* 266–277.

Feliz, J. (2017, August 23). *An open letter to the craftivism movement* [Blog post]. Retrieved from https://medium.com/@jd.feliz/an-open-letter-to-the-craftivism-movement-816ccb285b0

Franklin, B., Franklin, D., Franklin, S., Gore, L., Leone, L., Lopez, F., . . . Pajarillo, C. (2018). *Crafting change: Finding our way together.* Self-published, Blurb.com.

Freire, P. (1970). *Pedagogy of the oppressed.* New York, NY: Herder & Herder.

Garlock, L. R. (2016). Stories in the cloth: Art therapy and narrative textiles. *Art Therapy: Journal of the American Art Therapy Association, 33*(2), 58–66. doi:10.1080/07421656.2016.1164004

Gipson, L. (2017). Challenging neoliberalism and multicultural love in art therapy, *Art Therapy: Journal of the American Art Therapy Association, 34*(3), 112–117, doi: 10.1080/07421656.2017.1353326

Greer, B. (2011). Craftivist history. In M. A. Buszek (Ed.), *Extra/ordinary: Craft and contemporary art* (pp. 175–183). Durham, NC: Duke University Press.

Greer, B. (2019). Crafting a place in history: Creating subversion with handcrafts in modernity. In H. Mandell (Ed.), *Crafting dissent: Handicraft as protest from the American Revolution to the Pussyhats* (pp. 233–238). Lanham, MD: Rowman & Littlefield.

Han Sifuentes, A. (2017, April 23). Steps towards decolonizing craft [Blog post]. *Textile Society of America*. Retrieved from https://textilesocietyofamerica.org/6728/steps-towards-decolonizing-craft/

Herr, K., & Anderson, G. (2015). *The action research dissertation: A guide for students and faculty.* London, England: Sage Publications.

Homer, E. S. (2015). Piece work: Fabric collage as a neurodevelopmental approach to trauma treatment. *Art Therapy: Journal of the American Art Therapy Association, 32*(1), 20–26. doi:10.1080/07421656.2015.992824

Houpt, K., Balkin, L., Broom, R. H., Roth, A. G., & Selma. (2016). Anti-memoir: Creating alternate nursing home narratives through zine making. *Art Therapy: Journal of the American Art Therapy Association, 33*(3), 128–137. doi:10.1080/07421656.2016.1199243

Huss, E. (2010). Bedouin women's embroidery as female empowerment: Crafts as culturally embedded expression within art therapy. In C. H. Moon (Ed.), *Materials and media in art therapy: Critical understandings of diverse artistic vocabularies* (pp. 215–230). New York, NY: Routledge.

Ivey, D. (2019). Reshaping the narrative around people of color and craftivism. In H. Mandell (Ed.), *Crafting dissent: Handicraft as protest from the American Revolution to the Pussyhats* (pp. 309–318). Lanham, MD: Rowman & Littlefield.

Jones, A. (2005). The "sexual politics" of the dinner party. In N. Broude & M. D. Garrard (Eds.), *Reclaiming female agency: Feminist art history after postmodernism* (pp. 409–433). Berkeley: University of California Press.

Kapitan, L. (2014). Empowerment in art therapy: Whose point of view and determination? *Art Therapy: Journal of the American Art Therapy Association, 28*(1), 2–3. doi:10.1080/07421656.2014.876755

Kapitan, L. (2018). *An introduction to art therapy research* (2nd ed.). New York, NY: Routledge.

Kapitan, L., Litell, M., & Torres, A. (2011). Creative art therapy in a community's participatory research and social transformation. *Art Therapy: Journal of the American Art Therapy Association, 28*(2), 64–73. doi:10.1080/07421656.2011.578238

Kramer, E. (1975). Art and craft. In E. Ulman & P. Dachinger (Eds.), *Art therapy in theory and practice* (pp. 106–109). New York, NY: Schocken Books.

Leone, L. (2018). *Crafting change: Craft activism and community-based art therapy* (Doctoral dissertation). Mount Mary University. Retrieved from www.worldcat.org/oclc/1035718897

Leone, L. (2019). Crafting change: Craft activism for community-based art therapy. In H. Mandell (Ed.), *Crafting dissent: Handicraft as protest from the American Revolution to the Pussyhats* (pp. 247–262). Lanham, MD: Rowman & Littlefield.

Lufkin, F. (2019). The underground railroad quilt code myth and the culture of crafted experience. In H. Mandell (Ed.), *Crafting dissent: Handicraft as protest from the American Revolution to the Pussyhats* (pp. 77–94). Lanham, MD: Rowman & Littlefield.

McCulloguh, C. (2009). A child's use of transitional objects in art therapy to cope with divorce. *Art Therapy: Journal of the American Art Therapy Association, 26*(1), 19–25. doi:10.1080/07421656.2009.10129306

Morris, F. J., & Willis-Rauch, M. (2014). Join the art club: Exploring social empowerment in art therapy. *Art Therapy: Journal of the American Art Therapy Association, 31*(1), 28–36. doi:10.1080/07421656.2014.873694

Moxley, D. P., Feen-Calligan, H., Washington, O. G. M., & Garriott, L. (2011). Quilting in self-efficacy group work with older African American women leaving homelessness. *Art Therapy: Journal of the American Art Therapy Association, 28*(3), 113–122. doi:10.1080/07421656.2011.599729

Napoli, M., & Kirby, M. (2019). Crafting the "Vulva Quilt": A community response to being silenced. In H. Mandell (Ed.), *Crafting dissent: Handicraft as protest from the American Revolution to the Pussyhats* (pp. 279–290). Lanham, MD: Rowman & Littlefield.

Ottemiller, D. D., & Awais, Y. J. (2016). A model for art therapists in community-based practice. *Art Therapy: Journal of the American Art Therapy Association, 33*(3), 144–150. doi:10.1080/07421656.2016.1199245

Ouellette, L., & Hay, J. (2008). Makeover TV: Labors of reinvention. In L. Ouellette & J. Hay (Eds.), *Better living through reality TV: Television and post-welfare citizenship* (pp. 99–102). Malden, MA: Blackwell.

Portwood-Stacer, L. (2007, May). *Do-it-yourself feminism: Feminine individualism and the girlie backlash in the "craftivism" movement.* Paper presented at the annual meeting of the International Communication Association, San Francisco, CA. Retrieved from http://citation.allacademic.com/meta/p169635_index.html

Reed, T. V. (2005). *The art of protest.* Minneapolis: University of Minnesota Press.

Reynolds, F. (1999). Cognitive behavioral counseling of unresolved grief through the therapeutic adjunct of tapestry-making. *The Arts in Psychotherapy, 26*(3), 165–171.

Reynolds, F. (2000). Managing depression through needlecraft creative activities: A qualitative study. *The Arts in Psychotherapy, 27*(2), 107–114.

Reynolds, F. (2004). Textile art promoting well-being in long-term illness: Some general and specific influences. *Journal of Occupational Science, 11*(2), 58–67.

Robertson, K. (2011). Rebellious doilies and subversive stitches: Writing a craftivist history. In M. A. Buszek (Ed.), *Extra/ordinary: Craft and contemporary art* (pp. 184–203). Durham, NC: Duke University Press.

Robertson, K., & Vinebaum, L. (2016). Crafting community. *Textile, 14*(1), 2–13. doi:10.1080/14759756.2016.1084794

Roxbury Historical Society. (n.d.). *About Roxbury.* Retrieved from http://roxburyhistoricalsociety.org/about-roxbury/

Schmidt, S. (2019). Craft as a pedagogy of hope. In H. Mandell (Ed.), *Crafting dissent: Handicraft as protest from the American Revolution to the Pussyhats* (pp. 291–308). Lanham, MD: Rowman & Littlefield.

Sharma, R., & Bhaduri, G. (2019). How homespun cotton became the fabric of Indian political life. In H. Mandell (Ed.), *Crafting dissent: Handicraft as protest from the American Revolution to the Pussyhats* (pp. 123–137). Lanham, MD: Rowman & Littlefield.

Social Justice Sewing Academy. (n.d.). *What we do.* Retrieved from www.sjsacademy.com/what-we-do.html

Solomon, E. (2013). Craftivism and the professional-amateur: A literature review on do it yourself activist craft culture. *PsychNology Journal, 11*(1), 11–20.

Talwar, S. (2010). An intersectional framework for race, class, gender, and sexuality in art therapy. *Art Therapy: Journal of the American Art Therapy Association, 27*(1), 11–17. doi:10.1080/07421656.2010.10129567

Talwar, S. (2019). Beyond multiculturalism and cultural competence: A social justice vision in art therapy. In S. Talwar (Ed.), *Art therapy for social justice: Radical intersections* (pp. 3–16). New York, NY: Routledge.

Thompson, G. (2009). Artistic sensibility in the studio and gallery model: Revisiting process and product. *Art Therapy: Journal of the American Art Therapy Association, 26*(4), 159–166. doi:10.1080/07421656.2009.10129609

Timm-Bottos, J. (2017). Public practice art therapy: Enabling spaces across North America (La pratique publique de l'art-thérapie: Des espaces habilitants partout en Amérique du Nord). *Canadian Art Therapy Association Journal, 30*(2), 94–99. doi:10.1080/08322473.2017.1385215

Timm-Bottos, J., & Reilly, R. C. (2015). Learning in third spaces: Community art studio as storefront university classroom. *American Journal of Community Psychology, 55*, 102–114. doi:10.1007/s10464-014-9688-5

Ulman, E., Kramer, E., & Kwiatkowska, H. (1977). *Art therapy in the United States.* Craftsbury Commons, VT: Art Therapy Publications.

Walker, A. (1983). *In search of our mother's gardens: Womanist prose.* San Diego, CA: Harcourt Brace Jonanovich.

Watkins, M., & Shulman, H. (2008). *Towards psychologies of liberation.* New York, NY: Palgrave MacMillan.

Wheeler, E. (2012). *The political stitch: Voicing resistance in a suffrage textile.* Textile Society of America 13th Biennial Symposium Proceedings: Textiles and Politics, 758. Retrieved from https://digitalcommons.unl.edu/tsaconf/758/

Whittier Street Annual Report. (2016). Retrieved from www.wshc.org/assets/2016-Whittier-Street-Health-Center-Annual-Report.pdf

11

Zines, the DIY Ethic, and Empowering Marginalized Identities

JOE MAGEARY

Zines—or self-published, independent works of visual and/or written content—first came into my life when I was a teenaged punk. The socially critical, activist-oriented, and unabashedly unskilled (i.e. accessible to me) aspects of punk rock attracted me--but just listening to albums in my parents' basement left me with a sense of disconnection and otherness that contradicted the messages I was getting from the music. When I became aware of punk zines and saw how they demystified the musicians, the politics, and the practices of punk culture, I began to feel a connection to a community of activists and practitioners that inspired me to start my own bands and get involved in the various cultural aspects of the punk scene.

Over time, zines helped me learn how to expand my creative expression beyond just playing music, and they provided a template for how I could engage in activism of my own. After many years as a musician and scholar, I have come to view zines as emblematic of the do-it-yourself (DIY) ethos, inhabiting a niche at the intersection of DIY practices, crafting, and activism, which Orton-Johnson (2014) refers to as craftivism. In a craftivist frame, zines are activist tools that art therapists can use to support the empowerment of the people and communities they serve whose identities and perspectives are otherwise oppressed.

An important aspect of any discussion of power and oppression involves an acknowledgment of the identities, voices, and histories the author represents. Offering a note of transparency and contextualization in this regard allows the reader to both understand a little about the author's perspectives and to assess the merit of these perspectives. Transparency of this sort situates the research and ideas presented as something to be taken into consideration, as opposed to insinuating that the ideas are true for all people in all circumstances. In service of these ideas, I offer a brief note on who I am and what I represent, in relation to the topics of zines, art therapy, and craftivism.

I am a heterosexual, cisgender, white, able-bodied, male-identified, natural-born citizen of the United States whose professional identities include Licensed Mental Health Counselor, School Adjustment Counselor, and Professor of

Counseling and Psychology. Despite my position within many privileged spaces, I grew up inhabiting the fringes of my cultural groups, most visibly through my participation in the Boston punk rock scene. I was drawn to punk because of my personal struggles with anger, sadness, and isolation as well as because of a sense that many of the ways that my culture was enacted by people around me were unfair to others and misaligned with how I wanted to be in the world.

If the only people who are speaking up for social justice issues are those who have been marginalized then there is a risk that the pleas for equity and inclusion could get explained away by the dominant discourse as radical or overly sensitive viewpoints without merit. Consequently, I take the position of ally seriously. In the quest for inclusion it is important for those who hold positions of privilege to stand in solidarity with those whose statuses might otherwise not be given respect. I have used visual art in my clinical work and research (Mageary et al., 2015), and my clinical work with teens often utilizes music and visual art. Still, I come to the topic of art therapy from the outside. My training is in traditional counseling techniques and a holistic approach to promoting change, growth, and healing—but not explicitly in art therapy.

As a touring musician I have seen the benefit of zines in the promotion of music, events, and protests. Zines are one of the primary means of creating and maintaining punk cultural values, practices, and community across groups with little-to-no shared resources or organized affiliations (Moran, 2011). I documented the role that zines play in punk culture in a qualitative study of activist punk musicians (Mageary, 2018). Additionally, a thematic content analysis of punk zines played a significant role in my dissertation research on change-oriented punk culture (Mageary, 2012).

Anecdotally, my experience with zine engagement has led me to define zines as intentional, personalized, arts-based productions done for pleasure or with purpose, whose product can be duplicated, replicated, and produced in multiple editions. They serve the multiple purposes of creating, disseminating, and/or embodying sub- and countercultural beliefs, traditions, and practices as well as facilitating self-exploration, self-expression, and/or self-care. Zines also provide documentation of things that matter to people: a form of witnessing and history-keeping for people and movements. Together, these aspects of zine creation, consumption, and dissemination (collectively referred to from here forward as *zine engagement*) create a context for experiences of connection, exploration, and healing that do not require privileged statuses associated with formalized education or monetary investment.

Zine Engagement: Definition, History, and Examples

Short for "fanzine," which itself is short for "fan magazine," zines initially emerged as a distinct form of expression from science fiction fans in the U.S. between the 1930s and 1960s. Eager to take sci-fi stories beyond what was written, fans began writing, publishing, and trading their own stories; typically inspired by existing works of science fiction (Zobl, 2004, para. 3). In her concise history of zines, researcher of feminist self-publishing Elke Zobl (2004) argued that zines continue a legacy of self-publication that "[can] be traced back to 1517 when Martin Luther published his 'zine', the 'Ninety-five Theses,'" (para. 1). While self-publishing was a hallmark of several 20th-century art movements, the true emergence of the zine did not occur until the mid-20th century.

In the 1970s, punk rock culture seized onto zines as an enactment of the DIY ethos (Tiggs, 2006). Because of concurrent advancements in photocopying technologies, zines flourished and, due to their connection to counterculture, became platforms for activism (Ratto & Boler, 2014). Over time, zines have been associated with a range of social and artistic movements, from Dadaism and surrealism to anarchism and punk, as well as many feminist and liberation movements (Zobl, 2009). Between the 1970s and 90s, queer punks began using zines to challenge the norms of both the dominant culture and the punk scene itself (Morgan, 2015). As the ground covered by zines increased, their purpose became cemented as "literary appendages of a movement of youth unrest and social apprehension" (Liming, 2010, p. 121).

In one such example, Riot Grrrl, a third-wave feminist movement connected to the 1990s alternative and punk music scenes that began in the United States before spreading globally, used zines, music, and community to encourage authentic female expression and address issues of feminine empowerment, from sexuality to self-defense (Rosenberg & Garofalo, 1998). This movement took its name from a zine created by members of the punk band *Bikini Kill*, who aimed to "reclaim the vitality and power of youth with an added growl to replace the perceived passivity of 'girl'" (Rosenberg & Garofalo, 1998, p. 809). Much of what is discussed in this chapter is connected to Riot Grrrl's contributions to zine engagement. Here, a zine birthed a movement, which, in turn, breathed new life into zine culture. (For a more complete history of Riot Grrrl, see Radway, 2016.)

With the advent of the internet and online self-publishing came digital zines, or "e-zines" (Clark-Parsons, 2017; Liming, 2010). E-zines cover topics similar to those that can be found in print zines, and they serve the same purposes as their ink-and-paper counterparts. The main differences between the two variants are the creators' access to ways of expressing themselves (i.e., digital photograph alteration and web-based design) and the consumer's increased access to zine content from around the world. Many zinesters, however, continue to opt for printing physical zines (Clark-Parsons, 2017). This is due to the value of zines as cultural ephemera (Chidgey, 2014; Brouwer & Licona, 2016) but also because trading print zines is a useful way to build community (Licona, 2012). Similarly, the tactile, physical crafted nature of printed zines can provoke feelings and experiences that ezines cannot.

Zines cover as many topics and issues as there are authors. Zines can come in the form of distribution lists or distros, comic books, simple photocopied pamphlets, or intricate and involved magazines (Duncombe, 2008). They can be primarily word-oriented or primarily image-oriented but usually contain some combination of both. Some of the most common topics covered by zines are personal and political themes; music, especially punk; DIY arts, crafts, and hobbies; politics and activism; and feminist/queer/trans issues (Gabai, 2016; Ramdarshan Bold, 2017). Goulding (2015) argued that zines' connection to activist subcultures provides access for young women to engage in writing projects that resist traditional media values, particularly in countries where freedom of the press, freedom of expression, and access to information are limited (p. 162).

The continued creep toward ubiquity of internet access, coupled with the rise of maker culture (Sweeney, 2017), has blurred the lines between e-zines and other web content, including social media posting, blogging, and curating one's own website. In some contexts, the unique contributions of zines run the risk of being overshadowed. Ironically, activism, communication, and social justice researcher Clark-Parsons (2017) declared that the resurgence of zines over the last decade was fueled by the dramatic increase of blogging and social media use. Clark-Parsons explained that zines, as activist art and social media work in tandem because "zine-making is a *digitally networked feminist practice*, in which social media platforms act as porous yet protective boundaries, providing access to the zine community, but not to the actual content of zines themselves" (p. 3). In this spirit, I aim to shine a light on the transformative potential of zine engagement. I believe that zines belong in the conversation about ways the arts and art therapy can be used as activist tools, thanks to my own experiences of empowerment through zine engagement and the growing body of literature that supports viewing zines as a source of accessible activism.

De-Centralized and Transdisciplinary: Accessible Activism and the DIY Ethos

Short for *do-it-yourself*, the DIY ethical and practical stance emerged from mid- to late-20th-century countercultural movements in the United States and United Kingdom (Reitsamer & Zobl, 2014). Briefly, the purpose and goal of DIY is to free people from having to rely on capitalist and commercial entities, to engage creativity and learn skills for the purpose of personal and societal betterment, and to locally share resources in order to maintain networks capable of such independent production (Guerra, 2017). "For some, DIY is a financial necessity because it is often cheaper to 'do it yourself' than it is to pay for a service or product. Others embrace DIY practices in order to embody multiple fluid roles and identities in which "change means constantly evolving, questioning and exploring" (Trapese Collective, 2007, p. 5). DIY ethics are also seen as a political stance and a counterpoint to the consumer- and profit-driven elements of a dominant culture (Gabai, 2016).

Much of the existent literature on DIY culture and zines identifies the importance of adopting a critical feminist perspective due to its positioning in contrast or resistance to patriarchy. Interdisciplinary researcher Chidgey (2014) offers one of the most compelling arguments to the importance of such micropolitical acts of resistance. She observed that cheap, accessible, and hands-on publishing can serve as "antidotes to the excesses and apathies associated with consumer capitalism" (p. 104) and that

> several trajectories of DIY are being mobilized in the current moment—from the grassroots and participatory to the neoliberal and conservative—and that self-described DIY projects, wherever they take root, cannot necessarily guarantee liberating possibilities or outcomes by intention or declaration alone.
>
> (p. 102)

Referring to the critical consciousness that emerges from such intentional and focused resistance, Ratto and Boler (2014) highlighted the role that "DIY citizenship" and grassroots self-organization has played in everything from the 2011 Arab Spring uprisings to hacker culture. According to these authors, such applications result in "broadened concepts of citizenship [in which] creating community gardens, filming personal music videos, and even knitting can . . . be understood and evaluated as emergent modes of political activity" (p. 7).

Separately, Gibbens and Snake-Beings (2018) proposed a DIY educational pedagogy that takes a transdisciplinary approach to decentralizing knowledge creation that increases the diversity of perspectives that contribute to how communities prioritize what knowledge and skills need to be taught. This aligns with Bucciarelli's (2016) argument that art therapy as a discipline should move toward a transdisciplinary approach, a focus on both the individual and community, and an incorporation of diverse perspectives to engage in collaborative, holistic, and flexible problem solving. Shifts in definitions of citizenship and political engagement toward integrating the transdisciplinary use of craftivism beg the question of whether a DIY, activist-oriented approach to art therapy could have similarly significant therapeutic ramifications. In other words, if the lessons learned from DIY culture and practices are applied to the context of art therapy, then will new opportunities to empower, teach, and engage people and communities in creatively therapeutic experiences emerge?

The Therapeutic Potential of Zines: Art Therapy, Empowerment, Learning, and Community

Situating Zines in the Context of Art Therapy

To date, the formal body of academic literature discussing the use of zines in art therapy is limited but not without notable exemplars. Some authors have explicitly addressed the use of zines, and others have indirectly incorporated the values and cultures from which zines are produced into art therapy contexts. In one example of the latter, Drass (2016) included the use of punk's DIY ethos in her conceptualization of her art therapy practice, claiming that art therapy informed by punk culture can "create connection in four ways: collapse of hierarchy; search for authenticity and understanding; deconstruction/reconstruction; and empowerment through a DIY mindset" (p. 141).

Others like Chilton (2007) showed that there is precedent for using altered books in art therapy, and Lucas-Falk (2010) identified the blurring of visual and literary arts through comic creation as a useful medium for discussing personal experiences typically reserved for therapy. While zines, comics, and altered books are all different, each is an example of an application of Drass' (2016) DIY mindset. They are all means of artistic expression that intentionally prioritize accessibility over technique, training, or skill and that are highly adaptable to the person, topic, available materials, and setting.

There is also a precedent for arts activism within art therapy connected to performance-based activities that prioritize participation and occur in spaces not typically connected to established art-world venues, such as warehouses and street corners (Frostig, 2011, p. 54). The importance of this shift from individual- or office-based expressive therapies to activism is in its collaboration with others, reflection of a democratic paradigm, and the elicitation of viewpoints that challenge the dominant discourse. In a statement that is reminiscent of zine engagement, Frostig concluded that "arts activism is subversive by design and is not easily formulated for clinical practice. Aligned with grassroots organizing and the embrace of countercultural politics, activism may be viewed as institutionally suspect" (p. 55).

Among those who have explicitly written about zines as materials in art therapy, the most notable example is Houpt, Balkin, Broom, Roth, and Selma's (2016) use of zines in art therapy groups with elders in a skilled nursing facility. Houpt, who had previously used zines in her art therapy work, advocated for the development of a radical art therapy practice by inviting participants to be coauthors and co-presenters and "writing 'with' the art therapy participants, rather than 'about' them" (p. 129). Together, the co-researchers created a zine called *Anti-Memoir: Perspectives from the Literary Shipyard* as a "rejection of a single narrative [of people living in nursing facilities] based in the past as a sole sum of identity, rather stating that the story continues, it is complex, and it is made up of many stories, not one" (p. 130). The zine, the article itself, and the group's participation in the Chicago Zine Fest provided a counter-narrative to the generally accepted value of people living in nursing facilities. Illustrating the transformative and healing aspects of zine engagement, the authors declared that participating in the Chicago Zine Fest made the Anti-Memoir zine "a DIY voice against ageism" (p. 132).

In true DIY fashion, people around the world are creating self-care-oriented zines and calling them "mental health zines" or "therapy zines," and others are attributing therapeutic benefit to zine engagement. Some examples include a guide for how to create "mad maps" or self-created documents that illustrate a person's goals and values while acknowledging struggles and steps taken to counteract the influence of the struggles (The Icarus Project, 2015), a "round-up of zines and comics about women's mental health issues" (Rawhani, 2017), and an art therapy zine Twitter account (Art Therapy Zine, 2018). These are just a few examples of the many ways that people are engaging with zines in order to take agency over their own healing, make meaning, and find relief from suffering.

As these examples highlight, zines function outside of the medicalized models of therapy and thrive in community-based therapy spaces. Some examples of zine engagement outside the therapeutic literature involve empowering identity development (Mageary, 2012), DIY learning (Cordova, 2014), and community development and maintenance (Zobl, 2009). Together, these contributions result in experiences of empowerment, learning, and healing that often exist outside of or in contrast to traditional experiences of therapy.

Zines as Tools for Empowered Identity Development

There are many examples in the literature of how engaging with DIY practices can have transformative impacts on the individual (Del Pozo, 2017; Gibbens & Snake-Beings, 2018; Guerra, 2017; Lonsdale, 2015; Moran, 2011; Stockburger, 2011). One example, guided by my previous research, is in using zines as part of a preferred identity development process (Mageary, 2012). The notion of preferred identities comes from Social Constructionist ideas, inspired by Michel Foucault and adopted by the field of Narrative Therapy (White & Epston, 1990).

Preferred identities are definitions of self, co-constructed between the therapist and the person seeking counseling, that focus on who the person wants to be and why it is important for the person to claim that identity. These ideas stand outside of the models of fixed diagnoses and treatment geared toward a set standard of normalcy. They eschew culturally assigned roles and mores in favor of identification with values, behaviors, and people that are in harmony with how individuals want to live their lives (Monk, Winslade, Crocket, & Epston, 1997).

Narrative practitioners also prioritize connecting a person to a shared meaning-making within *communities of concern*: groups of people, either physically present or virtually connected, who, once aware of the choices being made by a person, can provide caring support for the maintenance and growth of these preferred ways of being (Madigan & Epston, 1995). The intent of developing these communities is to stand against exclusionary and degrading practices often associated with individual, pathologizing therapies. According to Narrative therapists, this combination of an individualized meaning-making process and community engagement can significantly influence the trajectory of a person's life (Freedman & Combs, 1996).

When considering applying the concept of preferred identity development to zine engagement, I questioned the potential implication that "preferred" identities are *chosen* over non-preferred alternatives when it is the experience of many marginalized people that societally prioritized aspects of a person's identity simply exist, rather than being an artifact of preference. This is not in any way Narrative Therapy's intention, but using the word "preferred" in this context conjures up unpleasant associations with ignorant arguments like "people choose their sexual orientation." I view zine engagement as an act of claiming, re-claiming, owning, and/or empowering one's authentic identity. To reconcile these perspectives, the term *preferred* identity development is replaced with *empowered* identity development here. Empowerment is a more fitting word because zine engagement can be emblematic of a sociopolitical activist stance. The highly nuanced, personalized nature of zine creation ties to engagement with social justice activism and the ways people enact the values, beliefs, and practices that matter to them and to their communities, which are often marginalized in some manner.

Additionally, in this context I propose a shift in language from my previous (Mageary, 2012) assertion that the DIY ethos promotes a "small-t" therapeutic experience, which I defined as "a self-constructed healing experience; a chance to acknowledge and confront old wounds and make progress on the path toward self-actualization without necessarily entering into the mental health system or engaging in the medical models of treatment" (p. 209). Although the essence of "small-t" therapeutic experiences resonated with this work, upon further reflection, the name did not adequately reflect the scope of zine engagement. The original intention of adopting the term "small-t" was to differentiate it from formal therapeutic practice, but doing so inadvertently set up a false power differential in which labeling these experiences as "small" infers that their benefits are inferior to traditional therapeutic experiences. Because this was not the original intent, I now offer the term *DIY learning and healing* as a revised descriptor for the transformative potential of engaging with DIY practices, such as zine engagement. In so doing, I also acknowledge Talwar's (2018) observation that art therapy can inadvertently adopt the neoliberal idea that healing is a personal responsibility. As Talwar notes, healing, trauma, and suffering should all be viewed through a societal and historical lens if we are to truly incorporate a social justice orientation in art therapy.

DIY Learning and Healing

Multiple scholars have portrayed zines as educational tools that "exist at the intersection of radical history, analog creativity, participatory culture, and community involvement" (Honma, 2016, p. 35). Chidgey (2014) stated that "even a cursory look at feminist zines would confirm the importance of 'creating', 'empowerment', 'skill-sharing', 'participation', and 'learning' within these networks" (p. 104). Zines, according to education scholar Rebekah Cordova (2014), are a part of a public pedagogy and are examples of performing one's ideologies. She conceptualized the learning that occurs during zine engagement as three types of educative spaces: *affinity spaces*, *free spaces*, and *transitional spaces* (p. 14).

As *affinity spaces*, zines act as a magnet for people with a wide range of experience who can learn from each other and even from the zines themselves in a non-hierarchical way. This lack of hierarchy or control, coupled with participants' voluntary engagement, constitute the *free space* for learning often associated with social movements and political activism. Zines also act as *transitional spaces* of learning because they promote new and creative ways of engaging with the self and others that need not be limited to zines themselves. In a similar vein, Chidgey (2014) notes that the DIY ethos prioritizes the production of alternatives spaces in which activism and community organizing can lead to learning and change. Many people who engage with DIY practices when they are young utilize the skills they learn from this grassroots work to create what Guerra (2017) calls DIY careers in fields that range from performance to politics and promotion.

Cordova (2014) conceptualized DIY creation as one of five steps toward healing from the wounds many people experience at the hands of formalized educational systems, the others being empowerment and inspiration; affirmation; ideals/convictions; and community (p. 128). The implications for zine engagement are clear: doing-it-yourself, in a way that is empowering and affirming of your identities and in line with your convictions, when shared with a community of concern, is a recipe for growth, change, and healing. In summarizing these points, Cordova invoked John Holt's (2004) suggestion that to engage people in education we must shift from identifying as "learners" to seeing ourselves as "do-ers" (p. 197). Being a do-er is clearly an integral aspect of the *do*-it-yourself ethic. Having said this, it must now be noted that doing-it-ourselves is not the same as going alone. The importance of community enactment of the DIY ethos cannot be overstated and warrants further discussion so as to more fully appreciate the scope of potential impact zine engagement carries.

Community Generation and Maintenance

Perhaps one of the most impactful aspects of zine engagement is the sense of community it imbues. Authors have highlighted the importance of participating in zine festivals, distros, and archives (Clark-Parsons, 2017; Houpt et al., 2016), suggested replacing the DIY moniker with DIT (do-it-together) (Chidgey, 2014), and explored the political implications of having power in numbers through DIY democracy (Chidgey, 2014). Across the spectrum, the value of connection with others experienced by zinesters is writ large within DIY circles.

Working with zines is more than just using materials and tools and is, in fact, a social practice inspired by the cultural contexts from which it emerges (Clark-Parsons, 2017). Chidgey (2014), calling zine engagement "a strategy further politicized by being shared" (p. 104), echoed Honma, who wrote that "individual action held within a collectivity" is "the basis of cultural resistance in these communities" (p. 103). Framing this collective cultural resistance as *networked feminist practice*, Clark-Parsons (2017) said that this networking creates "productive third spaces for authors" whose marginalized identities and statuses often result in a lack of representation within media and/or access to media outlets (p. 3). As an example, repurposing images from commercial print media enables zinesters to expose and critique encoded cultural norms, as well as to offer alternatives to the norms (Clark-Parsons, 2017). These practices help to contextualize images and symbols in ways that can prove fertile for art therapy.

Taking a global perspective, Reitsamer and Zobl (2014) introduced the concept of *transnational feminist alternative media*. The authors deemed participation in both critical content production and audience participation associated with feminist alternative media communities as essential for a type of active, critical engagement called *cultural citizenship*. An enacted learning process, cultural citizenship creates "spaces of civic engagement beyond consumption and intervene[s] in hegemonic discourses on neoliberal politics, feminism and migration" (p. 329). Similar to Cordova's (2014) views on DIY learning, Reitsamer and Zobl situated critical making and the acquisition of knowledge within contexts of informal learning and networking that coalesce around a common goal, which they call culturally productive affinity spaces (p. 335). Such investment in producing collective meaning provides participants with the chance to engage in a *DIY democracy* (Chidgey, 2014) where alternative networks, citizenship practices, and economies can be established and hyperlocal change-making is a reality.

Contrasting it with individualized, privatized models of art therapy, Talwar (2015) provided a parallel argument for a critical, community-focused orientation in art therapy, stating that the latter has the added benefit of addressing sociocultural oppression (p. 101). According to Talwar, the cultural competency of an approach is limited when not linked to a social justice framework. She urged all art therapists to "become allies in decolonizing art therapy . . . think beyond the narrowly defined, medicalized models of art therapy to envision ways to empower our clients, rather than pathologize the realities they cannot escape" (pp. 101–102).

Talwar (2015) envisioned new paradigms of care based in critical consciousness that emphasize empowering marginalized groups. This paradigm shift moves art making from "an intuitive process rooted in the unconscious [to] . . . one that is collective, critical, conscious, and communal" (p. 101). Such a shift from internalized, "thin" understanding to intentional "thickened" relationships parallels the empowered identity development process discussed earlier.

Adopting a critical consciousness in partnership with clients and colleagues who have experienced oppression allows art therapists to prioritize diversity frameworks as central to their practice. Incorporating zine engagement and craftivism into art therapy is one way to heed Talwar's call to action because, as Reitsamer and Zobl (2014) noted, the "constructive approach toward community that manifests itself in the production of local, transnational, and virtual networks . . . leads to a sense of community at a time when traditional security nets are disappearing" (p. 336). In the end, zines stand as documentation of ways in which the world can be different.

Conclusion

My hope is that you, the reader, will take away from this chapter both a declaration and an invitation. First, a declaration that zine engagement is providing transformative empowerment, learning, and healing opportunities for people around the world and, second, an invitation to adopt the DIY ethos in your own work: take up a creative and creation-oriented, community-focused mindset and consider that available resources and pre-existing definitions are only the starting point.

There is an idealism inherent in activism and acts of resistance. The actor(s) have identified an injustice or something in need of change. As the previous examples have argued, zines can be a potent context for empowering change because of their nature as tools for education, consciousness raising, alternate narrative creation, and development of communal knowledge. If nothing more, perhaps zine engagement and taking-up the DIY ethos can be acts of practicing creation, active engagement, and empowered change-making. Much of the magic in art therapy lies in its action-orientation. To be engaged in an expressive therapy is to *express* something, and, I contend, zine engagement is no different. Likewise, as Talwar (2018) noted, taking a social justice orientation to art therapy necessitates rethinking the purpose of art through challenging the systems and hierarchies of established therapeutic practice. Whether it is the zine itself that changes your life or the skills and perspectives gleaned from engaging with DIY practices that connect you to alternative ways of engaging with the world, zines stand as proof that there are diverse networks of people expressing their desires for a better world right now who have made room for you to join the conversation.

References

Art Therapy Zine [ArtTherapyZine]. (2018, January 24). [Twitter page]. Retrieved September 9, 2019, from https://twitter.com/arttherapyzine

Brouwer, D. C., & Licona, A. C. (2016). Trans(affective)mediation: Feeling our way from paper to digitized zines and back again. *Critical Studies in Media Communication, 33*(1), 70–83.

Bucciarelli, A. (2016). Art therapy: A transdisciplinary approach. *Art Therapy: Journal of the American Art Therapy Association, 33*(3), 151–155. doi:10.1080/07421656.2016.1199246

Chidgey, R. (2014). Developing communities of resistance? Maker pedagogies, do-it-yourself feminism, and DIY citizenship. In M. Ratto & M. Boler (Eds.), *DIY citizenship: Critical making and social media* (pp. 101–113). Cambridge, MA: MIT Press.

Chilton, G. (2007). Altered books in art therapy with adolescents. *Art Therapy: Journal of the American Art Therapy Association, 24*(2), 59–63.

Clark-Parsons, R. (2017). Feminist ephemera in a digital world: Theorizing zines as networked feminist practice. *Communication Culture & Critique, 10*(4), 557–573. doi:10.1111/cccr.12172

Cordova, R. (2014). *"Punk has always been my school": The educative experience of punk learners* (Doctoral dissertation). Retrieved from ProQuest Dissertations and Theses. (3641976).

del Pozo, J. G. (2017). Global social activism, DIY culture and lack of institutional help. *Journal of Urban Cultural Studies, 4*(3), 427–436.

Drass, J. M. (2016). Creating a culture of connection: A postmodern punk rock approach to art therapy. *Art Therapy, 33*(3), 138–143. doi:10.1080/07421656.2016.1199244

Duncombe, S. (2008). *Notes from underground: Zines and the politics of alternative culture* (2nd ed.). Bloomington, IN: Microcosm Publishing.

Freedman, J., & Combs, G. (1996). *Narrative therapy: The social construction of preferred realities.* New York, NY: W.W. Norton Company, Inc.

Frostig, K. (2011). Arts activism: Praxis in social justice, critical discourse, and radical modes of engagement. *Art Therapy: Journal of the American Art Therapy Association, 28*(2), 50–56.

Gabai, S. (2016). Teaching authorship, gender and identity through grrrl zines production. *Journal of International Women's Studies, 18*(1), 20–32.

Gibbens, A., & Snake-Beings, E. (2018). DiY (Do-it-Yourself) pedagogy: A future-less orientation to education. *Open Review of Educational Research, 5*(1), 28–42.

Goulding, C. (2015). The spaces in which we appear to each other: The pedagogy of resistance stories in zines by Asian American Riot Grrrls. *Journal of Cultural Research in Art Education, 32*, 161–189.

Guerra, P. (2017). "Just can't go to sleep": DIY cultures and alternative economies from the perspective of social theory. *Portuguese Journal of Social Science, 16*(3), 283–303.

Holt, J. (2004). *Instead of education: Ways to help people do things better.* Boulder, CO: Sentient Publications.

Honma, T. (2016). From archives to action: Zines, participatory culture, and community engagement in Asian America. *Radical Teacher, 105*, 33–43. doi:10.5195/rt.2016.277

Houpt, K., Balkin, L. A., Broom, R. H., Roth, A. G., & Selma. (2016). Anti-memoir: Creating alternate nursing home narratives through zine making. *Art Therapy: Journal of the American Art Therapy Association, 33*(3), 128–137.

Icarus Project, The (Eds.). (2015). *Madness and oppression: Paths to personal transformation & collective liberation.* New York, NY: Zine.

Licona, A. C. (2012). *Zines in third space: Radical cooperation and borderlands rhetoric.* Albany, NY: University of New York and SUNY Press.

Liming, S. (2010). Of anarchy and amateurism: Zine publication and print dissent. *The Journal of the Midwest Modern Language Association, 43*(2), 121–145.

Lonsdale, C. (2015). Engaging the "othered": Using zines to support student identities. *Language Arts Journal of Michigan, 30*(2), 8–16.

Lucas-Falk, K. (2010). Comic books, connection, and the artist identity. In C. H. Moon (Ed.), *Materials and media in art therapy: Critical understandings of diverse artistic vocabularies* (pp. 231–289). New York, NY: Routledge.

Madigan, S., & Epston, D. (1995). From "spy-chiatric gaze" to communities of concern: From professional monologue to dialogue. In S. Friedman (Ed.), *The reflecting team in action: Collaborative practice in family therapy* (pp. 257–276). New York, NY: Guilford.

Mageary, J. (2012). *"Rise above/we're gonna rise above": A qualitative inquiry into the use of hardcore culture as context for the development of preferred identities* (Doctoral dissertation). Retrieved from ProQuest Dissertations and Theses. (3508086).

Mageary, J. (2018). Now or never: A phenomenology of a political punk tour. *Interdisciplinary Humanities, 35*(2), 73–88.

Mageary, J., Glenn Wixson, J., Sivan, V., Roberts, R., Vlahakis, V. L., Rose, M., & Gaffney, D. (2015). Visual reflections: Taking outsider witnessing beyond words. *Journal of Systemic Therapies, 34*(3), 44–59.

Monk, G., Winslade, J., Crocket, K., & Epston, D. (1997). *Narrative therapy in practice: The archaeology of hope.* San Francisco, CA: Jossey-Bass.

Moran, I. (2011). Punk: The do-it-yourself subculture. *Social Sciences Journal, 10*(1), 1–8.

Morgan, C. L. (2015). Punk, DIY, and anarchy in archaeological thought and practice. *Online Journal in Public Archaeology, 5*, 123–146. doi:10.23914/ap.v5i0.67

Orton-Johnson, K. (2014). DIY citizenship, critical making, and community. In M. Ratto & M. Boler (Eds.), *DIY citizenship: Critical making and social media* (pp. 141–156). Cambridge, MA: MIT Press.

Radway, J. (2016). Girl zine networks, underground itineraries, and riot Grrrl history: Making sense of the struggle for new social forms in the 1990s and beyond. *Journal of American Studies, 50*(1), 1–31.

Ramdarshan Bold, M. (2017). Why diverse zines matter: A case study of the People of Color zines project. *Publishing Research Quarterly, 33*(3), 215–228. doi:10.1007/s12109-017-9533-4

Ratto, M., & Boler, M. (Eds.). (2014). *DIY citizenship: Critical making and social media.* Cambridge, MA: MIT Press.

Rawhani, A. (2017, October 24). *Round-up of zines and comics about women's mental health issues.* Retrieved from https://brokenpencil.com/news/round-up-of-zines-and-comics-about-womens-mental-health-issues/

Reitsamer, R., & Zobl, E. (2014). Alternative media production, feminism, and citizenship practices. In M. Ratto & M. Boler (Eds.), *DIY citizenship: Critical making and social media* (pp. 329–342). Cambridge, MA: MIT Press.

Rosenberg, J., & Garofalo, G. (1998). Riot grrrl: Revolutions from within. *Signs, 23*(3), 809–841.

Stockburger, I. Z. (2011). *Making zines, making selves: Identity construction in DIY autobiography* (Doctoral dissertation). Retrieved from ProQuest Dissertations and Theses. (3453547).

Sweeney, R. W. (2017). Makerspaces and art educational places. *Studies in Art Education: A Journal of Issues and Research, 58*(4), 351–359.

Talwar, S. K. (2015). Culture, diversity, and identity: From margins to center. *Art Therapy: Journal of the American Art Therapy Association, 32*(3), 100–103. doi:10.1080/07421656.2015.1060563

Talwar, S. K. (2018). Beyond multiculturalism and cultural competence: A social justice vision in art therapy. In S. K. Talwar (Ed.), *Art therapy for social justice: Radical intersections* (pp. 3–16). New York, NY: Routledge.

Tiggs, T. (2006). Scissors and glue: Punk fanzines and the creation of a DIY aesthetic. *Journal of Design History, 19*(1), 69–83.

Trapese Collective, The (Eds.). (2007). *Do it yourself: A handbook for changing our world.* New York, NY: Palgrave Macmillan.

White, M., & Epston, D. (1990). *Narrative means to therapeutic ends.* New York, NY: W.W. Norton & Company.

Zobl, E. (2004, April). *Zines: Zine history, the zine network, topics, and teaching zines in the classroom.* Retrieved from www.grrrlzines.net/overview.htm

Zobl, E. (2009). Cultural production, transnational networking, and critical reflection in Feminist zines. *Journal of Women in Culture and Society, 35*(1), 1–12.

12

Alone in the Desert

Making Sense of the Senseless Through Story Cloths

LISA RAYE GARLOCK

Throughout history and across cultures, people have used needle, thread, and fabric to tell stories. Stories of loss and memories, stories of triumphs and victories, stories of torture, death, and war, and stories of hope. Sewing together allows people to hear each other's stories in a slower, intimate—yet non-threatening—way and to process emotions through the rhythmic, repetitive, and bilateral movements of stitching. Deep emotions can be sewn into the cloth, transferring them from body to fabric in a way that makes meaning of confounding experiences and brings forth hidden or forgotten resiliency.

Narrative textiles often start as personal stories that need to be told and then become important statements about universal human rights and social justice issues. I am in a privileged position, working with young people who are training and entering the art therapy profession. As such, I feel a strong responsibility to encourage budding art therapists to look at the big picture of the world as it is, to not shy away from or avoid the difficult issues that concern us all, and to lean into issues we'd rather ignore. Living in the Washington, DC area, a center of political power, it is impossible to ignore the constant stream of news relating to human rights, climate change, inequality, and injustice.

Through my own process of making story cloths and leading story cloth groups since 2012, it's been revelatory to see how working with fabric and hand sewing contains and titrates strong emotions. Whether working with client sewing circles, art therapy students, or groups of professional therapists in the United States and abroad, I've experienced firsthand how narrative textiles and art therapy work powerfully together to inspire, express what needs to be known, and heal, both individually and collectively.

Introduction

One day, when the young goddess Persephone was playing outside, she saw a particularly beautiful and unusual flower. When she went to pick it, the ground opened and Hades, god of the underworld, abducted her. Her mother, Demeter, became panicked when she couldn't find Persephone. She looked everywhere and asked everyone, but no one had seen her. In her fury, Demeter scorched the earth, allowing nothing green to grow anywhere in the world. Eventually, Hades was forced to let Persephone go, but not before tricking her into eating pomegranate seeds in the underworld, which irrevocably tied them to each other for a portion of each year: for six months she is on Earth, and spring and summer prevail; for the other six months of the year, she must return below as Queen of the Underworld.

The story of Demeter and Persephone is a well-known Greek myth that on the surface explains the seasons. Similar to a number of myths, it speaks to ways men exerted their power, abducting and raping the women who often became their wives. I was reminded of the story when I heard about the 2014 abduction of almost 300 Nigerian school girls by Boko Haram. Many of those girls became the wives of their abductors and mothers to their children. Outraged, I created a story cloth that tells the Greek myth as a metaphorical response to the Boko Haram abduction (see Figure 12.1).

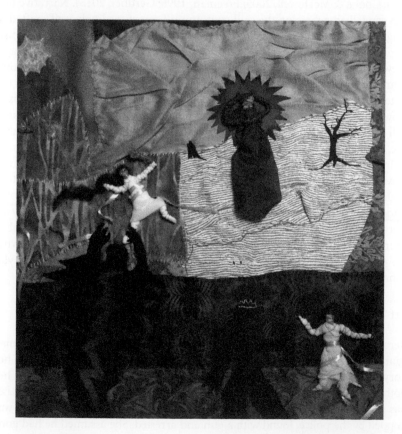

Figure 12.1 The Abduction of Persephone, detail, 2014

Source: Photo and story cloth by Lisa Raye Garlock. Courtesy Rachel Ann Cohen

What Is a Story Cloth?

Story cloths, *arpilleras*, narrative textiles, story quilts, memory quilts—all are names of figurative designs using fabric and threads to tell a story. A story cloth can be appliqued, embroidered, pieced together, batik, woven, painted, dyed, or any combination of techniques (Adams, 2014; Bacic, 2014; Barber, 1994; Cooke & McDowell, 2005; Gerdner, 2015; Grudin, 1990; Mazloomi, 2015). They can be flat, stuffed to create a bas relief, or made with three-dimensional fabric objects such as figures and objects of daily life. They are usually made with fabrics at hand—old towels and clothing, scraps leftover from other projects, found material, treasured scraps from childhood, shared stashes, thrift shop finds, and other inexpensive or free materials. Using such materials is economical, both assuring that materials are recognizable and making it more likely that they will carry meaning (Kalmanowitz, 1999; Moon, 2010). Some type of narrative textile can be found in virtually every culture, and may be figurative or symbolic (Adams, 2014; Cooke & McDowell, 2005; Freeman, 1996; Gerdner, 2015). Narrative textiles can fall anywhere on the skill continuum from exceedingly well-crafted to roughly or basically sewn together with little to no stitching skill. Art therapists let people know that they don't need to be artists to participate in art therapy; likewise with story cloths, people don't need to know how to sew to make one. In art therapy, it is part of the process to introduce and show people how to use materials, and when making story cloths, it is an integral part of the process to show and teach the techniques so the story can be the main focus, regardless of skill level with textiles. When working with a group, the members often collaborate, teaching and showing techniques and helping their peers develop skills.

In 2018 I created the Storycloth Database, which houses collections of narrative textiles related to human rights and shows a variety of styles of story cloths. The website shows work or links to work by professional artists, cloths made in trauma treatment, cultural work that falls in between, and work by art therapists-in-training. This database is a long-term project, with the goal of interesting more people in narrative textiles related to human rights. Viewing this database will give the reader an overview of some remarkable visual styles of narrative textiles (www.storyclothdatabase.org).

Art Therapy and Story Cloth Groups

Her red cloth was small, about eight inches square, and showed a large and a small figure, with a silhouette of a gun. Her stitches were large, raw and basic, and her story described an event that was equally raw: she described the figures in her cloth as herself and her baby. When she was in hospital to deliver, the baby's father was supposed to be on his way. He didn't show up, and she was told that he was stopped by the police, found with a gun and arrested. She assumed he had gone to jail, and she never saw him again. She whispered the story with an urgency that made it seem like she needed to tell it, to put it outside herself, to get rid of it.

A disparate group of women were sitting around the table in the transitional house basement, waiting. Most of them were tired from a day of job and house hunting, dealing with paperwork, and doing the other tasks necessary to reintegrate them into society after being released from prison. When I told them about story cloths—that this was an opportunity to tell their story—there were looks of concern around the room. They weren't at all sure they wanted to tell their stories about why they had been incarcerated or what it was like to be imprisoned. They wanted to leave those stories buried in the past and move on with their lives.

They were first asked to pick materials from a wide assortment of scraps, anything that caught their eye. This part of the process is always engaging. With a large pile of fabric in the middle of the table, it's easy to be in the present moment while at the same time transported by textures that are reminders of the past—a favorite dress from grade school, Grandma's sweater, or the baby blanket that lives under your pillow.

The room soon filled with conversations as the women admired pieces of cloth, found what they wanted, and helped each other find specific colors or patterns. Individual piles of cloth began to grow, and the room quieted as the women became lost in their own thoughts. Touching material, studying the patterns and colors, getting whiffs of different types of cloth, and collecting pieces that are visually compelling activates most of the senses, as well as tapping into subconscious emotions.

While the story cloth described earlier was made very quickly, another woman spent hours sewing her cloth with painstaking care. During groups she worked on her cloth quietly and intently. She seemed to pour her energy into it, and at the end of the group time, she appeared calm and ready to face her next challenge. She shared only that she was making a memory from her childhood and worked diligently on two trees that framed both sides of the fabric. Whether or not she completed her story cloth is a mystery; she found housing and stopped attending group. What struck me when she was working, however, was her passion to sew and create her story. As she stitched, she was lost in thought, possibly remembering things she'd forgotten, making sense of her experiences, and imagining a better future.

One of the interesting things that I've noticed in this group and many other story cloth groups I've facilitated is that each person goes deep into the making, the sewing, and the creative process of developing the visual story they want to tell. The materials and techniques used to create story cloths engage emotional, cognitive, and kinesthetic aspects simultaneously (Garlock, 2016; Homer, 2015) and tap into a shared heritage that has been forgotten (Barber, 1994; Gana & Jenkins, 2016). Working in a group adds a social element that may be somewhat foreign to young people coming from an individualistic culture, where art is usually made in solitude, but many people in story cloth groups and classes have noted how supporting and important it is to work together, to hear each story, and to feel connected to each other.

Story Cloths in Trauma Training

The story cloth showed a large ship on a choppy sea. Three figures in suits were in the stern, weighing down the ship, while in the bow a large group of people huddled. The boat was riddled with holes, reminiscent of the bullet holes still visible on the buildings throughout the country, reminders of the recent war. As she added details and worked on her cloth, its creator marveled at the depth of the process when she realized that what she thought was a political commentary was actually the story about her own personal life history.

The Common Threads Project (CTP) is an international organization that trains local therapists in an integrative trauma treatment method that includes making story cloths (Cohen, 2013). Rachel Cohen designed the program to work with survivors of gender-based violence, including domestic violence and sexual violence in conflict. The training takes the clinicians through an intensive two weeks where they learn the three phases of the program, including therapeutic art activities that lead into story cloth creation. Once trained, they facilitate therapy groups that are called women's circles or sewing circles. An important aspect of the training is that the clinicians and the circles bring in their own cultural traditions, group activities, songs, games, and materials. CTP is based on a sustainable model of working at a grassroots level, with people and resources that are available within communities. The trainees are encouraged to take the structure of CTP and make it their own.

In the first phase of the Common Threads Project the goals are developing strong group cohesion and trust, stabilization, psychoeducation, creative self-expression, and story cloth making. Phase II focuses on deepening group cohesion, processing traumatic memories, delving deeper into the story cloths, and building independence among the participants. They may make a group story cloth during this time. In Phase III, the circles continue meeting on their own. Having co-built this unique community, the group members can choose to exhibit their story cloths and enter the advocacy phase. Advocacy is about taking back power, standing up for self and others, and no longer being isolated, fearful, or intimidated. This aspect is left entirely up to each CTP group; only they can decide what feels right for them.

CTP training groups have been established in Ecuador, Nepal, Bosnia and Herzegovina (BiH), and the Democratic Republic of Congo (DRC). Of note is that in the DRC training cohorts, male clinicians have also been trained and become effective in working with women who have experienced severe sexual trauma. The CTP training group in BiH was comprised of women from four different women's organizations from around the country. Two of the organizations were only about four blocks apart, but they didn't know each other. The experience levels in this group varied from very new to seasoned therapists. The group was able to support each other and worked well together, despite their varied backgrounds, politics, and cultures. When it came time for story cloth making, they were given the same prompts that they would be offering their sewing circles, such as "This is what I need you to know," "This is what I did to survive," and "This is a moment I will never forget."

Some of the research findings regarding the success of Common Threads Project show quantitatively that women in the sewing circles found a significant reduction in depression, anxiety, and PTSD symptoms as shown from pre- and post-intervention Hopkins Symptoms Checklist and the PTSD Checklist (R. Cohen, personal communication, February 13, 2017). Participant comments related to how sewing helped them feel calmer—93.7% agreed or strongly agreed, 84% said that they or others noticed positive changes in themselves since they'd started CTP and making their story cloth helped in recovery from past trauma in 83% of respondents (R. Cohen, personal communication, March 16, 2017). Relating to their experience with the Common Threads Project, women said:

- "This was a unique thing that the story that we cannot speak about we could express it in pictures."
- "I used to be disturbed while recalling my past incidents. I always thought about it. But this made us express our stories into one textile and now I don't feel very disturbed when I express those things. We expressed it in a piece of cloth. That's it."
- "I used to get angry at the smallest things and would beat my daughters in frustration. Even though I used to feel guilty about it, I could not control myself . . . my anger's in check now, I don't fight with my husband and don't beat my daughters."

(R. Cohen, personal communication, March 16, 2017)

Story Cloths in Art Therapy Education

The white arm and hand across the top of the cloth draws the viewer's eye immediately. It is covered in dark red slashes, with lines of shiny red beads spilling like blood from the "wounds." Hypodermic needles and pills, a small figure in the fetal position, a crying woman, and the plaintive words "Where are you" tell a story of parental loss, addiction, abandonment, and also hope (see Figure 12.2). In the words of the story cloth maker:

I wanted to shed light on the topic of cutting and self-harm within the therapy field because I don't feel that therapists know enough about it—that was clear during a practicum supervision meeting at my university. Other mental health professionals seemed to pause when discussing the topic or weren't sure how to approach it with the client directly. The stigma against cutters only grows when we remain silent about it. By opening up about my own experiences that led to cutting, I hope to spread awareness and bridge the gap between our understanding of a cutter's experience and how we can better assist them in recovery.

(A.S., personal communication, June 30, 2019)

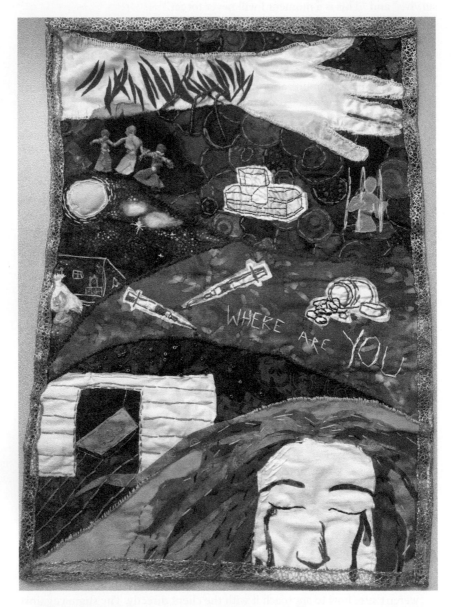

Figure 12.2 In the Life of a Cutter, 2019. Story cloth by A. C. S. Used with permission of the artist

Source: Photo by L. R. Garlock

Training future art therapists in story cloths adds another dimension to their education. Through narrative textiles, they deepen their self-knowledge, political awareness, and understanding of materials and process. Students in every story cloth class I've taught have created remarkable story cloths. As a result of stitching their stories, many were better able to understand how their own processing could translate into effective treatment for some of their clients. Two recent examples were particularly strong in terms of spotlighting human rights issues and illustrating how "the personal is political" (The Personal Is Political, n.d.).

The first story cloth, described earlier, is about an important therapy issue: self-harm, specifically cutting. This cloth is powerful and dramatic, personal in the knowledge about events that may lead to numbing of emotions and the socially unacceptable practice of cutting. Illuminating the issue of self-harm is essential to understanding and treating the causes and reasons people do it. This is a practice that is furtive, secretive, and destructive while at the same time provides an emotional outlet and allows the person to feel something, rather than nothing (Favazza, 1996). Creating this particular story cloth enabled the artist to clarify her own thoughts and feelings, make a strong public statement, and note the beginning of her role in educating colleagues within the therapy field.

Another story cloth tells of a cross-cultural friendship that had to end abruptly and emotionally (see Figure 12.3).

> I wasn't in Thailand to make a friend. I was there to help support a community organization. But over the course of a month spent together, she became just that, my friend. She showed me the brightest parts of her country and told me the darkest hurts of surviving there. Everything she did was to provide for her son and aging parents. The most lucrative thing she could offer was her own body. The night I went to say goodbye she was with a man . . . a customer. She and I cried and hugged each other one last time. The world stopped for a moment. Then she returned to work, and I to America . . . I hated having to leave feeling like I'd done nothing.
>
> (A.R., personal communication, June 26, 2019)

This cloth shows a bar in Thailand, though it could be almost anywhere in the world. In the background scantily clad women sit at the bar and pole dance. In the foreground are figures representing the two friends, one of whom is a sex worker; a third figure is a customer, money in hand. Many sex workers have limited choices or economic opportunities and are forced or tricked into becoming sex workers.

This story has a hopeful ending: two years after their parting, the Thai friend found A. R., the story cloth maker, through the Internet. She reported that she no longer worked at the bar, she and her son were okay, and she was very happy. She wrote the words, "Naver foget," which A. R. embroidered onto the story

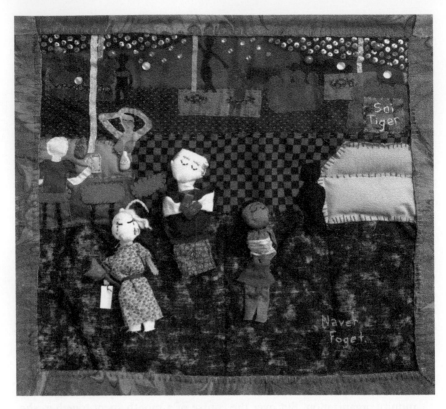

Figure 12.3 Never Forget, 2019. Story cloth by A. R. Used with permission of
the artist

Source: Photo by L. R. Garlock

cloth. This makes clear that the friendship had an important impact, despite the
original helpless feeling of having "done nothing."

In both stories, the art therapy students felt that the cloth and techniques of
creating a story presented the necessary medium for telling these disturbing yet
human stories. Working with fabric has a way of making it safe to approach difficult topics. Part of the power of working with fabric to create story cloths comes
from working with materials that have personal and universal meaning. Fabric is
literally all around us, familiar and intimate, ubiquitous, holding memories and
experiences, nourishing our senses. The textures are familiar and most humans
crave the comforting tactile sensations they bring. According to Jordana Munk
Martin of Blue: The Tatter Textile Library, "Textiles are an extension of our bodies and an essential part of human life—they connect us to our past, and to each
other" (as cited in Hong, 2019). Making story cloths epitomizes this idea particularly when working with trauma stories within a community. The physical act

of sewing—using both hands simultaneously, continually feeling the texture of cloth, and feeling the vibration of the thread pulling through the fabric—relaxes the autonomic nervous system and fosters peace, focus, and release of tension.

My Personal Story Cloth Process

Small golden-faced figures, swaddled in felt, are scattered on a patchwork of fabric, separated from each other and confined within different sections of cloth. In the background are patterned materials, one of which represents a satellite view of a reddish desert; small gold knots represent people who have died in the desert, lost on their journey to a better life. Feathers, which cannot fly without the bird, are tethered in two places; a turquoise net, white spirals, and a patterned circle triangulate to represent confusion, entrapment, and containment. Meandering lines criss-cross the fabric, disregarding the straight, sewn borders. Other found objects, man-made and natural, dot the image.

While I was creating this piece, a group of thousands of refugees from various Central American countries banded together as they made their way to the U.S. border. They were fleeing direct, physical threats to themselves or family members, the violence of poverty and starvation, or corrupt, repressive governments. This story cloth represents the U.S. government's horrific practice of separating children from their parents or guardian at the border and imprisoning them under inhumane conditions (see Figure 12.4, Color Plate 12).

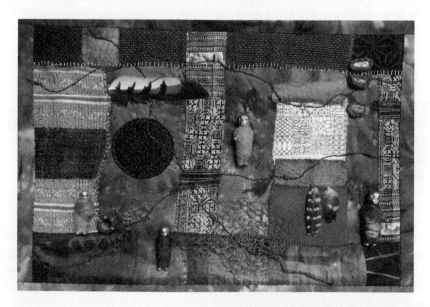

Figure 12.4 Separation I: Immigration Series, 2018

Source: Lisa Raye Garlock

During 2018, I created 12 story cloths that explored political themes that impassioned me: immigration, gender-based violence, and the environment. I started sewing together a mix of fabrics, rather than starting with a solid "canvas" and added objects I found on the street or while traveling, such as shards of tile, small, unidentifiable car parts, feathers, and other lost items. I discovered broken Victorian porcelain dolls online, salvaged from German manufacturing plants that made the dolls from 1850 to about 1920 (Fernandez, 2015). Using wool roving, which is soft and appealing to the touch, I felted around the broken figures—an attempt at caring for and nurturing the discarded dolls. In my story cloths, these dolls represent aspects of the human experiences of being hurt, broken, naked, traumatized; the blanketing of them in roving expresses the experience of nurturing, care-taking, healing, and loving. The pieced fabric shows straight borders and boundaries—attempts at control—while embroidered lines meander randomly across the cloth, showing that borders are generally arbitrary and easily crossed.

I found events in the news disturbing and difficult to tolerate. Stories about the U.S.-Mexico border wall, the rhetoric targeting immigrants, asylum seekers and refugees, families being separated, children dying, what happens to people's bodies when they die in the desert. In the past, it was easy for me to fall into a dark hole of anger and negativity. Creating the story cloth series helped me express my feelings of rage and frustration constructively and to use the slow process of piecing, sewing, felting, and embroidering to process emotions kinesthetically and bilaterally. This process provided calm and strength, helping me to see resiliency and focus on the strength of people who survive horrific experiences.

"Women's Work"

When people are oppressed or subjugated, stitching can become more than therapeutic; it can become an act of defiance (Bacic, 2014; Barber, 1994; Moya-Raggio, 1984). Messages have been graphically depicted on cloth images, woven into the fabric or hidden within abstract designs, the meaning and intent understood only by those who need to know (Fry, 1990; Gana & Jenkins, 2016; Huss, 2010). The images of a story cloth may, from a distance, appear charming or brightly colored and cheerful. Many Chilean *arpilleras*, for example, belie any initial thoughts of an idyllic-looking scene (Bacic, 2014). They may actually depict scenes of protest, occupation by the military, or kidnappings. Contrast that type of story cloth with some of the graphic images in the contemporary Threads of Resistance quilts, which were the reactions of artists to the results of the 2016 presidential election. There were political, angry, and visceral images that were so threatening that several venues canceled their exhibition after people staged boycotts at other sites (The Artist's Circle Alliance, 2017).

Work such as hand sewing, embroidering, knitting, and crocheting has historically been the kind of work that can be done while breast feeding and caring for children and other family members (Brown, cited in Barber, 1994). In patriarchal cultures, this work has been—and continues to be—undervalued, under-paid, or not paid at all. "Women's work" over time developed a pejorative tone, even though this work, including child bearing and rearing, was integral in ensuring collective survival. This discounting of labor done by women is one of the reasons that during Augusto Pinochet's dictatorship, women were able to make *arpilleras*, alerting the world to the atrocities that were happening in Chile (Adams, 2014; Agosín, 2008; Bacic, 2014). The military dictatorship did not take the women and their sewing projects seriously at first. When regime leaders realized what was being depicted and that the *arpilleras* were leaving the country, the cooperatives where the women worked were banned, but women continued to make them secretly and under the protection of the Catholic church (Adams, 2014; Agosín, 2008).

One of the things I've heard consistently from women in my classes and workshops is that they sewed when they were young. At some point, most got the impression from others that sewing was menial and old-fashioned. Making story cloths brought back memories of when they used to sew, and it got them thinking about the value of work, what our society considers valuable, and other personal but political issues. Many young people today are taking back "women's work" and rediscovering their own creativity and the influence textiles can have (Camhi, 2018; Chansky, 2010; Collier & Wayment, 2017; Greer, 2014; Mazloomi, 2015; Timm-Bottos, 2011).

Conclusion

Procne married Tereus, king of Thrace, and went to live with her new husband, leaving behind her sister, Philomela. Missing Philomela, Procne convinced Tereus to fetch her so they could be together. Rather than reuniting the sisters, Tereus took Philomela, raped her, cut out her tongue and imprisoned her, telling Procne that Philomela had died. Unable to speak, Philomela wove her story into a tapestry, and sent it to her sister. Procne freed Philomela and the sisters were reunited.

In the Greek myth of Philomela and Procne, the two sisters wreak terrible revenge on Tereus, and in the end the gods changed all three into birds. Rachel Cohen, founder of Common Threads, used this story as her introduction to a short video she made that helped launch the Common Threads Project. I also use it because it illustrates the silencing that happens with sexual assault and also shows the power of narrative textiles. Tereus's act of cutting out Philomela's tongue literally prevents her from speaking; trauma, fear, and shame can act in the same way. By weaving her story into a tapestry, Philomela finds a way to tell her story, to be heard even though she can no longer speak. Making sure the tapestry was delivered to her sister was self-advocacy, which saved her life. Healing from sexual assault involves finding one's stolen voice, transforming shame into defiance and strength, and rejecting victimhood for the power that comes with self-ownership.

Creating expressive cloth images of overwhelming current events, personal experiences, or meaningful memories helps people tell their own stories in their own time. Sewing stories facilitates a meditative state where memories surface, but rather than fixating on them, the physical actions of sewing calm the autonomic nervous system. That in turn allows the maker to review details that had been forgotten, view the story with a different perspective (Madigan, 2019), and begin to understand that what they did was what was necessary at the time. Connecting to the past means understanding what happened to us historically and how what happened still affects us. Narrative textiles have been made to document significant collective traumas, from slavery (Fry, 1990; Mazloomi, 2015) to the Holocaust (Krinitz & Steinhardt, 2005) and apartheid (Voices of Women-Amazwi Abesifazane-Museum, n.d.). Telling stories within a community connects people to each other, where they can trade experiences with trust and understanding and begin to advocate for themselves.

Making story cloths removes stories from a person's secret inner world where memories swirl and morph into monsters and releases them into the healing light of day. Seeing and hearing—and sharing—stories puts them into a broader context, enabling us to discover that what we were ashamed or afraid of has lost its power, that our weaknesses have been transformed into strengths, just as patched cloth is stronger than the original. Making textiles connects us with our heritage and those who came before, our ancestors who passed on the skills to make everyday, necessary objects; clothing, blankets, linens. Sewing story cloths offers another powerful tool in art therapy, where working with our hands and telling our stories in community can help us become healthier individuals, so that we in turn can build healthier communities.

References

Adams, J. (2014). *Art against dictatorship: Making and exporting arpilleras under Pinochet*. Austin, TX: University of Texas Press.

Agosín, M. (Ed.). (2014). *Stitching resistance: Women, creativity, and fiber arts*. Kent, England: Solis Press.

Agosín, M. (2008). *Tapestries of hope, threads of love: The arpillera movement in Chile* (2nd ed.). Lanham, MD: Rowman & Littlefield Publishers.

The Artist Circle Alliance, LCC. (2017). *Threads of resistance: A juried exhibition created to protest the Trump administration's actions and policies*. Catalog, designed by Perez, I. and Perez, J.C. Retrieved from www.threadsofresistance.com

Bacic, R. (2014). The art of resistance, memory, and testimony in political arpilleras. In M. Agosín (Ed.), *Stitching resistance: Women, creativity, and fiber arts*. Kent, England: Solis Press.

Barber, E. W. (1994). *Women's work: The first 20,000 years: Women, cloth, and society in early times*. New York, NY: WW Norton & Co.

Camhi, L. (2018). Some of the most provocative political art is made with fibers. *The York Times*. Retrieved July 4, 2019, from www.nytimes.com/2018/03/14/t-magazine/art/fiber-knitting-weaving-politics.html

Chansky, R. A. (2010). A stitch in time: Third-wave feminist reclamation of needled imagery. *Popular Culture, 43*(4), 681–700.

Cohen, R. A. (2013). Common Threads: A recovery programme for survivors of gender based violence. *Intervention: Journal of Mental Health and Psychosocial Support in Conflict Affected Areas, 11*(2), 157–168.

Collier, A. D., & Wayment, H. A. (2017). Psychological benefits of the "Maker" or do-it-yourself movement in young adults: A pathway towards subjective well-being. *Journal of Happiness Studies, Online,* 1–23.

Cooke, A., & MacDowell, M. (Eds.). (2005). *Weavings of war: Fabrics of memory: An exhibition catalogue.* Lansing, MI: Michigan State University Museum.

Favazza, A. (1996). *Bodies under siege: Self-mutilation and body modification in culture and psychiatry* (2nd ed.). Baltimore, MD: The Johns Hopkins University Press.

Fernandez, E. (2015). *"Still she never stirred": Frozen Charlotte dolls of the Victorian era.* Retrieved from July 4, 2019, from academia.edu/12251298/_Still_She_Never_Stirred_Frozen_Charlotte_Dolls_of_the_Victorian_Era

Freeman, R. (1996). *A communion of spirits: African-American quilters, preservers, and their stories.* Nashville, TN: Rutledge Hill Press.

Fry, G. (1990). *Stitched from the soul: Slave quilts from the Antebellum South.* New York, NY: Dutton Studio Books.

Gana, C. P., & Jenkins, L. M. (2016). *Resilient threads: Telling our stories (Hilos resilientes: Cosiendo nuestras historias).* Textile Society of America Symposium Proceedings, 981. Retrieved from http://digitalcommons.unl.edu/tsaconf/981

Garlock, L. R. (2016). Stories in the cloth: Art therapy and narrative textiles. *Art Therapy: Journal of the American Art Therapy Association, 33*(2), 58–66.

Gerdner, L. A. (2015). *Hmong story cloths: Preserving historical and cultural treasures.* Atglen, PA: Schiffer Publishing, Ltd.

Greer, B. (2014). *Craftivism: The art of craft and activism.* Vancouver, BC: Arsenal Pulp Press.

Grudin, E. U. (1990). *Stitching memories: African American story quilts.* Williamstown, MA: Williams College Museum of Art.

Homer, E. (2015). Piece work: Fabric collage as a neurodevelopmental approach to trauma treatment. *Art Therapy: Journal of the American Art Therapy Association, 32*(1), 20–26.

Hong, C. (2019). The Tatter Textile Library is a crafter's paradise. *Martha Stewart.* Retrieved July 5, 2019, from www.marthastewart.com/1535318/tour-blue-the-tatter-textile-library

Huss, E. (2010). Bedoin women's embroidery as female empowerment. In C. Moon (Ed.), *Materials & medial in art therapy: Critical understanding of diverse artistic vocabularies* (Kindle for iPad version 4.8). Retrieved from Amazon.com

Kalmanowitz, D., & Lloyd, B. (1999). Fragments of art at work: Art therapy in the former Yugoslavia. *The Arts in Psychotherapy, 26*(1), 15–25.

Krinitz, E., & Steinhardt, B. (2005). *Memories of survival.* Washington, DC: Bernice Steinhardt & Helene McQuade.

Madigan, S. (2019). *Narrative therapy* (2nd ed.). Washington, DC: American Psychological Association.

Mazloomi, C. (2015). *And still we rise: Race, culture, and visual conversations.* Atglen, PA: Schiffer Publishing.

Moon, C. (2010). *Materials & media in art therapy: Critical understanding of diverse artistic vocabularies* (Kindle for iPad version 4.8). Retrieved from Amazon.com

Moya-Raggio, E. (1984). "Arpilleras": Chilean culture of resistance. *Feminist Studies, 10*(2), 277–290.

The Personal Is Political. (n.d.). *Wikipedia.* Retrieved October 12, 2019, from https://en.wikipedia.org/wiki/The_personal_is_political

Timm-Bottos, J. (2011). Endangered threads: Socially committed community art action. *Art Therapy: Journal of the American Art Therapy Association, 28*(2), 57–63.

The Voices of Women (Amazwi Abesifazane) Musuem. (n.d.). Retrieved from www.amazwi-voicesofwomen.com/archives

13

Empowerment Through Mentorship
Peer-Led Craft Workshops in a Forensic Psychiatric Hospital

JAIMIE PETERSON AND ALISON ETTER

People with mental health conditions and a criminal history face a dual stigma. Individuals with mental health conditions are also often stereotyped as dangerous or potentially violent, which makes social interaction difficult (Cleary, Deacon, Jackson, Andrew, & Chan, 2012). Wolfensberger's (2000) social role valorization theory states that an individual's value is determined by what a person has to offer society, making it difficult for society to see value in those facing this dual stigma. In our work with people who have been committed to a psychiatric hospital by the criminal justice system, we found that art mentorship through peer-led craft workshops assisted in reducing stigma, creating community, and providing valuable social roles.

Introduction

Kerrville State Hospital (KSH) is a 217-bed forensic psychiatric hospital located in a rural Texas community. The residents are under a "forensic commitment," meaning they have committed or have been accused of committing a crime linked to their mental health condition. The hospital treats both individuals who are considered mentally unstable ("incompetent") to stand trial and those who have received a verdict of "not guilty by reason of insanity" (NGRI) in a court of law. All of the residents are living with severe mental health conditions such as schizophrenia, bipolar disorders, postpartum depression, psychosis, and mood disorders. They are living not only with a psychiatric condition but also the implications related to allegedly committing serious and violent crimes. The average length of stay at the facility is between two and seven years.

In a correctional institution such as Kerrville State Hospital, therapeutic programming can include therapy groups, substance abuse classes, medication education, community reintegration programming, and creative arts therapy. All off-campus outings must have a therapeutic purpose and require approval by both a treatment team and a judge. According to Reisman (2016), "The mental health system frequently forces patients to give up their power and relate to the world only through their illnesses, reinforcing the experience of social defeat" (p. 92). The residents of KSH not only face severe stigmatization due to their diagnoses and the crimes they have been accused of but also frequently feel guilt, shame, discord with family, and internalized stigma. Self-stigma, defined as the internalization of negative stereotypes about mental illness and self-blame, can be reduced significantly by supporting individuals in empowering themselves (Reisman, 2016).

Within a forensic psychiatric hospital community, the medical model is often the dominant paradigm. However, creative arts therapy can focus on the stigma of mental health conditions and forensic commitments through a social justice lens. Corrigan, Watson, Byrne, and Davis (2005) stated that "framing mental illness stigma as a social justice issue reminds us that people with mental illnesses are just that—people" (p. 363). By shifting this focus, it allows the community outside the hospital to view these individuals as people, rather than a diagnosis or crime. Members of the community outside KSH do not often get a chance to interact with the residents, but thanks to the hospital's artist collective they may have a chance to view their artwork in the community. This focus allows the community to interact with the art of those who are hospitalized rather than focusing on the stigma.

Open studio approaches and community-based studios focus on artistic identity and personal strengths while de-emphasizing diagnosis (Moon, 2002). Viewing individuals as artists rather than patients focuses on strength-based treatment and person-centered care. KSH models this approach through an artist collective. When I (Jaimie) was in graduate school, I interned at Project Onward, a studio for artists with mental and developmental disabilities, under the supervision of Randy Vick. This experience made a profound impact on my art therapy practice and how I organized the art studio and artist collective at KSH. Although KSH is a unique community because of the forensic component, many of its goals are similar to those at Project Onward. Both programs promote creating art in a safe environment, connecting artists to the larger community, and inspiring change by bringing their art into the world. In community-based art studios for people with disabilities, the focus is on strengths and identity (Vick, 2016). Contemporary art can influence art therapy and the cultivation of the artistic self and creative insight into life's challenges. When an individual develops an artistic identity, it can help the individual find acceptance, confidence, freedom, and empathy (Thompson, 2009). In the Social Empowerment Art Therapy model by Morris and Willis-Rauch (2014), which was developed in an inpatient psychiatric hospital, the focus is on personal empowerment as an artist, group empowerment through collaboration and decision-making, and reduction of stigma in the community through art exhibition. This gives participants an opportunity to reframe themselves as artists within their environment and community (Morris & Willis-Rauch, 2014). The artist collective at KSH embraces personal empowerment, utilizing collaborative work such as large-scale sculpture, paintings, and musical ensembles in group work; personal freedom for individuals to choose the way they express themselves; and musical performance and art exhibition within the hospital community and the outside community to cultivate the artist identity.

Social Roles and the Artist Collective

Through involvement in the arts, individuals can develop positive qualities such as strength and resilience, which effectively contrast with adverse qualities and stigma associated with their diagnosis and/or alleged crime. According to the social role valorization theory, individuals who fulfill positive social roles are viewed as valuable in society, while individuals who fulfill negative ones are socially devalued (Wolfensberger, 2000).

Open art studios, exhibitions, peer mentorship, and the refinement of artistic skills and identities provide valuable social roles for marginalized people. Artist collectives such as the one at KSH place an emphasis on the artist or mentor identity rather than social differences or disabilities (Moon, 2016). Using person-first language such as "artist," "musician," "mentor," "teacher," and "individual" may contribute to breaking down barriers. A community of artists can create a safer space, reduces anxiety, and facilitates an accepting culture (Howells & Zelnik, 2009). For individuals experiencing marginalization and stigma, this creative community can provide a refuge for expression.

The artist collective at Kerrville State Hospital is a creative community of artists and musicians who work side by side in the studio, exhibit their talents in exhibitions and concerts, and mentor each other in workshops. The art studio offers open studio time five days a week, a pottery studio, a painting studio, digital photography classes, a sewing class, a sewing circle, and an artist-led art magazine. Crafting in the studio is very popular and has become an important part of our community. Crafts are often passed down by family members and learned while growing up, and artists often reminisce about these memories of learning specific skills. Interaction, collaboration, and informal mentorship occur when passing down stories about crafting and skills to friends and fellow artists. Many crafts have a utilitarian purpose, whether wearable or usable in the home, which holds significance at our hospital. Many residents have lost their home along with all of their possessions and mementos when faced with long-term hospitalization. Being able to make things for their room, things to wear, and gifts for loved ones becomes empowering as they try to rebuild their lives within the hospital walls.

The music therapy studio offers open music studio time twice a week, guitar classes, Recovery Radio (a group that allows residents to collaborate and share their interests through prerecorded segments), and a ukulele club and also facilitates multiple bands and music history classes. To make this artist collective possible, the studio needs to facilitate a collaborative space. One way to address this is by referring to individuals as artists when they enter the hospital studio space. This creates a unique identity in this creative space as individuals are typically referred to as patients or residents by medical and care staff. The artists are encouraged to obtain their supplies from the cabinets and make their own creative decisions. The residents do not have many freedoms when confined to a forensic institution, but the art and music studios attempt to foster some independence within the creative space. The artist collective is run like a community studio where artists come to work, make art and music, and learn new skills. All residents are welcome in the art studio. Some treatment teams refer the residents to the studio, but many individuals drop in to explore the space and become engaged independently. Eventually, the resident artists begin to interact, collaborate, and help one another naturally. We encourage this in the studios by reminding the artists of their skills when they are around newcomers to the studio, often casually encouraging the experienced artists to orient the new ones. If an artist is working on a new project in the studio, using media or a process in which another resident artist has experience, I (Jaimie) will introduce the two artists and suggest they collaborate and learn from each other. Often this will instill confidence in the experienced artists, and they will begin engaging with fellow artists in an informal mentor role.

Mentorship

Stimulating interaction and creating valuable social roles can also be obtained through volunteerism within the hospital. Because this community resides within the confines of the hospital, artists often find opportunities in the studio. Volunteerism and mentorship are ways for artists to feel ownership in the studio and collapse hierarchies. Timm-Bottos and Reilly (2015) described this type of community as a level playing field where everyone is welcome to share with their peers. By focusing on the collective, artists are valued for what they contribute to the community rather than their roles outside of the studio such as resident or staff (Moon, 2016). Many artists in the studio work alongside each other or collaborate on a project regardless of their role at the hospital. As artists take on a new role as peer mentors, they move from the role of helpee to a helper, which promotes recovery and self-esteem (Dunn, Wewiorski, & Rogers, 2008). Volunteering, through mentorship in this case, fosters a social environment and gives those with a disability an opportunity to demonstrate that they are reliable and capable individuals in a society that may not regularly see these traits due to stigma (Mjelde-Mossey, 2006). In a community, volunteers are people who give their time and talents to make their community a better place and therefore display valuable social roles.

Mentorship began in the music therapy program when a resident offered to teach piano lessons to his peers. This resident spent much of his life before hospitalization performing and teaching piano lessons and saw an opportunity to give back to his community by providing this service. He developed a simple method to teach rhythm and chords to beginners and began teaching his peers with minimal supervision from staff. One of his students, who was also learning to play the guitar, was inspired by the leadership exhibited by his piano teacher. This student eventually began leading bible study groups for his peers. He used the guitar to lead songs during worship on the unit.

Another resident volunteered her time and talents as a mentor to teach voice lessons to her peers. I (Alison) began to notice the unique relationship forming between the teachers and students within the artist collective. As other musicians and artists observed these interactions, a culture of mentorship and volunteering began to spread throughout the artist collective.

In the art studio, mentorship naturally started to occur when the artists began building a holiday float for a community parade. The float was created to raise awareness of the hospital in the larger community and reduce the stigma of mental illness. One resident artist became very knowledgeable about papier-mâché and sculpture while at the hospital. He started teaching the other resident artists and the staff how to build pieces for the float. Eventually, he became the informal "float director" and mentored new artists in the studio, teaching them the art of papier-mâché.

The mentoring also spread to the pottery studio and leatherworking class. Individuals who had been in the studio and mastered various skills began assisting with teaching their peers. The opportunity to mentor changes the residents' role in the community from patient to teacher and empowers the individual. I (Jaimie) noticed that artists started taking on the role of expert in their art media and opening up to other artists, teaching informally in the studio. The artists also often brought their treatment team members to the studio to show and teach them their skills. This was the beginning of the shifting role for the resident artist as the expert and mentor.

One of the earliest workshops was on creating origami cranes. An artist had the goal of making 1,000 paper cranes because he learned of a Japanese legend that in doing so a wish may come true. He learned the steps and informally started teaching staff and residents on his unit. He made a diagram of the process and asked if he could hold a workshop to teach more artists. All artists were welcome to sign up for the workshop. When introducing the project, he asked all the participants to write their wishes on the papers before folding them, clearly describing the steps and helping his peers.

At the end of the session, the group started discussing their wishes, and every participant had written that they wished to go home or see their family again. It was a humbling and eye-opening experience for me (Jaimie) to witness this unanimous, heartbreaking wish. It brought up the themes of strength, resilience, sadness, frustration, and hope for the participants. This really struck a chord with me, personally. I often think about my privilege when working with the artists at the hospital. On my drive to and from work, I frequently reflect on my personal freedom and how I am able to leave the hospital each day, while the artists I work with cannot. I try to be aware of these privileges of being able to come and go and to see my family and friends whenever I want. The origami crane is a daily visual reminder in the studio for me to be conscious of my privilege as I work with our artists.

The origami-making mentor taught the craft throughout the hospital informally and was able to obtain 1,000 cranes. With these cranes, he created an installation in the studio (Figure 13.1, Color Plate 13). The artist strung the cranes in groups of 50 and hung them from the ceiling, surrounding a pillar.

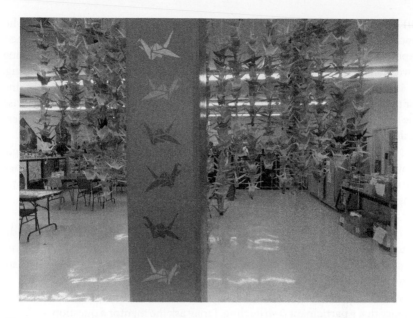

Figure 13.1 An installation of 1,000 paper cranes on display in the art studio
following a workshop taught by a resident mentor

He painted the pillar and created a stencil of the crane, repeating the image on all sides. As one walks around the cranes, they softly flutter, and through the folds, the word *home* reveals itself many times. Now as I walk by the origami cranes and they sway with my movements through the studio, I am constantly reminded of my privilege and freedom relative to those hundreds of wishes to go home. This workshop and installation has become a symbol of hope in the studio and is eye-catching to all who enter the space.

Following the workshops in the artist collective, I noticed that many of the mentors were exhibiting more confidence. Peer-led programming increases feelings of empowerment, self-confidence, and builds on relationships with others (Hodgson, Stuart, Train, Foster, & Lloyd, 2018). This programming creates a community for artists of varying abilities and an area and role for all in the studio where everyone is valued and included. After observing the impacts of mentor-led workshops, we developed a mentorship survey to document the benefits of mentors within the artist collective.

Peer-Led Craft Workshops

After two years of informal mentorship within the studio, we started noticing the profound positive impact that mentorship had on resident artists. The art studio staff and the art therapist began a peer-led craft workshop program in

2017. Peer-led workshops feature a volunteer resident artist each month who teaches a class on a craft that they have mastered, allowing them to share their expertise with others. A variety of craft workshops have been taught, including jewelry making, embroidery, sewing, card making, origami, and leatherworking.

I (Jaimie) act as an advisor to the mentor when coordinating and preparing for the workshops. I collaborate with the mentor on creating a flyer to advertise the workshop and decide on the number of participants. The mentor gathers materials and decides what supplies need to be purchased for the workshop.

Next, I schedule a time to meet with the mentor to do a practice run-through, in which the mentor teaches the project if there are steps or specific skills they are instructing. The mentor utilizes me for assistance in creating handouts and diagrams for teaching aids and is responsible for setting up the space and materials for the workshop.

During the workshops, I will introduce the mentor to the group, if the individual asks me to do so, but then I assume the role of assistant and observer. Occasionally I and other art studio staff will assume the role of participant depending on the perceived comfort level of the mentor.

If I observe that the mentor is having a difficult time explaining something or I notice that a participant is struggling, I may ask the mentor a question to clarify. If the project involves multiple steps such as origami and multiple participants need assistance, studio staff and I ask to be of assistance to the mentor before jumping in to help teach. The studio staff's role is as an active participant and assistant as needed, but the role of the teacher is given entirely to the mentor. During the craft workshops, the mentor takes ownership of the creative space.

Workshop Examples

Mr. L.: Mr. L is a leather artist who received an NGRI acquittal. He usually has a flat affect and is very quiet. After excelling in leatherworking classes taught by studio staff, I (Jaimie) asked Mr. L to be an art mentor and assist in teaching the introductory leatherworking class. Mr. L quietly assisted the new students but often needed prompting to engage with them at first. I observed how, once he started assisting, Mr. L was attentive to his peers and became more expressive when instructing.

Mr. L was working toward discharge into the community. The date was approaching and was to fall before Christmas. I asked him if he would like to teach an art workshop before he left. Mr. L excitedly agreed, smiling widely. He planned a leather ornament workshop, in which he would teach basic stamping techniques open to anyone, even those without leatherworking experience. Mr. L practiced by teaching me the techniques and came up with a plan to safely set up all the tools for the class.

The workshop had a full attendance, and Mr. L did an excellent job teaching his peers. He confidently stood over the participants the entire time, carefully watching the artists and instructing them on how to use the tools. He was friendly and attentive. This workshop had sparked the interest of Mr. L's treatment team, and his psychiatric nurse practitioner had asked me if they could drop by to observe. I had asked Mr. L ahead of time if this would be okay and had assured him it was okay to decline, but he had expressed excitement at the idea of the treatment team attending. He did not show any signs of anxiety and was fully engrossed in his workshop. It appeared as if he did not notice the staff around him. The participants were delighted with their ornaments and expressed gratitude toward Mr. L for his class. Afterward, Mr. L was beaming. He stated, "I never thought I could do something like that." Staff members were surprised at his animation and strengths in teaching others.

Shortly after leading the workshop, Mr. L applied for an artist scholarship through the hospital's volunteer services. I started this program to allow artists to receive funds or art supplies to continue their art practice outside of the hospital. Mr. L said:

> Art helps me forget mental illness, makes me proud that I learned how to do leather—I'm no longer defined as mental illness, but seen as an artist. You guys taught me leather—it's now who I am, it's a part of me. I am a mentor now!

Mr. L received the inaugural scholarship at the hospital and was able to receive funds to purchase leather tools and supplies to use after discharge to continue the art form that was so beneficial to his recovery.

Ms. B.: Ms. B is a mixed media artist who has been judged legally incompetent to stand trial. I (Jaimie) have worked with her for over ten years. Ms. B often engages in negative self-talk and struggles with her self-image.

She is very active in the studio and enjoys creating collages, writing poetry, weaving, and drawing. Ms. B started creating altered books to express her poetry visually. I saw her struggle with self-esteem and some social interactions but also noticed Ms. B's natural way of helping others in the studio when they asked about her techniques.

I suggested to Ms. B that she try teaching a workshop on altered books. Ms. B agreed tentatively, and we agreed on a two-hour workshop. Ms. B was anxious about the workshop, often calling the studio multiple times a day for reassurance outside of her studio time. I continually encouraged her but was worried she might back down from the workshop or become too stressed. She was extremely focused on planning and perfecting her workshop, despite her continued self-doubt and negativity.

On the day of the workshop, Ms. B came to the studio early to set up the tables and pull out all the materials she needed. She appeared calm and focused on her tasks. She personally greeted everyone as they entered the studio and made sure everyone was comfortable in their seats for art making. Ms. B introduced herself to the group and introduced each member to one another.

I was surprised by Ms. B's confidence and lecture skills. Ms. B handed out a compilation of resources, images, and lists of ideas she put together about altered books and then started demonstrating the beginning process. During the workshop, I realized that due to time constraints, the artists would only be able to begin the process, and many of Ms. B's techniques would not be demonstrated. The fellow artists picked up on this quickly, and an artist commented, "Ms. B, this workshop is so fantastic, you are going to have to hold a Part Two!" The other artists agreed, and they scheduled a time for a second, follow-up workshop.

In preparation for the next class, Ms. B enlisted the assistance of other artists to help demonstrate skills. She stopped calling the studio continuously and did not mention the second workshop when in the studio. The day of the workshop, Ms. B arrived in time to set up and was calm and prepared. The second workshop went very well, and Ms. B reported to staff that she felt more confident during the second workshop. Ms. B continued to check in with workshop participants on the progress of their books and proceeded to mentor in the studio after her workshops.

Mr. O: Mr. O is an origami artist who is at KSH due to an NGRI acquittal. He does not attend the art studio often but visited during a *Pathways to Community Re-entry* class on recreation. *Pathways to Community Re-entry* is a six-month curriculum developed by the hospital's Rehabilitation Services Department that NGRI residents take to prepare for discharge. The recreation class educates the residents on healthy ways to spend leisure time, and the class comes to the studio for one session to talk about art. I (Jaimie) engage the students of the class, and they share any creative hobbies they may have. Some artists get their work out and share with their classmates.

During the class Mr. O expressed his love for origami. He asked for a piece of paper and quickly made an origami jumping frog for the class, impressing everyone. He told everyone he used to fold them in school and make them jump into his teachers' coffee mugs. He joked and said it often landed him in detention. After the session, Mr. O continued to return to the studio to look at origami books and fold more frogs.

One of Mr. O's peers suggested that he teach an origami workshop, and he loved the idea. After asking me, we worked together to plan the workshop, and he taught me the steps of how to fold the frog. I am not very good at origami and struggled with the process. Mr. O returned to the studio and made a diagram (Figure 13.2) on a poster board of all the steps for everyone to reference.

Mr. O was very excited about the class and invited all his friends. The workshop classes are usually small, six to eight participants depending on the craft, but the day of the workshop, 12 participants arrived! Fortunately, I had practiced the steps multiple times and could assist with artists seated on one side of the long table of origami folders. Mr. O exhibited great patience in teaching the craft of origami to so many people. He walked around the table and made sure the participants were following along with his instructions. At the end of the session, everyone made their frogs jump. There were lots of laughs and fun in this workshop. When finishing up, I congratulated Mr. O and asked him to tell the class why he loves to make origami frogs so much. He told the group that his mom used to make them all the time and even went to one of his classes when he was a child and taught his classroom how to make them. He loved that memory, and

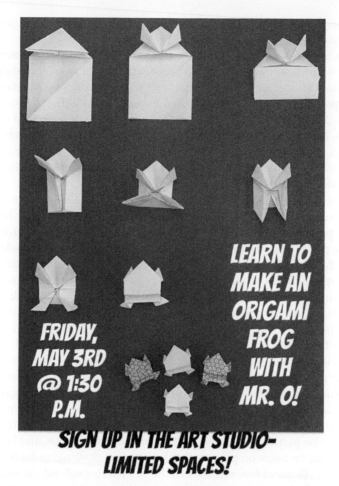

Figure 13.2 An advertisement for an origami frog workshop taught by a resident mentor displays the steps on how to make an origami frog

that is why he continues to make them. One workshop participant commented, "I bet your mom is so proud of you now that you are teaching this too!" Mr. O smiled and later informed me that he had called his mother to tell her about his workshop. Mr. O took his diagram to his *Pathways* class the following week with some origami paper. He taught the recreation class how to make origami frogs as well. The frogs have spread around the hospital campus as more and more individuals learn this craft. The little paper frogs scattered throughout the hospital remind our community of the impact of art mentorship.

Ms. S.: Ms. S is a fiber artist who received an NGRI acquittal and is working toward discharge. She is very active, participating in the pottery studio, photography, and sewing circle, as well as attending the open studio three times a week.

Art making was not part of her life before hospitalization, but since coming to KSH she has made it a daily ritual.

When she was first admitted to the hospital, Ms. S did not interact much with fellow residents but was comfortable with the staff. The art studio gave her a safer space to interact with other residents with the common ground of art. She enjoyed embroidery and even started helping others in the studio to learn this craft. Ms. S made lots of friends in the studio and is often looked up to by her peers. After making several embroidery pieces, Ms. S taught an embroidery workshop, where participants learned to stitch designs on a pre-made tote bag. Her first workshop was a success, and she often acts as a resource to other artists in the studio who take up embroidery and sewing.

Ms. S and another staff member learned how to make a no-sew pillow from a nurse on their unit and asked if she could teach a workshop, as residents could all probably use an extra pillow. The project used fleece material and a pre-made pillow form. The studio did not have any fleece, so some needed to be purchased. Ms. S was transitioning into the community and was getting ready to discharge soon. All residents in the hospital who received NGRI acquittals must go through a pass committee as part of their reintegration back into the community. Most of the passes given by the hospital are part of the *Pathways to Reintegration* course curriculum. I (Jaimie) and another art studio staff member were able to propose a pass that would help Ms. S learn about purchasing art materials in the community and how to price compare. The plan was to price pre-made pillows and calculate the yardage of fleece needed for the project.

Ms. S utilized the week before the workshop to prepare by cutting material and practicing the steps involved in the project. The workshop was limited to five participants due to the number of steps and materials involved. During the workshop, one participant had difficulty focusing, was anxious, and had a history of giving up easily on projects that became too challenging for her. Ms. S sat with her, reassured her, and assisted the woman throughout the workshop. Because of Ms. S's patience and attentiveness, the participant stayed for two hours and finished her project. Everyone praised the participant for finishing the project. Ms. S stated that she learned a lot from the participants and that it made her more observant when working with people.

Mentorship Surveys

We created a survey for the mentors to fill out before and after workshops for quality assurance purposes for the hospital and to gather data on their self-perceptions in this mentoring role. The five survey questions each utilize a five-point Likert scale and assess the self-perceptions of artistic skill level, confidence in public speaking, preparedness for leading a group, patience, and skill level as a mentor/instructor.

When introducing the survey, we used it after the craft workshops, but since February 2019, we have started providing identical pre- and post-workshop surveys to see if the artists' perceptions had changed (Figure 13.3). In that time,

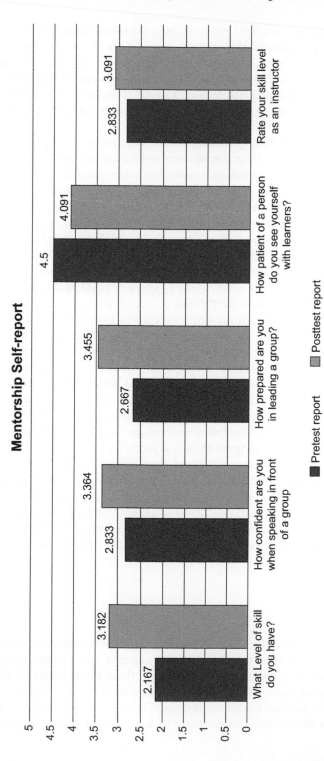

Figure 13.3 Self-perceptions of mentors based on pretest and posttest data

six mentors have completed pre- and post-workshop surveys, and five mentors completed post-workshop surveys only. Of the six surveys that included pre- and post-workshop data, four mentors rated their skill level as higher following their completed workshop. Three reported increased confidence. Four stated that they feel prepared to lead a group. Two mentors stated that they were patient with learners, and three reported an increase in skill level as an instructor.

While some mentors reported the same score for pre- and post-workshop data, it should be noted that two of them rated their patience with learners as lower following their workshop. In addition to the quantitative data, mentors can provide comments about their workshop in the pre- and post-workshop survey. One individual scored herself low on her perception of herself as an instructor and level of skill and commented "It went well except I was hearing voices at the time of the workshop. My peers helped fill in when I wasn't able to, and we helped each other out." Another workshop leader wrote, "I really thank you all for letting me take this giant leap of faith for me in teaching a workshop." When debriefing with us, most mentors expressed pride, and many discussed how surprised they were in their abilities.

The participants of each workshop were asked to complete a questionnaire with open-ended questions following the workshop. The questionnaire asked what the participant learned, what their favorite part was, changes they would make to the workshop, and take-away points from the workshop. Additionally, participants can provide comments or feedback for the peer instructor. The comments from peers were very positive and encouraging, praising their peer mentor. The suggestions thus far have included things such as playing music in the background and providing more materials to choose from; overall, the peers have been very encouraging toward and grateful for their mentors.

Following each workshop, I (Jaimie) meet with the mentor to discuss their thoughts about the workshop, and ask if they would like to receive survey comments from their peers about the workshop. The data from these surveys is helpful to me and the studio staff as we assist with future peer-led workshops. The artist collective plans to collect this data over a more extended period for quality assurance purposes and to further look at the effects of peer mentorship and peer-led craft workshops.

Conclusion

Mentorship opportunities such as peer-led craft workshops allow residents of Kerrville State Hospital to assume a social role as a peer mentor. Mentors are able to share their talents and expertise with their fellow artists. Within this artist collective, many of the mentors also take on the role of learners as they support new mentors in their workshops. The artist collective is a supportive community that creates an environment for learning and shared ideas and skills.

In reviewing the mentorship surveys, the mentors rated their self-perceptions of their skill level, confidence, and ability as an instructor higher in post-workshop surveys. The mentors expressed pride and surprise in their abilities when debriefing with us and received positive feedback and encouragement from their peers. While the creative arts can be an essential part of an individual's recovery, volunteer opportunities allow members of the artist collective to learn from and inspire each other. In this way, the artist collective at Kerrville State Hospital aids in reducing stigma, creating community, and providing valuable social roles. Creating social roles through peer mentorship and artist collectives can inform art therapy with individuals with stigmatized and/or marginalized identities in a range of settings.

References

Cleary, M., Deacon, M., Jackson, D., Andrew, S., & Chan, S. (2012). Stigma in mental illness: A continuing concern. *Contemporary Nurse: A Journal for the Australian Nursing Profession, 40*(1), 48–50.

Corrigan, P. W., Watson, A. C., Byrne, P., & Davis, K. E. (2005). Mental illness stigma: Problem of public health or social justice? *Social Work, 50*(4), 363–368. doi:10.1093/sw/50.4.363

Dunn, E. C., Wewiorski, N. J., & Rogers, E. S. (2008). The meaning and importance of employment to people in recovery from serious mental illness: Results of a qualitative study. *Psychiatric Rehabilitation Journal, 32*(1), 59–62.

Hodgson, E., Stuart, J. R., Train, C., Foster, M., & Lloyd, L. (2018). A qualitative study of an employment scheme for mentors with lived experience of offending within a multi-agency mental health project for excluded young people. *The Journal of Behavioral Health Services & Research.* https://doi.org/10.1007/s11414-018-9615-x

Howells, V., & Zelnik, T. (2009). Making art: A qualitative study of personal and group transformation in a community arts studio. *Psychiatric Rehabilitation Journal, 32*(3), 215–222. doi:10.2975/32.3.2009.215.222

Mjelde-Mossey, L. A. (2006). Involving people with disabilities in volunteer roles. *Journal of Social Work in Disability & Rehabilitation, 5*(2), 19–30. doi:10.1300/j198v05n02_02

Moon, C. H. (2002). *Studio art therapy: Cultivating the artist identity in the art therapist.* London, England: Jessica Kingsley.

Moon, C. H. (2016). Open studio approach to art therapy. In D. E. Gussak & M. L. Rosal (Eds.), *The wiley handbook of art therapy* (pp. 829–839). West Sussex, England: John Wiley & Sons.

Morris, F. J., & Willis-Rauch, M. (2014). Join the art club: Exploring social empowerment in art therapy. *Art Therapy: Journal of the American Art Therapy Association, 31*(1), 28–36. doi:10.1080/07421656.2014.873694

Reisman, M. D. (2016). Drama therapy to empower patients with schizophrenia: Is justice possible? *The Arts in Psychotherapy, 50,* 91–100. doi:10.1016/j.aip.2016.06.001

Thompson, G. (2009). Artistic sensibility in the studio and gallery model: Revisiting process and product. *Art Therapy: Journal of the American Art Therapy Association, 26*(4), 159–166. doi :10.1080/07421656.2009.10129609

Timm-Bottos, J., & Reilly, R. C. (2015). Learning in third spaces: Community art studio as storefront university classroom. *American Journal of Community Psychology, 55*(1), 102–114. doi:10.1007/s10464-014-9688-5

Vick, R. (2016). Community-based disability studios: Being and becoming. In D. E. Gussak & M. L. Rosal (Eds.), *The wiley handbook of art therapy* (pp. 829–839). West Sussex, England: John Wiley & Sons.

Wolfensberger, W. (2000). A brief overview of social role valorization. *Mental Retardation, 38*(2), 105–123.

14

Queer Ethos in Art Therapy

MIKEY ANDERSON

As I carefully organize my playful craft supplies filled with glitter, sparkling gems, decorative buttons, sequins, shimmery ribbon, fabric paint, and sewing materials, I'm excited by how campy, queer, and exaggerated my craft supply choices are. I am preparing materials for my Story Quilts group with my partnership with SAIC at Homan Square in Chicago's North Lawndale neighborhood. SAIC at Homan Square hosts a collaborative program with SAIC artists and the North Lawndale community to promote collective art making grounded in social justice. The North Lawndale community is predominantly African American and has a rich history of civic action.

I find parking near the Senior Center and awkwardly carry a large suitcase full of craft supplies, while clutching a stack full of large cardboard sheets. I enter a small building with "Senior Center" written on the entrance of the door. The Senior Center is nestled alongside large buildings occupied by other Lawndale Christian Health Center locations. The Senior Center is home to Senior Day Program of Lawndale Christian Health Center, which offers activities, meals, socialization, and medical support for elders.

I begin setting up the bedazzled materials and fabric scraps on two long tables facing the community members who are finishing up breakfast. They are seated along a wall with five small tables, talking amongst themselves. The space has two larger windows that brightly light up the small space. I find the space to be cozy and accessible, which gives me the opportunity to pass materials out to each table quickly.

In the space, I present as a Queer, white, able-bodied, male, femme-of-center individual. I am surrounded by 15 older adult residents of North Lawndale who have the option to participate in my Story Quilts group after breakfast. Joining them are three of their direct support staff. Almost immediately on my first day, I observe confused looks and receive a variety of questions and comments about my Queer body in the space from the participants. *You sew, young man? Where did you learn to sew? Did your mother teach you?* I begin to notice my own feelings of nervousness and discomfort about my Queer identity. *Will I be judged? Am I assumed to be straight? Is it okay for me to be teaching quilting in a religious organization?* I also recognize that I am a young white person among a roomful of older adults of color.

I engage with the participants by answering their questions in earnest and returning with my own. *Who here has sewn before? Who taught you? What are your experiences with sewing? What memories come up for you?* The group begins to share about their memories and histories with sewing and craft. Their stories are evidence of the powerful way in which the act of sewing can summon up memories of family and culture.

I am amidst a group of Black and Brown participants who have a robust history with sewing and who trust me to sew their artworks together. I feel humble and grateful in this moment as the room of participants pass their fabrics off to me to sew. With each exchange of fabric I continue to learn something new about participants. As a Queer-identifying artist and art therapist, my Queerness in community groups I run is a political and performative act that often disturbs the gendered notions of crafts and quilting. My body unravels the gendered history related to crafts, domesticity, and my Queer identity. Simultaneously, the participants share about the racism they've experienced and how it intersects with sexism, ageism, and heterosexism they've faced in their workplaces, homes, and communities. Our quilts are evidence of their stories and highlight their dynamic voices. It feels crucial as a white, male presenting, femme-of-center, able bodied art therapist to listen to their stories and use their quilts to amplify their voices in the community through their lens. As with many other groups I facilitate, in this group we begin to build cross-cultural and intergenerational connections among one another through the use of craft.

As I describe in the previous narrative, my crafts are informed by my community-driven art therapy practice, through which I integrate art, art therapy, Queer theory, and activism. Through crafts, I forefront accountability for understanding Queer folks' experiences through an intersectional lens and for working with the Queer community in an ethically responsible way. I do this by creating collective community-based art-making groups and workshops as a form of social activism by Queering the spaces I enter (Ahmed, 2016). Through the performative actions of crafting, I disrupt the seemingly ordinary heteronormativity established in these spaces and offer the community a new radically Queer form of kinship (Halberstam, 2011). These groups help participants discover new community support networks, develop strong social connections, and encourage LGBTQ+ individuals to open up about their experiences and use art to heal themselves and our communities. I have facilitated these groups at LGBTQ+ assisted living facilities, memory care units, Queer youth therapy groups, middle schools, high schools, and art centers.

My engagement in fiber crafting is informed by the Queer theorists Jack Halberstam, Judith Butler, Alison Kafer, and Michael Warner—I manifest the potential of their research and techniques to disrupt dominant notions of gender and to reclaim and reimagine gender as performative (Butler, 1990). I'm drawn to craft materials that invoke a campy aesthetic and bring to mind the many Queer fiber artists I find inspirational, such as Ben Cuevas, L. J. Robert, and Nick Cave (Chaich & Oldham, 2018). We use our crafts as political fuel to emancipate ourselves and our viewers from a heteronormative society, and we use art exhibitions to challenge binary categorizations of gender and sexuality (Butler, 1990). By rejecting individualism, I aim to foster a community of art therapists around a collective crafting movement where we use tools, such as embroidery floss or needles, to intentionally remake and rewrite dominant narratives stitched throughout our culture (Halberstam, 2011).

In everything I do, I ask myself: am I effectively interweaving my identities as a Queer artist, art therapist, and activist to best support the diverse communities I work in across Chicago? How does my Queer, white male presenting, femme-of-center, artist-art therapist self Queer the practice of art therapy? These are the central questions that I work to interrogate from a Queer lens. Grounding my research in critical arts-based inquiry, I engage deeply in self-reflexivity (Talwar, 2019), which has taken several material forms, including: creation of a quilt; reflections on community Queer groups I lead that are inspired by my art practice; reflections on vending opportunities for Yarnies—the line of plush toys I design—at Queer events; self-reflexive writings; and the creation of an informational zine for art therapists.

My multi-faceted approach feels attuned to the current political climate in the U.S., which is marked by a rise in hate crimes and the passage of anti-LBGTQ+ laws threatening the LGBTQ+ community (Karcher, 2017). In addition, in 2017 the American Art Therapy Association Board made the decision to align with Second Lady Karen Pence, an antagonist of LGBTQ+ rights, on her Healing with the HeART initiative, which has been critiqued by other art therapists (Talwar, 2017; Kaiser, 2018). Faced with such challenges, I work to bring attention to the structural inequalities facing the LGBTQ+ community, collective trauma, which results in a higher risk of mental health problems, substance abuse, suicide, and homelessness (McDermott, Roen, & Scourfield, 2008).

Throughout this text, I use the terms Queer and LGBTQ+ to represent anyone who identifies as lesbian, gay, bisexual, transgender, gender-expansive, non-binary, Queer, questioning, intersex, and/or asexual. My intention is not to exclude anyone. I am aware of the essentializing nature of the term Queer, as well as the impact it has on our LGBTQ+ elders. I capitalize Queer as a noun and adjective to interrupt conventional writing standards shaped by a racist, classist, and ableist society and to highlight how our Queer lives exist outside conventional narrative experiences (Bianco, 2014). I use Queer(ing) as a verb to describe the actions I am taking as an artist-art therapist to disrupt the naturalization of heteronormativity (Kafer, 2003) in the art therapy profession.

Queer Crafting: Sewing as Research

I was drawn to create a *Queer quilt* to hold the homophobic slurs that have been thrown against my body while crafting in community spaces where I was practicing as an art therapist. I stitched the words community members said to me directly and passively (Figure 14.1) when they rejected the idea to sew with our craft groups. Through the creative process of making the *Queer quilt*, I engaged

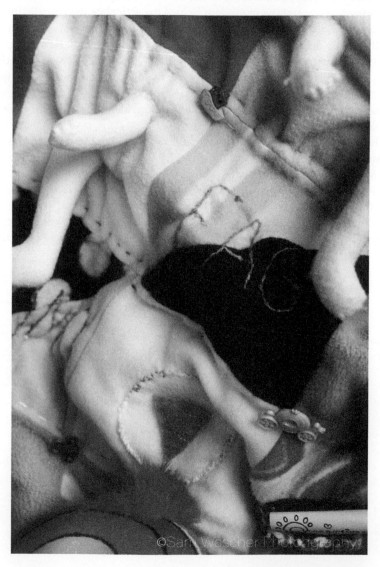

Figure 14.1 Mikey Anderson, *Queer quilt*—mix media fiber crafts

in a deep self-reflexive examination regarding my power, privilege, bias, and trauma history, all of which have shaped my identity. The process of defining and claiming my social locations is ongoing, and thus my identity is continually in flux, a fluid experience that has been affirmed by Queer theorists (Fawaz & Smalls, 2018). The *Queer quilt* (Figure 14.2, Color Plate 14) is a formal engagement with this kind of personal-social examination and informs my research of Queer identities, theory, and narrative, all of which help me locate myself within the art therapy community as a Queer art therapist.

Sewing and researching in tandem helped me articulate the complexities of my identity, which has been shaped by layers of trauma, societal assumptions, and the biases that have been enacted upon my body. These layers of experiences are represented in the three layers of the *Queer quilt*, all sewn together. Complexities play out in my *Queer quilt* via the disruption of traditional quilt patterns. I incorporated knitted pockets, soft sculptures, and embroidery in my piece in order to Queer the normative and gendered practices of quilting (Chaich & Oldham, 2016).

The Queer, campy aesthetic of my quilt deconstructs the process of quilting and, in turn, serves to Queer my quilt. I looked to Queer fiber craft artists like Melanie Braverman, Hayden Phipps, Jade Yumang, and Maria Piñeres (Chaich & Oldham, 2016) who use their crafts to open up spaces for fantasy and imagination (Halberstam, 2011) in a world that is shaped by laws and policy that stigmatize the Queer community (Warner, 2000). These interpretive spaces are necessary for reimagining human identities that were previously

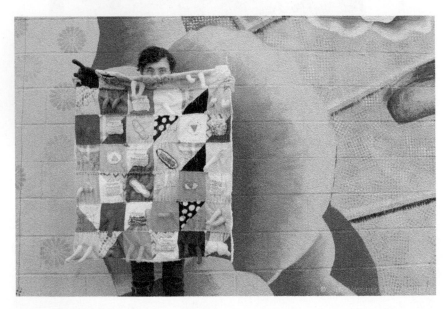

Figure 14.2 Mikey Anderson, *Queer quilt*—mix media fiber crafts

fixed by representations of race, gender, or sexuality (Salley, 2012). These artists employ crafting as a means to liberate the Queer community from oppressive, heterosexist social forces, particularly through making their work visible via exhibitions, performances, and publications.

Fiber craft processes such as knitting, crocheting, embroidery, and sewing have historically been associated with femininity or women's work, which has contributed to the reification of binary notions of gender (Talwar, 2019). Also, within a broad social context, crafts have been considered less prestigious or legitimate than fine arts (Chaich & Oldham, 2016; Moon, 2010).

By engaging in the performative action of fiber crafting in public spaces I'm Queering the potential for materials and techniques to shatter dominant notions of gender and to reclaim and reimagine gender as existing outside of hegemonic societal norms (Halberstam, 2011). In turn, I use the quilting process to disrupt the claim that art therapy is apolitical or that quilting is a gender-specific practice. My practice of quilting in public spaces makes visible my Queer identity, how this identity innately influences the way I practice as an art therapist, and how my participants and I bring our intersecting identities into our therapy encounters.

My *Queer quilt* is soft and cuddly, inviting people to come closer and engage. I allow people to touch and hold my artwork. I perceive the *Queer quilt* as a bridge that enables people to approach me both emotionally and physically, through responding to its softness while holding and touching it. The *Queer quilt* invites reciprocal engagement through actions like holding and wrapping oneself inside it or treating it with care. It is a testament to radical care practices in relation to both how it was created—turning inward to fight for myself—and how I receive emotional strength when other people respond to it in a caring manner. In general, radical care practices through art making and art sharing allow me to grow emotionally and physically closer to people, leading me to the knowledge that my emotional well-being is fundamental to the health and sustainability of my art therapy practice (Feng, 2018; Ravichandran, 2019). At the same time, after the viewer looks beyond the cuteness of the *Queer quilt*, they begin to recognize the pain I have experienced as a Queer art therapist navigating a homophobic culture stitched within art therapy. When I observe people registering this awareness, sometimes they hold on to the quilt longer, with greater care. Others seem to react with shock at seeing such vulnerability, immediately setting the quilt down.

The *Queer quilt* bears scar-like stitched shapes, each embellished with glitter as inspired by the Queer graphic novel *Gaylord Phoenix* (Fake, 2010; Figure 14.3). This visual narrative suggests that the willful reopening of Queer scars can be a means of reclaiming them and subsequently releasing into the world the unexpected, magical energies they contain (Fawaz & Smalls, 2018). The stitched glitter shapes on my quilt represent the scars of my past experiences—some of which were traumatic—that have shaped my personality. Instead of trying to subsume these experiences, I find strength in them through my ongoing development as a Queer artist-art therapist.

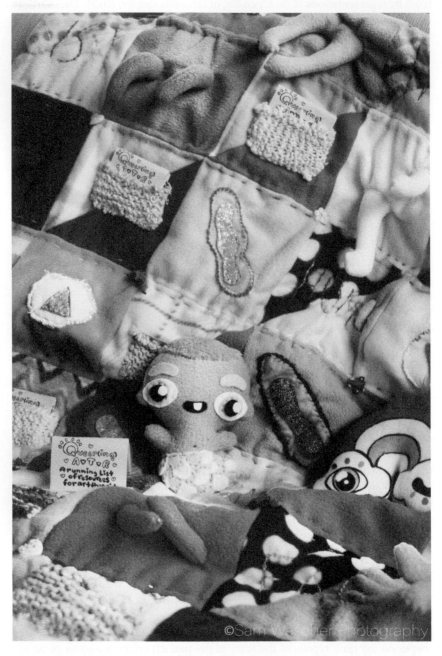

Figure 14.3 Mikey Anderson, *Queer quilt, Queering Art Therapy Zine, Yarnie Plushies*—mix media fiber crafts

The *Queer quilt* served as a way for me to express my identity as a Queer quilter and to push the boundaries of normativity, troubling the norms of art therapy practice. Art making has provided a means of strength and resilience for me to confront my innermost struggles through my art practice.

Queering the Art Therapy Field

My experience as an art therapist at a women's shelter when a community member shouted in my face "FAGGOT" led me to examine how homophobia in art therapy is harmful to both clinicians and participants. Being a Queer, white, male presenting, femme-of-center artist-art therapist has led me to examine how my lived experiences and scholarly research might coalesce in approaching art therapy from a Queer perspective. I have looked to Queer culture, theory, history, fiber crafts, music, zines, activists, and archivists to spark ideas for Queering art therapy. In doing so, I have considered how the process of Queering art therapy can disrupt the dynamics of power that persist in both heterosexist institutions (Young, 2012) and art therapy practices.

I aim to represent the pain other Queer art therapists and I feel due to the lack of Queer research in art therapy and the American Art Therapy Association's alignment with Karen Pence's initiative, Healing with the HeArt (Kaiser, 2018), which promotes contested ideas related to normalization (Warner, 2000) and healing and thus further marginalizes communities who don't comply with the standards and expectations of a heteronormative world. In defense of their decision to associate with Pence, AATA leaders maintained that the organization does not take political stands (Potash, 2019); still Pence cannot be disentangled from the toxic Trump administration, which has directly harmed art therapists and art therapy clients who are LGBTQ+, people of color, female, immigrants, and/or disabled. The Trump-Pence administration has cultivated an increasingly hostile cultural environment for the U.S. Queer community, particularly those members who are not wealthy, white, male, heterosexual, cisgender (non-trans), able-bodied, and/or Christian (Karcher, 2017). Since day one, the administration has negatively impacted the Queer community, including: discontinuing the LGBTQ+ section of the White House website; rescinding Title IX protection for transgender students (Lopez, 2018); appointing anti-LGBTQ+ activist Roger Severino to lead the Health and Human Services Civil Rights office; cutting HIV/AIDS research funds; implementing an Executive Order on Religious Liberty; failing to acknowledge Pride month; and extending invitations from the U.S. Department of Education to the anti-LGBTQ+ organizations Focus on the Family and the Family Research Council as part of The Trump Accountability Project of 2017 (Glaad, 2018, May 1). The list of harmful policies and practices continues to grow and directly affects Queer therapists and participants in art therapy.

The actions of the Trump-Pence administration have emboldened people prone to anti-LGBTQ+ hate speech (Karcher, 2017). In response, many Queer individuals have felt forced, or out of safety concerns, many of us have altered and censored our appearances to blend in with the larger hegemonic society, what is sometimes called "compulsory heterosexuality" (Kedley & Spiering, 2017). Out Queer individuals have found ourselves retreating back to the closet. Compared to heterosexual individuals, we are more susceptible to physical and emotional violence, perpetrated by a heterosexist society that expects adherence to socially constructed behavioral and attitudinal norms (McDermott et al., 2008).

This pain has been incorporated into my *Queer quilt*, conveyed through limbs that protrude from the flat plane (Figure 14.4). They push against the

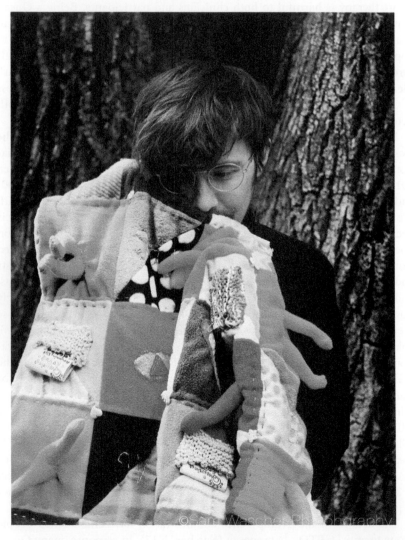

Figure 14.4 Mikey Anderson, *Queer quilt*—mix media fiber crafts

surface, refusing to conform to a traditional quilt design. I see these limbs as representative of the pain born by myself and other Queer individuals from the past and into the present, masked and made inviting by the tender appearance of the *Queer quilt*. It is pain born from struggling against the constant violence of a homophobic culture limiting Queers' sexual freedom through shame, laws, stigma, and idealist moralism (Warner, 2000, p. 17).

This pain has been amplified by the lack of adequate resources for Queer art therapists, who are sometimes left vulnerable within the communities in which we work. Too often, service organizations lack nondiscriminatory hiring practices and inclusive policies for their staff and members, which means that Queer therapists come to embody the harmful effects of homophobia enacted upon us. We must constantly seek out community and self-care resources that exist outside of those authored from a heterocentric perspective (van Dernoot Lipsky & Burk, 2009).

I look to other Queer therapists, artists, and scholars for inspiration related to expanding the limits of my gender identity and expression. Critically engaging with my position of power as a mental health worker means not separating myself from the Queer community, showing how the personal is political, and being unapologetically Queer in all spaces (hooks, 2000; Taylor, 2018). Doing so allows me to use my privilege as an art therapist to help unsilence the voices of the Queer therapy participants with whom I craft and converse.

Within art therapy literature, several key texts consider Queer theory and intersectionality in relation to working with the LGBTQ+ community; not surprisingly, the most relevant works have all been published in the United States in the last few years, responding to the political trauma pervading the country. Karcher (2017) spoke to the impact of collective trauma on communities, specifically the impact of the Trump-Pence administration on the U.S. Queer community. Zappa (2017) held art therapists ethically accountable to practices informed by an understanding of Queer participants' intersectional identities, including their racial and cultural locations. Both Karcher and Zappa challenged homophobic practices in art therapy and asked art therapists to address structures of oppression that are based on race, class, gender, ethnicity, and immigration status. Clinton explored their genderqueer identity to confront their internalized shame using a critical arts-based inquiry to explore their narratives from personal, social, and political perspectives (Talwar, Clinton, Sit, & Ospina, 2019). The work of these scholars has strengthened my commitment to practicing art therapy through a social justice framework. These scholars are working toward expanding art therapy to include many different voices in the field who have historically experienced marginalization and silencing (Gipson, 2017). Collectively, we are pushing back against the U.S. art therapy field's national alignment with Karen Pence and its history of silencing LGBTQ+ voices.

While the work of the previously mentioned scholars in the field of art therapy is notable, there remains a lack of publications that focus on the experiences and needs of Queer individuals. There is abundant literature reflecting the historical pathologization of Queerness within the U.S. mental health system, including within the art therapy field, as well as the continued pathologization that trans and gender-expansive individuals face in order to access services. Unfortunately, though many art therapy journal articles appear to have good intentions, they nevertheless cause harm by promoting antiquated psycho-therapeutic practices; problematic art interventions created for Queer clients by heterosexual, cisgender art therapists; or unfounded hypotheses to design therapeutic interventions "targeting" Queer individuals (Beaumont, 2012).

When Queer art therapists look to their field for affirming research and best practices, what they find instead is a preponderance of literature that reinforces gender stereotypes, buttresses traumatizing narratives, and aligns with hetero-sexist social norms. In offering a critique of art therapy literature written about working with LGBTQ+ participants, I acknowledge that all of the research and writing occurred within specific historic periods, including moments when mainstream understanding of gender differed greatly from today's currently evolving understandings (Zappa, 2017). Overall, however, art therapy litera-ture presents an objectified image of Queer individuals by generalizing our experiences. It would benefit art therapy scholars and the individuals and com-munities they serve to include Queer voices in their research and to ground their ideas *in* Queer experience, not *about* Queer experience; harm comes from oversimplified approaches to treatment based on case studies that are not rep-resentative of the diversity of Queer individuals.

Queer Approaches to Art Therapy

It's crucial for an art therapist to be aware of social stigma, discrimination, homophobia, and transphobia and the ways in which these conditions threaten the emotional and physical health of Queer clients (Pelton-Sweet & Sherry, 2008). Through storytelling, art therapists can begin to bring in more Queer voices—particularly QTPOC (Queer and trans people of color) voices—into the art therapy community. Specifically, this could support art therapists in understanding how racial differences may affect QTPOC in reference to their developmental milestones, including when they disclose their sexual and/or gender identity. Additionally, when working with Queer clients, art therapists should offer culturally sound services and abide by the most basic fundamental ethical principle of "do no harm." Art therapists working with QTPOC commu-nities must be accountable for understanding landmark and current theories of sexual and gender identity development. Also, art therapists should support the entire Queer community with comprehensive care through the conscious use of Queer affirmative language.

King and Rose (2016) took an archivist approach to documenting the experi-ences of QTPOC across disciplines through interviews about their history and identity development. This archival approach dismantles the whitewashing that too often occurs in literature, media, and art therapy, which both directly and incidentally erases the work and voices of QTPOC from history. King and Rose (2016) highlighted the roles QTPOC play in shaping our society and demand representation of their rich and influential history within archives. Bringing a Queering framework to art therapy can be supported through the use of such archival resources by non-QTPOC art therapists to educate themselves and contextualize the experiences of the QTPOC clients and colleagues with whom they work.

In my efforts to Queer my approach to art therapy I have sought out literature that incorporates personal narratives to deepen the reader's understanding of the systemic injustices experienced by QTPOC. These narratives are centered in the current U.S. political climate, wherein transgender women of color are experiencing frequent, horrific attacks that rarely receive attention or response. These hate crimes hang heavy over QTPOC community members, who must navigate nearly constant physical and symbolic threats of violence (King & Rose, 2016). For transgender women of color, social media and the use of hashtags like #SayHerName and #Time4BlackTransWomen have served as a platform to demand recognition and justice. In its efforts to meaningfully serve QTPOC communities, the art therapy community must expand its awareness of and response to the daily social, legal, and physical realities of QTPOC.

Art therapists must adopt a broad, intersectional framework that considers ability, immigration status, gender identity, sexuality, class, and race, as well as the lack of visibility experienced by the Queer community in a political climate fraught with violence and animosity (Talwar, 2010). Queering art therapy will help ensure the health, well-being, self-care, and community care for Queers—everyone who sees themselves outside the conventional heteronormative narrative. In this way, Queering art therapy can be understood as an act of service that will enable the field to better support individuals and communities that historically have been denied the luxuries of time, space, and self-care. It can also be understood as an act of resistance against inequitable political structures in art therapy. For intersectional LGBTQ+ communities that have long lacked political recognition and action, social services that adequately meet their needs, and inclusion in historically white LGBTQ+ organizations (Kline & Cuevas, 2018), the Queering of art therapy is not optional. It is critical.

To manifest this clarion call within my own work, I nested my Queering Art Therapy resource zine (Figure 14.5) within knitted pockets stitched into my *Queer quilt.* These knitted pieces were created from the material remnants of my internship as an art therapist at a women's shelter. Incorporating these scraps into the quilt seemed like a fitting presence within my presentation because our knitting groups had allowed for intergenerational and transcultural connections through our shared passion for crafting. The Queering Art Therapy zines[1] (Figures 14.6 and 14.7) contain an illustrated list of LGBTQ+ resources for art therapists that expands beyond art therapy literature (Anderson, 2019).

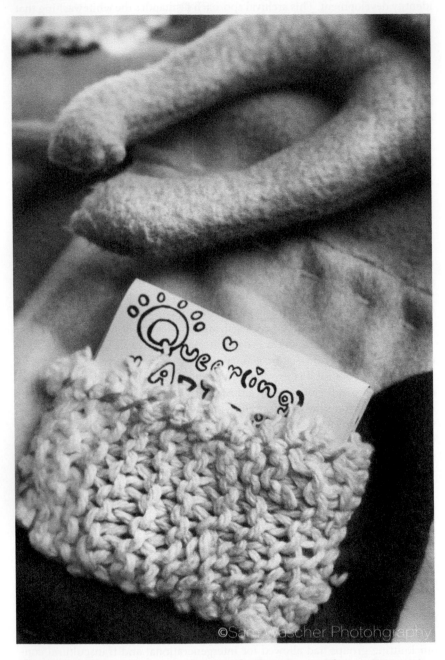

Figure 14.5 Mikey Anderson, *Queer quilt, Queering Art Therapy Zine*—mix media fiber crafts

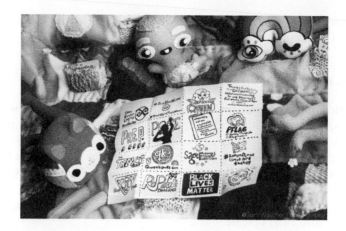

Figure 14.6 Mikey Anderson, *Queer quilt, Queering Art Therapy Zine*—mix media fiber crafts

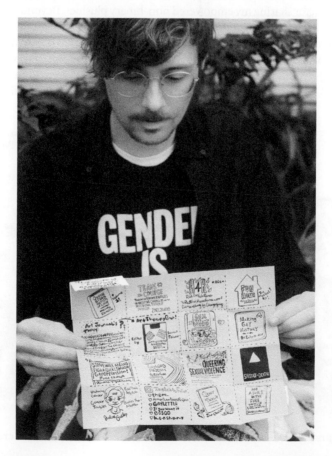

Figure 14.7 Mikey Anderson, *Queer quilt, Queering Art Therapy Zine*—mix media fiber crafts

Furthermore, the zine makes the political demand that art therapists must see and hear Queers (Eichhorn, 2016).

Crafting as a Queer Artist-Art Therapist

I approach my art practice as a way to model and share new narratives of Queerness with the Queer community. Through my art practice, I work to convey the trauma of being Queer in a heteronormative world (Hackford-Peer, 2010), offering to others what art has done for me through self-reflexive projects like my *Queer quilt*. I see this process of Queering myself through crafts as a way to extend LGBTQ+ awareness into the art therapy sessions I run, the community art projects I'm involved in, and the Yarnies (Figure 14.8) I create.

I have found many outlets for my approach. For example, I sold my Yarnies as a vendor at a free event for children, teens, and their caregivers that was focused on exploring gender through curiosity, creativity, and community (Figure 14.9)—a perfect event for sharing my empowered non-binary plushies. Beyond supporting the event through participation, I found inspiration in the resilience of LGBTQ+ families and in witnessing Queer youth allowing themselves to play in a safe environment. Another example is the Queering Puppetry art group I facilitated with an LGBTQ+ youth group. Prior to my involvement, the group had been talking about LGBTQ+ history and Queer icons they admired. The group facilitator and

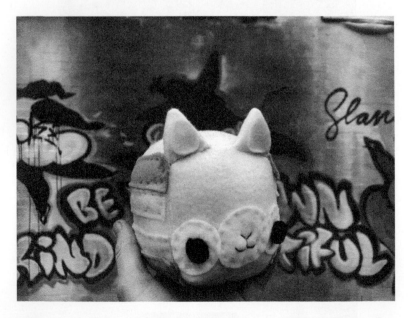

Figure 14.8 Mikey Anderson, *Yarnie Plushie*—mix media fiber crafts

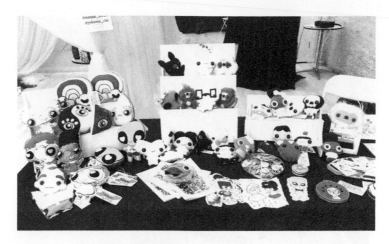

Figure 14.9 Mikey Anderson, *Yarnie display*—mix media fiber crafts

I created an LGBTQ+ icons puppetry workshop for the youth. We discussed past and present icons who have worked as pioneers for equal rights for Queers in the U.S. We discussed how their puppets could serve as extensions of themselves, objects that could hold their intersectional identities and invite conversations about their cultural backgrounds. The excitement that resulted from learning about Queer history was matched by the group's playfulness in animating their puppets during the sharing portion of the group. My Pride Quilts (Figure 14.10) workshops brought to light the intersection of memory impairment and the LGBTQ+ community and the need to support our elders who continue to pave the way for the Queer community. For example, a participant created a square he titled *Late Bloomer* and then shared his story of coming out as a septuagenarian. I spoke to the members about our quilts being a form of "craftivism," to highlight that their personal stories shaped our Chicago community and continue to resonate in the current expression of Pride.

Using my craft practice to Queer art therapy spaces and places, I have challenged traditional conceptions of art therapy groups in which the art therapist holds all the power. In a Queered approach, the power within a session is shared through skill shares and collaborative art-making experiences in which people learn from one another. I also consider how these Queer groups are sites of resistance that enable comfort, security, and freedom of expression for the participants. My community art practice resists the silencing of Queer voices and erasures of our identities through collective crafting. My art therapy practice responds to and resists the U.S. art therapy field's national alignment with the Trump-Pence administration. An all-Queer space creates a sense of safety, which can support the expression of gender and sexual identity at any age. The unconditional love and support fostered by these spaces encourage participatory engagement, which, in turn, leads to new forms of meaning-making for the Queer community (Frostig, 2011).

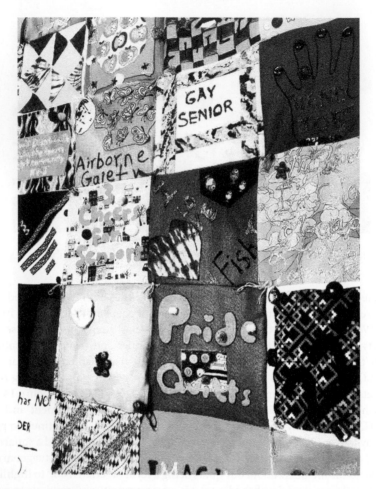

Figure 14.10 Mikey Anderson and Center on Addison community, *Pride Quilt*—mix media fiber crafts

What Do I Know So Far as a Queer Artist-Art Therapist?

My long-term mission as an art therapist is to create courageous, affirming Queer spaces for the LGBTQ+ community, where both practitioners and participants can freely explore their gender expressions, build awareness of Queer identities, and advocate for themselves. By Queering art therapy and thereby asserting the personal as the political (hooks, 2000), my art practice can become a form of social critique that supports the creation of a radical ethical Queer aesthetic (Warner, 2000). This radical Queer aesthetic has taken the form of my *Queer quilt*, community quilts, Queer puppetry workshops, art shows, and events. By combining fiber crafts, social art practice, and art therapy, I am contributing to the deconstruction of gender stereotypes developed by mass media and oppressive social norms. Art making has helped me imagine radical Queer spaces in which I can practice intersectional art therapy. It is an acknowledgment to art therapists; to those who participate in individual, group, and community art therapy contexts; and to myself that we all bring our intersecting identities and our personal and social histories with us into the therapy space.

In Queering art therapy, I seek to dismantle visible and invisible power structures to disturb the heteronormativity in art therapy practice and education. Art therapists have an opportunity and a responsibility to counter the dominant narrative of heteronormativity and to choose Queer inclusion (Middleton, 2017). Queering is a political act I am undertaking with my fiber crafts and Yarnies in hand, to create spaces of resistance and healing for the Queer community.

Note

1. A downloadable copy of the *Queering Art Therapy Zine* is available at http://mikey-anderson.com/art-therapy-work#/new-page-72/

References

Ahmed, S. (2016). *Living a feminist life*. Durham, NC: Duke University Press.

Anderson, M. (2019). *Queering art therapy Zine*. Retrieved from http://mikey-anderson.com/art-therapy-work#/new-page-72/

Beaumont, S. L. (2012). Art therapy for gender-variant individuals: A compassion-oriented approach. *Canadian Art Therapy Association Journal, 25*(2), 1–6. doi:10.1080/08322473.2012.11415565

Bianco, M. (2014). Queer writing and the structures of identity politics. *Lambda Literary*. Retrieved from www.lambdaliterary.org/features/02/04/queer-writing-and-the-strictures-of-identity-politics/

Butler, J. (1990). *Gender trouble: Feminism and the subversion of identity*. New York, NY: Routledge, Taylor & Francis Group.

Chaich, J., & Oldham, T. (2016). *Queer threads: Crafting identity and community*. Los Angeles: Ammo.

Eichhorn, K. (2016). *Adjusted margin: Xerography, art, and activism in the late twentieth century*. London, England: The MIT Press.

Fake, E. (2010). *Gaylord Phoenix*. Jackson Heights, NY: Secret Acres.

Fawaz, R., & Smalls, S. P. (2018). Queers read this! *GLQ: A Journal of Lesbian and Gay Studies, 24*(2–3), 169–187. doi:10.1215/10642684-4324765

Feng, J. (2018, June 9). Practicing radical self-love: Why you need self care the most when it seems impossible. Retrieved November 7, 2018, from https://thebodyisnotanapology.com/magazine/radical-self-love-means-radical-self-care/

Frostig, K. (2011). Arts activism: Praxis in social justice, critical discourse, and radical modes of engagement. *Art Therapy: Journal of the American Art Therapy Association, 28*(2), 50–56. doi:10.1080/07421656.2011.578028

Gipson, L. (2017). Challenging neoliberalism and multicultural love in art therapy. *Art Therapy: Journal of the American Art Therapy Association, 34*(3), 112–117. doi:10.1080/07421656.2017.1353326

Glaad (2018, May 1). Retrieved from www.glaad.org/tap/mike-pence

Halberstam, J. (2011). *The queer art of failure*. Durham, NC: Duke University Press.

hooks, b. (2000). *Feminism is for everybody: Passionate politics*. Brantford, ON: W. Ross MacDonald School Resource Services Library.

Hackford-Peer, K. (2010). In the name of safety: Discursive positioning's of queer youth. *Studies in Philosophy and Education, 29*(6), 541–556. doi:10.1007/s11217-010-9197-4

Kafer, A. (2003). Compulsory bodies: Reflections on heterosexuality and able-bodiedness. *Journal of Women's History*, *15*(3), 77–89. doi:10.1353/jowh.2003.0071

Kaiser, D. H. (2018). What do structural racism and oppression have to do with scholarship, research, and practice in art therapy? *Art Therapy: Journal of the American Art Therapy Association*, *34*(4), 154–156. doi:10.1080/07421656.2017.1420124

Karcher, O. P. (2017). Sociopolitical oppression, trauma, and healing: Moving toward a social justice art therapy framework. *Art Therapy: Journal of the American Art Therapy Association*, *34*(3), 123–128. doi:10.1080/07421656.2017.1358024

Kedley, K. E., & Spiering, J. (2017, September). Using LGBTQ graphic novels to dispel myths about gender and sexuality in ELA classrooms. *English Journal*, 54–60. doi:107.1(2017):54-60

King, N., & Rose, E. (2016). *Queer and trans artists of color* (Vol. 2). Place of publication not identified: Biyuti Publishing.

Kline, N., & Cuevas, C. (2018). Resisting identity erasure after Pulse: Intersectional LGBTQ Latinx Activism in Orlando, FL. *Chiricú Journal: Latina/o Literatures, Arts, and Cultures*, *2*(2), 68. doi:10.2979/chiricu.2.2.06

Lopez. (2018, October 22). *The Trump administration's latest anti-transgender action, explained*. Retrieved November 25, 2018, from www.vox.com/policy-and-politics/2018/10/22/18007978/trump-administration-lgbtq-transgender-discrimination-civil-rights

McDermott, E., Roen, K., & Scourfield, J. (2008). Avoiding shame: Young LGBT people, homophobia and self-destructive behaviors. *Culture, Health & Sexuality*, *10*(8), 815–829. doi:10.1080/13691050802380974

Middleton, M. (2017). The queer-inclusive museum. *National Association for Museum Exhibition*. Retrieved from static1.squarespace.com/static/58fa260a725e25c4f30020f3/t/5bdfab81032b e42558d5521c/1541385091673/15_Exhibition_QueerInclusiveMuseum.pdf

Moon, C. H. (2010). *Materials & media in art therapy*. New York, NY: Routledge.

Pelton-Sweet, L. M., & Sherry, A. (2008). Coming out through art: A review of art therapy with LGBT clients. *Art Therapy: Journal of the American Art Therapy Association*, *25*(4), 170–176. doi:10.1080/07421656.2008.10129546

Potash, J. S. (2019). Relational social justice ethics for art therapists. *Art Therapy: Journal of the American Art Therapy Association*, *35*(4), 202–210. doi:10.1080/07421656.2018.1554019

Ravichandran, S. (2019). Radical caring and art therapy: Decolonizing immigration and gender violence services. In S. K. Talwar (Ed.), *Art therapy for social justice: Radical intersections* (pp. 144–160). New York, NY: Routledge.

Salley, R. J. (2012). Zanele Muholis elements of survival. *African Arts*, *45*(4), 58–69. doi:10.1162/afar_a_00028

Talwar, S. K. (2010). An Intersectional framework for race, class, gender, and sexuality in art therapy. *Art Therapy: Journal of the American Art Therapy Association*, *27*(1), 11–17.

Talwar, S. K. (2017). Ethics, law, and cultural competence in art therapy. *Art Therapy: Journal of the American Art Therapy Association*, *34*(3), 102–105. doi:10.1080/07421656.2017.1358026

Talwar, S. K. (2019). *Art therapy for social justice: Radical intersections*. New York, NY: Routledge.

Talwar, S. K., Clinton, R., Sit, T., & Ospina, L. (2019). Intersectional reflexivity: Considering identities and responsibility for art therapists. In S. K. Talwar (Ed.), *Art therapy for social justice: Radical intersections* (pp. 123–143). New York, NY: Routledge.

Taylor, S. R. (2018). *The body is not an apology: The power of radical self-love*. Oakland, CA: Berrett-Koehler.

van Dernoot Lipsky, L., & Burk, C. (2009). *Trauma stewardship: An everyday guide to caring for self while caring for others*. Oakland, CA: Berrett-Koehler.

Warner, M. (2000). *The trouble with normal: Sex, politics, and the ethics of queer life*. Cambridge, MA: Harvard University Press.

Young, T. (2012). Queering "the human situation". *Journal of Feminist Studies in Religion*, *28*(1), 126. doi:10.2979/jfemistudreli.28.1.126

Zappa, A. (2017). Beyond erasure: The Ethics of art therapy research with trans and gender-independent people. *Art Therapy*, *34*(3), 129–134. doi:10.1080/07421656.2017.1343074

15

Quilting Across Prison Walls
Craftwork, Social Practice,
and Radical Empathy

SAVNEET TALWAR AND RACHEL WALLIS

In this chapter, as authors, we are interested in how the current field of social practice can intersect with ethics of care and well-being, especially when making happens with and for others. At the same time, we are interested in the performative nature of collaboration to engender "radical empathy" (Caswel & Cifor, 2016). This chapter examines how social practice—or socially engaged art—can contribute to the practice of art therapy and vice versa, using an ethics of care methodology to contextualize "radical empathy" in public and private crafting spaces, such as the project that tells stories of incarcerated mothers. We begin by examining what constitutes socially engaged art and the critiques that surround it to question if such art and collaboration can effect change within a neoliberal social order. As collaborators, we are both interested in exploring the potential of craft to raise awareness of structural injustice, in this case incarceration and criminal justice. Focusing on the ethics of care, we attempt to explore the messiness of radical empathy when crafting for a social cause. Elaborating on the *Inheritance: Quilting Across Prison Walls* project, we argue for shifting the focus of art making from uncovering pathology, as in art therapy, to crafting in public spaces to produce socially inclusive dialogue and increase awareness of structural inequity. For us, the performative function of making has the potential to challenge the contradictions of crafting to highlight structural injustices. The chapter ends with the ethical concerns and the responsibility of artists and art therapists who engage in community-based settings or socially engaged art.

Socially Engaged Art and Neoliberalism: Connections and Contradictions

The current resurgence of making and crafting offers a new platform for examining feminism and its complex history. Being heralded as a form of "new domesticity" or "feminist sensibility," the current feminist craft movement reengages the repudiation of the home and the domestic sphere by second wave feminists and has been embraced by third wave feminists as a subversive and political place (Talwar, 2019a, 2019b). Cvetkovich (2012) wrote that craft has always been part of women's culture as a form of slow living, recognizing, as she does, that manual labor has always informed women's way of knowing. Robertson and Vinebaum (2016), as editors of the special issue of *Crafting Community*, stated that "the prevalence of collaborative and participatory, performative, and publicly sited approaches in fiber today, are connected to earlier strategies deployed by craftspeople, designers, curators, activists, and of course—artists" (p. 3). For them, public crafting, also known as socially engaged art, has generated a new discourse for the audience, viewers, and collaborators. As authors we are interested in what happens when crafting practices are moved from the private to the public sphere. How does public or community crafting create social bonds? Do the performative strategies of crafting and its materiality offer an avenue for personal and political change? Can the craft objects and their materiality have a performative function to challenge unjust policies?

Social practice—or socially engaged art practice—emerged in the last 20 years and "cultivated a productive environment for artists, art therapists, and educators to explore activism in the professional sector" (Gipson, 2017, p. 112). It can encompass a wide range of practices to raise awareness of human rights, engage the public in response to neoliberal polices, or disrupt notions of individualism and autonomy (Chul Kim, 2017; Kester, 2011). Kester (2011) argued that social practice emerges as a form of collective or civic action to engage citizens in conversations about inequality and structural injustice. Enigbokan (2015), Bishop (2012), and Helguera (2011) have questioned the missionary vision that socially engaged art will solve longtime social injustices. Rather, Bishop (2012) is more interested in how socially engaged art calls attention to the contradictions of social discourse without claims of transforming society. For her, the goal of socially engaged art is to challenge the inherent contradictions of socially unjust laws and policies in order to disrupt the perceptions of viewers and participants.

Craft has increasingly gained a foothold in the art world to reposition the social value of embroidery, knitting, and crocheting (Robertson, 2011). Feminist artists in the 1970s and 80s used craft to create spaces for dialogue. For example, Judy Chicago's installation *The Dinner Party*, created between 1974 and 1979, draws upon traditional fiber crafts to symbolize and memorialize the erasure of women in Western civilization (Cvetkovich, 2012). Faith Wilding's 1972 *Crocheted Environments*, also referred to as "womb rooms," part of the *Womanhouse* project, drew out the contradictions inherent to the domestic pursuit of crocheting in order to open a conversation about reproduction (Cvetkovich, 2012). Janet Morton used old knitted sweaters to cover furniture and household objects, calling attention to the "home as a site of comfort, as well as of excess and misplaced sentimentality" (Turney, 2009, p. 22). Morton's focus is the invisible labor of everyday life connected to domestic work. She draws the viewers' attention to the monotony of domesticity through lamps, tables, telephones, vacuum cleaners, and other household objects covered with knitted fabric. Examining the history of textiles and feminism, Robertson and Vinebaum (2016) write about feminist artists, such as Faith Ringgold, Miriam Schapiro, Faith Wilding, and others, who turned to the political potential of fiber crafts to critique the patriarchal hegemony of the fine art world.

The political potential of fiber crafts is also seen in the example of quilting during the abolitionist movement in the United States, when quilts were sewn both to illustrate the injustice of slavery and to raise money for the cause (World Quilts, n.d.). In the early 1900s hand-embroidered banners created by suffragists, stitched with the participation of hundreds of women, were used in protests. Similarly, in 1976, the Madres de la Plaza de Mayo made scarfs, hand embroidered with the names of their disappeared children, to protest the "dirty war" of the Argentinian military dictatorship. Their head scarfs became a symbol of protest and resistance.

Drawing on fiber traditions like sewing, quilting, and knitting, socially engaged artists are increasingly creating spaces for dialogue to draw attention to oppression and social injustice, thus politicizing the private/public sphere duality (Robertson, 2011). But socially engaged practice is not without contradictions. The popularity of crafting and craftivist projects has taken social media by storm. Articles insisting that crafting is good for health, helps deal with depression and anxiety, and reduces cognitive decline have gained popularity in the medical community and art therapy. Studies now show that the medical community considers crafting and art a "natural anti-depressant" for trauma survivors dealing with depression and anxiety (Geda et al., 2011; Riley, Corkhill, & Morris, 2012). Although knitting and embroidery are being considered a radical act, Robertson (2011) argued that such acts are largely made redundant by the politics of neoliberalism. Han Sifuentes (n.d.), a fiber artist, cautioned against the celebratory nature of crafts; she argues for a distinction between the labor of artisans for whom craft is a way of making a living and crafting as a Western leisure activity that "fetishiz[es] traditional crafts and their practitioners" (as cited in Talwar, 2019b, p. 181).

The free market and the individualistic ideologies of neoliberalism and capitalism perpetuate the idea that individual acts can contribute to social change. In similar ways social practice and craftivism have had to contend with veiled neoliberalism and what Robertson (2011) called the "conservative edge" of the resurgence of crafting. Although crafting for political causes can contribute to a sense of individual fulfillment, it is often largely disconnected from policies that need to be changed. Furthermore, movements that began to address political and structural injustices have been coopted by large corporations. Several companies in the craft industry now use popular political causes to market their products. Companies like Hobby Lobby directly benefit from DIY and craft projects but actively oppose women's reproductive rights on religious grounds. In 2014 the U.S. Supreme Court ruled in favor of Hobby Lobby, exempting it from observing the contraceptive mandate of the Affordable Care Act on the basis of the Religious Freedom Restoration Act (Liptak, 2014). The same company benefitted from yarn sales across the U.S. when scores of women made their "pussyhats" to protest against Donald Trump's election in 2016. From the start, the Pussyhat Project came under criticism as exclusionary, the hats a symbol only meaningful to cisgender white women (Shamus, 2018). While a sea of white women marched across the U.S., Angela Peoples, the co-director of GetEQUAL, a lesbian, gay, bisexual, transgender, and queer (LGBTQ) equality organization in Washington, DC, used the Women's March as a participatory moment. She had a friend take photos of her posing as a protester in front of groups of white people in pink hats taking selfies and posting them on social media. Sucking a lollipop, she holds a sign saying, "Don't forget: White women voted for Trump," and wears a hat that says "stop killing Black people" (Obie, 2017).

A "participatory turn" in crafting practices is nothing new. Crafting and textile practices "have always operated at the intersection of individual and group activity" (Robertson & Vinebaum, 2016, p. 7). Thus, on an individual level, a craftivist project like the Pussyhat Project worked for groups of people across the gender spectrum to show their solidarity for human rights and women's rights. On a collective level, the millions of people marching in pink hats on January 22, 2017, had little effect; under the Trump administration an unprecedented number of states have passed the most restrictive reproductive laws—endangering women's bodies and their reproductive health—since *Roe v. Wade* was decided in 1973.

At the same time many socially engaged artists also distance their practices from art therapy. Although social practice artists and art therapists may both engage in questions of individual and community trauma, artists are rarely held accountable by the communities from which they take their subjects. And they may be less concerned with the ethics of their work than its level of visibility and recognition. For example, in the lead up to Art Basel 2019, Artnet News identified Andrea Bowers's *Open Secret* as the biggest conversation piece of the show (Kinsella, 2019). The sprawling installation, priced at $300,000, documented the history of the #MeToo movement. But it was soon reported that the piece included sexual violence survivors' names and photographs used without their knowledge or consent (Arnold, 2019). Bowers's piece was not the first artwork accused of profiting from the trauma of others. Although the artist's aim was to reassert the voices of the #MeToo movement, her means and disregard for the right of privacy opens a window to important questions raised by feminist scholars about ethics of care in archival practices (Caswel & Cifor, 2016). The next section elaborates on an ethics of care methodology to contextualize how a "radical empathy" approach is needed in order for socially engaged art to offer effective public platforms for engagement.

Crafting and Ethics of Care: Comfort and Discomfort

Feminist scholar Rudrappa (2004) and art therapist Ravichandran (2019) have written about using an ethics of care to consider "radical care" in helping those who have experienced gender-based violence. Caswel and Cifor (2016) proposed the use of radical empathy to examine the structural forces at play when activists and researchers enter communities to do research. A radical ethics of care means understanding one's obligations toward communities as "central focal points" in all aspects of social practice and research (Caswel & Cifor, 2016, p. 81). In a framework like radical empathy and care, social practitioners are seen as participants who engage with communities through mutual care and responsibility. Yet an ethics of care or radical empathy is not enough to produce powerful and effective social practice work. Comfort often comes at the expense of conflict or confrontation, which are necessary to address the root causes of inequality and injustice. The embrace of socially engaged art by large institutions and government bodies often produces art more interested in community building and "raising awareness" than in the organizing and movement building necessary to create structural change. Bishop (2012) touched on this tension in her book *Artificial Hells*, where she argued that by conflating ethics and goodness, "neoliberal states have effectively harnessed much of the field of social practice for their own ends" (p. 275), defanging its potential for effective criticism and change making. Effective and powerful socially engaged art must confront both comfort and discomfort. It should create accountable spaces for participants to engage in creative endeavors but be wary of "feel good" undertakings that do not move us closer to justice.

Artist and quilter Sarah Nishiura shared her thoughts at a quilting workshop:

> You don't make a quilt for someone to keep them warm. There are faster, cheaper, and easier ways to do that. You make a quilt for someone to show them that you care for them. That they were remembered and thought of during the hours and weeks and months that you worked on the quilt.
>
> (personal communication, July 14, 2018)

Although many communities have made quilts out of necessity, binding together scraps and salvaging blankets to keep warm, Nishiura touched on something fundamental about the power and meaning of handmade textiles, especially when making them for others. For centuries, textiles have been used to mark important moments in the lives of families and communities. People have sewn to celebrate births and weddings and to mourn deaths. It is no surprise, then, that people have utilized the metaphorical power of textiles, that physical manifestation of love and care, to reach beyond their immediate families and address suffering farther removed from their day-to-day lives.

Craft also allows us to bring an ethics of care to situations where it is easy to get overwhelmed or paralyzed in the face of massive injustice or devastation. An ethics of care asks us to consider whether our labor is benefiting or comforting anyone other than ourselves. When considering community-engaged textile projects, the cautionary tale of the penguin sweaters is important to remember. After a devastating oil spill coated nearly 500 penguins at the Phillip Island Nature Park in Australia in 2000, a call went out for people to knit sweaters for baby penguins who had been impacted by the oil spill. To this day people continue to share the appeal for knitters to make sweaters and the Phillip Island

Conservation Foundation has received upwards of 15,000 tiny sweaters since the spill. Not only has the immediate need long passed, but many people who work with marine wildlife argue that putting a sweater on an oil-covered penguin would unnecessarily stress the bird and trap potentially toxic chemicals close to its skin (Halcomb, 2011). Yet nearly two decades later, well-meaning knitters continue to churn out tiny sweaters, likely feeling pleased with their good deed and unaware with whether their actions are helpful or needed.

Next, we discuss the *Inheritance* quilt project that Wallis facilitated after receiving an Envisioning Justice Grant in 2019. As a socially engaged art project with a focus on radical empathy, we discuss the limitations, challenges, and contradictions of doing the project in the Cook County jail to highlight the implications of criminalization and incarceration on families and children.

Envisioning Justice—*Inheritance: Quilting Across Prison Walls*

In the last decade, artists, cultural workers, and activists in Chicago have worked tirelessly for criminal justice reform. Responding to the efforts of abolitionists, artists, and activists, the Illinois Humanities and Safety + Justice Challenge (2018–2019) called for a radical revisioning of the criminal justice system. Through its Envisioning Justice initiative, the project focused on highlighting the impact of criminalization and incarceration using the arts and humanities. The initiative represented artists, activists, and community-based organizations working to shift the conversation from "punishment" to alternative models of health and care in Illinois and the Chicagoland area. "Envisioning Justice seeks to strengthen efforts to reimagine our criminal legal system and is inspired by the goals of justice, accountability, safety, support, and restoration for all people" (Envisioning Justice, 2016a).

In 2018 and 2019, the Illinois Humanities offered grants to create dialogue on mass incarceration. The grants focused on three areas: "arts programs within jails and prisons, communications efforts, and stories meant to grow awareness and civic dialogue" (Envisioning Justice, 2016b). Wallis was awarded a grant for the *Inheritance* quilt project that tells stories of incarcerated mothers (outlined later), one of the projects to be funded by the Envisioning Justice grant.

Initiatives like Envisioning Justice reveal the gross injustices perpetuated by the carceral state. The United States of American is home to 5% of the world's population, but 25% of its population is in prisons, the largest in any country in the world (Wagner & Rabuy, 2017). Research indicates that there is relatively little positive impact of incarceration, but incarceration has severely affected the lives of people of color and low-income communities. People from Black communities are five times more likely to end up in prisons than people from white communities (Wagner & Rabuy, 2017).

In their book *The Long Term: Resisting Life Sentence, Working Toward Freedom*, Kim et al. (2018) outlined the impact of criminalization and incarceration on low-income communities and communities of color in Illinois. Illinois is one of six states where "life sentences are imposed without the possibility of parole"

(p. 2). Sixty-eight percent of those incarcerated are Black people, although the total Black population of Illinois is only 14.7%. Policies framed to restore "law and order" have been deployed by politicians since the 1960s. In 1968 Richard Nixon declared the so-called War on Drugs and pushed for mandatory sentencing and "no-knock" warrants to curb the Black Power and Civil Rights movements. Subsequently, Ronald and Nancy Regan started the "Just Say No" campaign, increasing hysteria and incarceration rates. In 1994, Bill Clinton's crime bill (Kim et al., 2018) devastated communities of color through long-term sentences with no option for parole. Such policies have led to a massive system of surveillance, detention centers, jails, and the privatization of prisons, thus shifting money from education toward criminalization and policing, which, in Chicago, particularly impacted the West and Southside. Clinton's 1994 Violent Crime Control and Law Enforcement Act also eliminated Pell Grants for incarcerated students. Only recently have local universities (Northeastern and Northwestern University) and nonprofits partnered with the Department of Corrections to slowly restore some educational programs for incarcerated individuals, but these opportunities are not offered to individuals who have "long-term" sentences.

Deconstructing the concept of criminalization and incarceration, Black scholars like Beth Richie have elaborated on the concept of "prison nation." Richie (2012) argued that the prison nation reflects the "dimensions of civil society that use the power of law, public policy, and institutional practices in strategic ways to advance hegemonic values and to overpower efforts by individuals and groups that challenge the status quo" (p. 3). Similarly, Michelle Alexander's (2012) book *The New Jim Crow: Mass Incarceration in the Age of Colorblindness* examined the history of racism and targeting of Black men through laws and programs like the War on Drugs and the 1994 Violent Crime Control and Law Enforcement Act; she demonstrated how the U.S. criminal justice system functions as a contemporary system of racial control though criminalization and incarceration.

The curators of Envisioning Justice (Illinois Humanities, 2019), Alexandia Eregbu and Danny Orendroff, challenged the visitors of the exhibition to consider three questions: "What do we mean when we ask for and speak for justice?," "How does the creative process and task of the artist play a role in facilitating vision and new forums towards liberation?," and "What is needed or necessary among a common people to imagine a balanced and harmonious society?" (Illinois Humanities, 2019 "Curatorial Vision," para. 1). What follows as one response is the story of the *Inheritance* quilt project.

The Inheritance *Quilt Project*

After months of emails and meetings with jail administrators, negotiating over every pencil and piece of paper we can carry with us, we drive to the Cook County Jail. The landscape changes drastically as we approach the jail, which covers 96 acres of land at 2700 South California Avenue. Rows and rows of tall buildings house 6,500 prisoners, and the jail employs about 4,000 law enforcement officers with about 7,000 civilian employees (Cook County Jail, Chicago, IL, n.d.). It is the largest single-site jail in the country. As we walk from the parking lot to the building, we are carded three times, and all our materials go through a scanner. We carry a see-through backpack so all items we bring are visible. No objects with sharp edges are allowed for fear that a participant could steal them or harm themselves. Despite being textile artists working on a quilting project, we have not been permitted to bring any sewing tools with us into the jail. We approach the building where we are going to hold our group, showing the guards a copy of the letter that allows us into the building. We wait for the supervisor to come and get us and escort us to the room where we will meet the participants in our group. It is a small platform with a few tables and chairs, surrounded by an out of use cellblock with empty cells. There is a white board but no markers, and trash is littered across the space.

Our students are from the THRIVE tier, a unit in the jail housing women sentenced to drug rehab. Although this is technically a diversion program, they still serve time under the same restrictive settings as everyone else in the jail. The age of the participants in the sessions varies from early 20s to 60s, and they come from diverse racial and class backgrounds. For some it is their first time in Cook County Jail; others have been through this rehab program multiple times. They are all serving 30–90 day sentences, but their release date depends on their progress through the program, and the reports from their counselors go to the court.

Inheritance began as a project that drew on the history of care, craft, and collaboration to create a socially engaged textile project that attempts to address the deeper structural forces at work behind prisons and policing that need urgent attention. Focusing on connecting incarcerated mothers to their children and grandchildren, *Inheritance* is about creating broader conversations about mass incarceration and its impact on families. Studies have repeatedly suggested that parental incarceration adversely affects attachment and leads to a high risk of mental health issues for children with an incarcerated mother (Shlafer & Poehlman, 2010). For us as crafters, quilts serve to mark and commemorate relationships in families. They are made for celebrating births, weddings, and to mourn deaths. They have been passed down within families from generation to generation for hundreds of years. For millions of families, however, the relationships between generations have been ruptured by incarceration. *Inheritance* attempts to address the issue of family separation and mass incarceration in three ways: first, by working with incarcerated mothers to design quilts for their children; second, by using volunteer quilters to translate the designs and make the quilts that are then mailed to the children to promote remembrance and connection; and third, by using community quilting circles outside of the prison walls to foster public conversations about mass incarceration.

The *Inheritance* workshops have been conducted twice at the Cook County Jail in Chicago. The first iteration was as a five-week series in summer and fall 2018 with Savneet Talwar, an art therapist. The second session was taught over six weeks with Melissa Blount, a psychologist. We adjusted to the challenge of not having scissors or needles by focusing the workshops on storytelling and using design exercises to explore the theme of inheritance. Guided by specific questions, the women wrote and shared stories about their family relationships, what was passed down to them, and what they wanted to pass along to their children. In the workshop, we studied the history of quilts, the changes in their designs, and the role they played in communities. In one session we brought in precut felt pieces so the participants could experiment with quilting shapes. Each of the participants designed an original quilt for someone in their family, such as a child, a grand-child, or a niece or nephew. Each of the participants was given graph paper and colored pencils to design a quilt with instructions (Figure 15.1). Volunteer quilters[1] outside of the jail sewed each woman's vision into a quilt based on her design; the finished quilts were then mailed to the chosen recipients (Figure 15.2). At the same time, the community quilting circles produced one large quilt based on all of the women's designs, including embroidered excerpts from their writings (Figure 15.3, Color Plate 15). The quilt is now a part of the Illinois Humanities *Envisioning Justice* show (Illinois Humanities, 2019). The public community quilting circles (Figure 15.4, Color Plate 16) served as a time for the larger public to engage with quilting and learn about the impact of mass incarceration on women and families; to connect with organizations working to support incarcerated people who are women, gender nonconforming, and/or trans; and to strategize about how to take action to end mass incarceration and family separation.

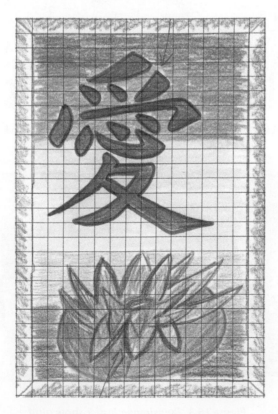

Figure 15.1 Asia's quilt design

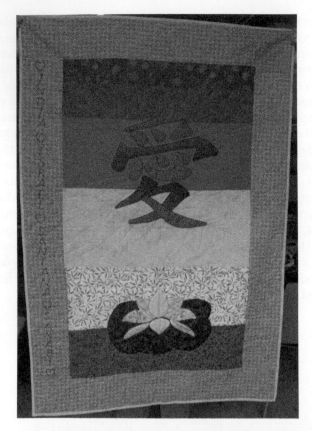

Figure 15.2 Asia's quilt completed by volunteer Chanelle Polk

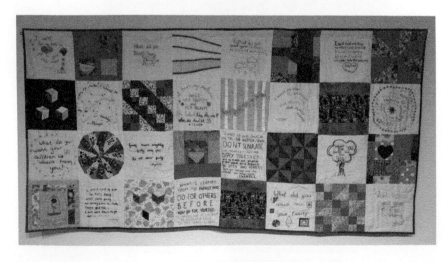

Figure 15.3 *Envisioning Justice* show quilt

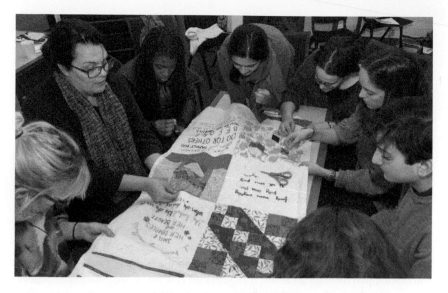

Figure 15.4 Quilting Circle

Source: Photo by The Pozen Family Center for Human Rights at the University of Chicago

Radical Empathy: Problematizing Art Therapy

The Envisioning Justice initiative poses new questions for the practice of art therapy. There are a number of art therapists who work in jails, juvenile detention centers, and prisons but mostly as part of a mental health team in collaboration with psychiatrists and psychologists. A quick review of the art therapy literature indicates that the research and writing about work in prisons focuses on diagnosis and treatment that "fosters frustration tolerance, alleviates depression, and increases problem solving and socialization skills" (Breiner, Tuomisto, Bouyea, Gussak, & Aufderheide, 2011, p. 3), all issues that arise as a result of incarceration. Art therapy services provide art materials to "inmates" for self-expression, to promote self-regulation, manage anger, and to treat other behavioral symptoms (Gussak, 2009). What is evident in these publications is that there is no systemic analysis of the effects of criminalization and incarceration. The focus remains on the individual's ability to participate in treatment that arises from a diagnosis, observation of behavior, and, finally, the use of drawings as a normative framework to analyze the psychological disposition of "inmates" for treatment. The language used, such as "inmates," "offenders," and "perpetrators" strips the incarcerated individual of dignity and respect. When the effects of incarceration are examined only through a psychological lens, criminality becomes a fixed concept divorced from poverty, class, race, or gender. When an individual is viewed only as a criminal undergoing punishment and rehabilitation, while the host of laws and policies that have systematically targeted communities of color are ignored, the only result is a reinforcement of the status quo.

Although the *Inheritance* project draws on the love, comfort, and care associated with quilting to raise awareness and empathy for incarcerated people, the project also lends itself to a critique: that it serves as a "feel good" project for white, bourgeois women. While there is a certain truth to that, spreading an understanding of the impact of incarceration on local communities is a valuable service. *Inheritance* asks the volunteer participants to consider the strategies for transforming the "criminal legal system away from dependence on incarceration and towards goals of justice, accountability, safety, support and restoration" (Illinois Humanities, 2019, "An Overview of the Envisioning Justice Initiative," para. 1). In extending the warmth and concern for the families and children whose lives have been shattered by the systemic injustice enacted by unjust policies through incarceration, the abolitionist artists have been working toward ending prisons and policing as institutions. To do this, the work of abolitionist artists is to discomfort the audience and participants as an act of radical empathy—reminding the audience of our complicity in systems of mass incarceration while providing opportunities to build movements and take action. Although prison abolition will not happen through art alone, it requires an epic act of imagination to believe that people are worth more than their worst act—that no one is disposable. The radical empathy engendered by sitting in community and enacting the labor of love inherent in quilting is a crucial first step toward building a more just future.

Ethics of Care: Questions for Collaboration, Community Art Therapy, and Social Practice

While craft can be an powerful tool to heal trauma, build community, and strengthen movements, there are key concepts that we need to consider so that as "well meaning" practitioners we don't end up adding to the pile of penguin sweaters in the world or stereotyping coping skills and behavioral interventions without contextualizing the systemic nature of structural injustice. An ethics of care methodology asks key questions before beginning projects in communities that we do not belong to, such as:

- What is consent and the power of language?
- How is the project centering the voices of the community?
- Who benefits from the project?
- What is the risk of harm to those being represented by the project or participating in the project? What policies and systemic view does the project address?

Consent and the Power of Language

Often in community settings, participation is considered voluntary. Despite the voluntary nature of these projects, close attention needs to be paid to what the participants are consenting to and what the project is about. In many cases where art therapists are involved in community settings, language about how to talk about the participants is key. Suspending clinical frameworks and refraining from diagnosis and the use of clinical observations is important, as the framework in a community setting is about social engagement rather than frameworks of treatment (L. Gipson, personal conversation, August 15, 2019). Thus, engaging in a cross-disciplinary setting means responding to the needs of the community and carefully choosing the language used in addressing participants that supports mutual respect and integrity (Talwar, 2019a). For example, a few art therapy programs have considered the use of language to address their participants. *A Long Walk Home* uses "Girl/Friends" (Tillet & Tillet, 2019), *CEW (Creatively Empowered Women) Design Studio* "members," (Talwar, 2019b), *Apna Ghar* uses "community members" (Ravichandran, 2019), and *Access Living* uses "consumers" (Yi, 2019) to address membership to community-based projects.

Centering Community Voices

Building intentional relationships with individuals and communities on the front lines from the very beginning of a project ensures that the messaging of the piece doesn't simply reflect the project's understanding of an issue and its solutions. It is critical to actively engage with the voices of the community as collaborators at every stage of the project. For example, in the case of the *Gone But Not Forgotten* quilt project, community members directly impacted by police violence, incarceration, racism, and family separation were invited to facilitate quilting circles, direct the content or design of the quilting project, speak at openings and public events, and, to accompany the work, create zines that included the stories and analysis by the community. In collaborative projects like the *Inheritance quilt*, the role of the art therapist shifts from "expert" or "leader" to one of collaborator (Ottermiller & Awais, 2016; Talwar, 2016).

Acknowledging Benefits and Ownership

Whenever possible, ensure that the collaborators benefit materially from the work. That means paying stipends or honorariums to facilitators or speakers, directing space rental fees and donations to grassroots groups doing important work on the ground, and hiring artists and activists of color for tasks like editing, documentation, or graphic design related to the project. It is critical to share credit, naming the individuals, organizations, or communities who contribute labor, stories, or experience to the project. And when working with people who cannot be paid, for example because they are incarcerated, it's important to compensate them in other ways.

Self-Reflexivity and Assessing the Potential for Harm

At their worst, social practice and art therapy can often involve practitioners parachuting into communities, engaging around deep trauma and community conflict, and leaving disappointment and fractured relationships in their wake. Although there are always unanticipated outcomes to any project, it is essential to try to limit the potential for harm. Spend time reaching out to the community members to host meetings and discuss the project. For example, Rachel Wallis reached out to families of individuals killed by the police before launching *Gone But Not Forgotten*, a memorial quilt project that names individuals who lost their lives to police brutality, asking for their feedback and offering to remove their family member's name from the project if they wished. She engaged with trained restorative justice practitioners to facilitate quilting circles and to manage any conflict or emotions that might arise during the conversations. During the *Inheritance* quilt project, she worked to protect the incarcerated collaborators' identities, offering them the option of using just their first names, nicknames, or leaving them off altogether in materials about the project. She partnered with mental health practitioners when engaging collaborators on issues like incarceration and family separation, which might trigger deep and unresolved trauma.

Promoting a Systemic Understanding of Injustice

The goals of socially engaged art often begin and end with "raising awareness" or "starting a conversation" about issues of injustice. Although we don't believe that a quilt is going to end mass incarceration, we try to bring a deeper structural analysis into the root causes of criminalization and incarceration through making and doing. Thus, partnering with organizations working at the grassroots level and engaging the community partners in opportunities to turn their newfound "awareness" into ongoing activism is the potential goal of socially engaged art projects.

Conclusion

To conclude, a call for "radical empathy" means bringing a critical understanding of political structures that have produced a carceral state and reflecting on our complicity in structural injustices. A structural analysis is primarily concerned with how social inequalities are formed and then maintained. Identities and their politics are, therefore, products of historically entrenched systems (Grzanka, 2014). A critical methodology of care asks that we question our "feel good" intentions as artists, cultural workers, art therapists, and service providers when we engage in communities that we do not belong to. Our knowledge and experiences informed by a critical methodology of care means that art making is not just an "intuitive and unconscious process" but a "collaborative process, one that is socially conscious, open to public discourse and invested in social change" (Talwar, 2016, p. 846). Thus, in collaborations where communities become invested in collective participation that is critical and communal, a radical empathy approach means that "art" is not just an object of contemplation; it is a subversive practice that reveals the contradictions of everyday life.

Note

1. Mary Scott Boria, Savneet Talwar, Sophie Canade, Marie Shebeck, Pamela Calvert, Sarah Nishi-ura, Hope Williams, Dana Jones, Molly Kafka, Karen Gilbert, Sarz Maxwell, Laurie Griffith Bernard, Megan Bernard, Stacy Ratner, and Kara Jacob all created quilts for the participants in the workshops.

References

Alexander, M. (2012). *The new Jim Crow: Mass incarceration in the age of colorblindness*. New York, NY: New Press.

Arnold, A. (2019). Artist apologizes over tone-deaf #MeToo piece at Art Basel. *The Cut*. Retrieved from www.thecut.com/2019/06/art-basel-andrea-bowers-me-too-sexual-assault.html

Bishop, C. (2012). *Artificial hells: Participatory art and the politics of spectatorship*. London, UK: Verso.

Breiner, J. B., Tuomisto, L., Bouyea, E., Gussak, D., & Aufderheide, D. (2011). Creating an art therapy anger management protocol for male inmates through a collaborative relationship. *International Journal of Offender Therapy and Comparative Criminology*, 1–20.

Caswel, M., & Cifor, M. (2016). From human rights to feminist ethics: Radical empathy in the archives. *Archivaria, 81*(Spring), 23–43.

Chul Kim, H. (2017). A challenge to the social work profession? The rise of socially engaged art and a call to radical social work. *Social Work, 6*(4), 305–311.

Cook County Jail, Chicago, IL. (n.d.). Retrieved from www.jailguitardoors.org/fullscreen-page/comp-jeiye3ip/212dda50-69b3-4351-a643-718dbf6e3a11/10/%3Fi%3D10%26p%3Dvglvp%26s%3Dstyle-jeyvm8vr

Cvetkovich, A. (2003). *An archive of feelings: Trauma, sexuality and lesbian cultures*. Durham, NC: Duke University Press.

Cvetkovich, A. (2012). *Depression: A public feeling*. Durham, NC: Duke University Press.

Enigbokan, A. (2015). Work ethics: On fair labour practices in a socially engaged art world. *Art & the Public Sphere, 4*(1+2), 11–22. doi:10.1386/aps.4.1–2.11_1

Envisioning Justice: A resource guide from Illinois Humanities. (2016a). Retrieved from https://envisioningjustice.org/app/uploads/2019/08/Envisioning-Justice-Web300.pdf

Envisioning Justice: A resource guide from Illinois Humanities. (2016b). Retrieved from https://envisioningjustice.org/app/uploads/2019/08/Envisioning-Justice-Web300.pdf

Geda, Y., Topazian, H., Roberts, L., Roberts, R., Knopman, D., Pankratz, V. S., . . . Petersen, R. (2011). Engaging in cognitive activities, aging and mild cognitive impairment: A population based study. *Journal of Neuropsychiatry and Clinical Neurosciences, 23*(2): 149–154. doi:10.1176/appi.neuropsych.23.2.149

Gipson, L. (2017). Challenging neoliberalism and multicultural love in art therapy. *Art Therapy: Journal of the American Art Therapy Association, 34*(3), 112–117. doi:10.1080/07421656.2017.1353326

Grzanka, P. (Ed.). (2014). *Intersectionality: A foundations and frontier reader*. Boulder, CO: Westview Press.

Gussak, D. (2009). The effects of art therapy on male and female inmates: Advancing the research base. *The Arts in Psychotherapy, 36*, 5–12.

Halcomb, J. (2011). Sweaters on oiled penguins? *International Bird Rescue: Every Bird Matters*. Retrieved from http://blog.bird-rescue.org/index.php/2011/10/sweaters-on-penguins/

Han Sifuentes, A. (n.d.). Steps towards decolonizing craft. *Textile Society of America*. Retrieved from https://textilesocietyofamerica.org/6728/steps-towards-decolonizing-craft/

Helguera, P. (2011). *Education for socially engaged art: A materials and techniques handbook*. New York, NY: Jorge Pinto Books.

Illinois Humanities. (2019). *Envisioning justice: A resource guide from Illinois Humanities*. Retrieved from https://envisioningjustice.org/app/uploads/2019/08/Envisioning-Justice-Web300.pdf

Kester, G. (2011). *The one and the many: Contemporary collaborative art in a global context*. Durham, NC: Duke University Press.

Kim, A., Meiners, E., Petty, J., Petty, A., Richie, B., & Ross, S. (2018). *The long term: Resisting life sentence, working toward freedom.* Chicago, IL: Haymarket Press.

Kinsella, E. (2019). The #MeToo movement will headline Art Basel unlimited this year with Andrea Bowers's epic account of America's harassment reckoning. *Art Fairs.* Retrieved from https:// news.artnet.com/market/andrea-bowers-art-basel-1517467

Liptak, A. (2014, June 30). 2014 the U.S. supreme court ruled in favor of Hobby Lobby. *The New York Times.* Retrieved from www.nytimes.com/2014/07/01/us/hobby-lobby-case-supreme-court-contraception.html

Obie, B. (2017). Woman in viral photo from Women's March to White female allies: "Listen to a Black Woman". *The Root: Black News, Opinions, Politics and Culture.* Retrieved from www. theroot.com/woman-in-viral-photo-from-women-s-march-to-white-female-1791524613

Ottermiller, D., & Awais, Y. (2016). A model for art therapists in community based practice. *Art Therapy: Journal of the American Art Therapy Association, 33*(3), 144–150.

Ravichandran, S. (2019). Radical caring and art therapy: Decolonizing immigration and gender violence services. In S. K. Talwar (Ed.), *Art therapy for social justice: Radical intersections* (pp. 144–160). New York, NY: Routledge.

Richie, B. (2012). *Arrested justice black women, violence, and America's prison nation.* New York, NY: New York University Press.

Riley, J., Corkhill, B., & Morris, C. (2012). The benefits of knitting for personal and social wellbeing in adulthood: Findings from an international survey. *The British Journal of Occupation Therapy, 76*(2), 50–58.

Robertson, K. (2011). Rebellious dollies and subversive stitches: Writing a craftivist history. In M. E. Buzek (Ed.), *Extra/ordinary: Craft and contemporary* (pp. 184–203). Durham, NC: Duke University Press.

Robertson, K., & Vinebaum, L. (2016). Crafting community. *Textile, 14*(1), 2–13. doi:10.1080/147 59756.2016.1084794

Rudrappa, S. (2004). Radical caring in an ethnic shelter: South Asian American women workers at Apna Ghar, Chicago. *Gender & Society, 18*(5), 588–609.

Shamus, K. J. (2018, January 12). Pink pussyhats: The reason feminists are ditching them. *Detroit Free Press.* Retrieved from https://eu.freep.com/story/news/2018/01/10/pink-pussyhats-feminists-hats-womens-march/1013630001/

Shlafer, R. J., & Poehlman, J. (2010). Attachment and caregiving relationships in families affected by parental incarceration. *Attachment & Human Development, 12*(4), 395–415. doi:10.1080/14616730903417052

Talwar, S. K. (2016). Creating alternative public spaces: Community-based art practice, critical consciousness and social justice. In D. Gussak & M. Rosal (Eds.), *The Wiley-Blackwell handbook of art therapy* (pp. 840–847). Oxford, UK: Wiley Blackwell.

Talwar, S. K. (2019a). Feminism as practice: Craft, labor, and art therapy. In S. Hogan (Ed.), *Inscribed on the body: Gender and difference in the arts therapies* (pp. 13–23). New York, NY: Routledge.

Talwar, S. K. (2019b). "The sweetness of money": The Creatively Empowered Women (CEW) design studio, feminist pedagogy and art therapy. In S. K. Talwar (Ed.), *Art therapy for social justice: Radical intersections* (pp. 178–193). New York, NY: Routledge.

Tillet, S., & Tillet, S. (2019). "You want to be well?" Self-care as a black feminist intervention in art therapy. In S. K. Talwar (Ed.), *Art therapy for social justice: Radical intersections* (pp. 123–143). New York, NY: Routledge.

Turney, J. (2009). *Culture of knitting.* Oxford, England: Berg Publishers.

Wagner & Rabuy. (2017). *Following the money of mass incarceration, prison policy initiative.* Retrieved from www.prisonpolicy.org/reports/money.html

World Quilts. (n.d.). *Abolition.* Retrieved from http://worldquilts.quiltstudy.org/americanstory/engagement/abolition

Yi, S. (2019). Res(crip)ting art therapy: Disability culture as a social justice intervention. In S. K. Talwar (Ed.), *Art therapy for social justice: Radical intersections* (pp. 161–177). New York, NY: Routledge.

Index

Note: Page numbers in *italics* indicate figures and in **bold** indicate tables on the corresponding pages.

Printed and bound by CPI Group (UK) Ltd, Croydon, CR0 4YY

23/10/2024

01778263-0006